Molecular and Clinical Advances in Anticancer Drug Resistance

Cancer Treatment and Research

WILLIAM L MCGUIRE, *series editor*

Paulson D.F. (ed): Genitourinary Cancer 1. 1982. ISBN 90-247-2480-5.
Muggia F.M. (ed): Cancer Chemotherapy 1. 1983. ISBN 90-247-2713-8.
Humphrey G.B., Grindey G.B. (eds): Pancreatic Tumors in Children. 1982. ISBN 90-247-2702-2.
Costanzi J.J. (ed): Malignant Melanoma 1. 1983. ISBN 90-247-2706-5.
Griffiths C.T., Fuller A.F. (eds): Gynecologic Oncology. 1983. ISBN 0-89838-555-5.
Greco A.F. (ed): Biology and Management of Lung Cancer. 1983. ISBN 0-89838-554-7.
Walker M.D. (ed): Oncology of the Nervous System. 1983. ISBN 0-89838-567-9.
Higby D.J. (ed): Supportive Care in Cancer Therapy. 1983. ISBN 0-89838-579-5.
Herberman R.B. (ed): Basic and Clinical Tumor Immunology. 1983. ISBN 0-89838-579-2.
Baker L.H. (ed): Soft Tissue Sarcomas. 1983. ISBN 0-89838-584-9.
Bennett J.M. (ed): Controversies in the Management of Lymphomas. 1983. ISBN 0-89838-586-5.
Humphrey G.B., Grindey G.B. (eds): Adrenal and Endocrine Tumors in Children. 1983. ISBN 0-89838-590-3.
DeCosse J.J., Sherlock P. (eds): Clinical Management of Gastrointestinal Cancer. 1984. ISBN 0-89838-601-2.
Catalona W.J., Ratliff T.L. (eds): Urologic Oncology. 1984. ISBN 0-89838-628-4.
Santen R.J., Manni A. (eds): Diagnosis and Management of Endocrine-Related Tumors. 1984. ISBN 0-89838-636-5.
Costanzi J.J. (ed): Clinical Management of Malignant Melanoma. 1984. ISBN 0-89838-656-X.
Wolf G.T. (ed): Head and Neck Oncology. 1984. ISBN 0-89838-657-8.
Alberts D.S., Surwit E.A. (eds): Ovarian Cancer. 1985. ISBN 0-89838-676-4.
Muggia F.M. (ed): Experimental and Clinical Progress in Cancer Chemotherapy. 1985. ISBN 0-89838-679-9.
Higby D.J. (ed): Issues in Supportive Care of Cancer Patients. 1986. ISBN 0-89838-816-3.
Surwit E.A., Alberts D.S. (eds): Cervix Cancer. 1987. ISBN 0-89838-822-8.
Jacobs C. (ed): Cancers of the Head and Neck. 1987. ISBN 0-89838-825-2.
MacDonald J.S. (ed): Gastrointestinal Oncology. 1987. ISBN 0-89838-829-5.
Ratliff T.L., Catalona W.J. (eds): Genitourinary Cancer. 1987. ISBN 0-89838-830-9.
Nathanson L. (ed): Basic and Clinical Aspects of Malignant Melanoma. 1987. ISBN 0-89838-856-2.
Muggia F.M. (ed): Concepts, Clinical Developments, and Therapeutic Advances in Cancer Chemotherapy. 1987. ISBN 0-89838-879-5.
Frankel A.E. (ed): Immunotoxins. 1988. ISBN 0-89838-984-4.
Bennett J.M., Foon K.A. (eds): Immunologic Approaches to the Classification and Management of Lymphomas and Leukemias. 1988. ISBN 0-89838-355-2.
Osborne C.K. (ed): Endocrine Therapies in Breast and Prostate Cancer. 1988. ISBN 0-89838-365-X.
Lippman M.E., Dickson R. (eds): Breast Cancer: Cellular and Molecular Biology. 1988. ISBN 0-89838-368-4.
Kamps W.A., Humphrey G.B., Poppema S. (eds): Hodgkin's Disease in Children: Controversies and Current Practice. 1988. ISBN 0-89838-372-2.
Muggia F.M. (ed): Cancer Chemotherapy: Concepts, Clinical Investigations and Therapeutic Advances. 1988. ISBN 0-89838-381-1.
Nathanson L. (ed): Malignant Melanoma: Biology, Diagnosis, and Therapy. 1988. ISBN 0-89838-384-6.
Pinedo H.M., Verweij J. (eds): Treatment of Soft Tissue Sarcomas. 1989. ISBN 0-89838-391-9.
Hansen H.H. (ed): Basic and Clinical Concepts of Lung Cancer. 1989. ISBN 0-7923-0153-6.
Lepor H., Ratliff T.L. (eds): Urologic Oncology. 1989. ISBN 0-7923-0161-7.
Benz C., Liu E. (eds): Oncogenes. 1989. ISBN 0-7923-0237-0.
Ozols R.F. (ed): Drug Resistance in Cancer Therapy. 1989. ISBN 0-7923-0244-3.
Surwit E.A., Alberts D.S. (eds): Endometrial Cancer. 1989. ISBN 0-7923-0286-9.
Champlin R. (ed): Bone Marrow Transplantation. 1990. ISBN 0-7923-0612-0.
Goldenberg D. (ed): Cancer Imaging with Radiolabeled Antibodies. 1990. ISBN 0-7923-0631-7.
Jacobs C. (ed): Carcinomas of the Head and Neck. 1990. ISBN 0-7923-0668-6.
Lippman M.E., Dickson R. (eds): Regulatory Mechanisms in Breast Cancer: Advances in Cellular and Molecular Biology of Breast Cancer. 1990. ISBN 0-7923-0868-9.
Nathanson, L. (ed): Maligant Melanoma: Genetics, Growth Factors, Metastases, and Antigens. 1991. ISBN 0-7923-0895-6.
Sugarbaker, P.H. (ed): Management of Gastric Cancer. 1991. ISBN 0-7923-1102-7.
Pinedo H.M., Verweij J., Suit, H.D., (eds): Soft Tissue Sarcomas: New Developments in the Multidisciplinary Approach to Treatment. ISBN.
Ozols, R.F., (ed): Molecular and Clinical Advances in Anticancer Drug Resistance. 1991. ISBN.

Molecular and Clinical Advances in Anticancer Drug Resistance

edited by

Robert F. Ozols
Fox Chase Cancer Center

1991 **KLUWER ACADEMIC PUBLISHERS**
BOSTON / DORDRECHT / LONDON

Distributors

for North America: Kluwer Academic Publishers, 101 Philip Drive, Assinippi Park, Norwell, Massachusetts 02061 USA
for all other countries: Kluwer Academic Publishers Group, Distribution Centre, Post Office Box 322, 3300 AH Dordrecht, The Netherlands

Cancer Treatment and Reasearch is indexed in the National Library of Medicine MEDLARS system.

Library of Congress Cataloging-in-Publication Data

Molecular and clinical advances in anticancer drug resistance / edited by
    Robert F. Ozols.
        p.   cm. — (Cancer treatment and research; 57)
    Includes bibliographical references and index.
    ISBN 0-7923-1212-0
    1. Drug resistance in cancer cells.   I. Ozols, Robert F.   II. Series:
Cancer treatment and research; v. 57.
    [DNLM: 1. Alkylating Agents — pharmacology.   2. Doxorubicin —
pharmacology.   3. Drug Resistance — genetics.   4. Membrane
Glycoproteins — genetics.   5. Neoplasms — drug therapy.
    6. Vinblastine — pharmacology. W1 CA693 v. 57 / QZ 267 M7184]
    RC271.C5M644 1991
    616.99'4061 — dc20
    DNLM/DLC
    for Library of Congress   91-7026
                                                                      CIP

Copyright

© 1991 by Kluwer Academic Publishers

Printed on acid-free paper.

PRINTED IN THE UNITED STATES OF AMERICA.

Table of Contents

Foreword to the series

Where do you begin to look for a recent, authoritative article on the diagnosis or management of a particular malignancy? The few general oncology textbooks are generally out of date. Single papers in specialized journals are informative but seldom comprehensive; these are more often preliminary reports on a very limited number of patients. Certain general journals frequently publish good in-depth reviews of cancer topics, and published symposium lectures are often the best overviews available. Unfortunately, these reviews and supplements appear sporadically, and the reader can never be sure when a topic of special interest will be covered.

Cancer Treatment and Research is a series of authoritative volumes that aim to meet this need. It is an attempt to establish a critical mass of oncology literature covering virtually all oncology topics, revised frequently to keep the coverage up to date, and easily available on a single library shelf or by a single personal subscription.

We have approached the problem in the following fashion: first, by dividing the oncology literature into specific subdivisions, such as lung cancer, genitourinary cancer, pediatric oncology, etc.; and second, by asking eminent authorities in each of these areas to edit a volume on the specific topic on an annual or biannual basis. Each topic and tumor type is covered in a volume appearing frequently and predictably, discussing current diagnosis, staging, markers, all forms of treatment modalities, basic biology, and more.

In *Cancer Treatment and Research*, we have an outstanding group of editors, each having made a major commitment to bring to this new series the very best literature in his or her field. Kluwer Academic Publishers has made an equally major commitment to the rapid publication of high-quality books and to worldwide distribution.

Where can you go to find quickly a recent authoritative article on any major oncology problem? We hope that *Cancer Treatment and Research* provides an answer.

WILLIAM L. MCGUIRE
Series Editor

List of contributors

BAHNSON, ROBERT R. Division of Urologic Surgery, University of Pittsburgh School of Medicine and the Pittsburgh Cancer Institute, Pittsburgh, PA 15213

BAKER, RAYMOND M. Grace Cancer Drug Center and Dept. of Experimental Therapeutics, Roswell Park Cancer Institute, Buffalo, NY 14263

BASU, ALAKANANDA. Department of Pharmacology, University of Pittsburgh School of Medicine and the Pittsburgh Cancer Institute, Pittsburgh, PA 15261

BECK, WILLIAM T. Department of Biochemical and Clinical Pharmacology, St. Jude Children's Research Hospital, 332 N. Lauderdale, Memphis, TN 38101

BOHR, VILHELM A. Laboratory of Molecular Pharmacology, Division of Cancer Treatment, National Cancer Institute, Bethesda, MD 20892

CHEN, YANFENG. Grace Cancer Drug Center and Dept. of Experimental Therapeutics, Roswell Park Cancer Institute, Buffalo, NY 14263

CORNWELL, MARILYN M. Department of Human Oncology, University of Wisconsin Medical School, 600 N. Highland Avenue, Madison, WI 53792

DALTON, WILLIAM S. University of Arizonia Cancer Center, Tuscon, AZ 85724

EASTMAN, ALAN. Department of Pharmacology and Toxicology, Dartmouth Medical School, Hanover, NH 03756

FORNACE, ALBERT J. Laboratory of Molecular Pharmacology, NCI, NIH, Bethesda, MA 20892

FREDERICKS, WILLIAM J. Grace Cancer Drug Center and Dept. of Experimental Therapeutics, Roswell Park Cancer Institute, Buffalo, NY 14263

FREI, EMIL III. Dana-Farber Cancer Institute, Boston, MA 02115

GOLDSTEIN, LORI J. Laboratory of Molecular Biology, National Cancer Institute, National Institutes of Health, Bethesda, MD 20892

GOTTESMAN, MICHAEL M. Laboratory of Cell Biology, National Cancer Institute, National Institutes of Health, Bethesda, MD 20892

GROGAN, THOMAS M. University of Arizona Cancer Center, Tuscon, AZ 85724

LAZO, JOHN S. Department of Pharmacology, University of Pittsburgh School of Medicine and the Pittsburgh Cancer Institute, Pittsburgh, PA 15261

LINK, CHARLES, J. Laboratory of Molecular Pharmacology, Division of Cancer Treatment, National Cancer Institute, Bethesda, MD 20892

MILLER, THOMAS P. University of Arizona Cancer Center, Tuscon, AZ 85724

PAPATHANASIOU, MATILDA A. Laboratory of Molecular Pharmacology, NCI, NIH, Bethesda, MA 20892

PASTAN, IRA. Laboratory of Molecular Biology, National Cancer Institute National Institutes of Health, Bethesda, MD 20892

PINEDO, HERBERT M. Netherlands Cancer Institute and The University Hospital, Free University, Amsterdam, The Netherlands

ROSS, WARREN E. College of Medicine, University of Florida, Gainesville. FL 32610

SULLIVAN, DANIEL M. J.G. Brown Cancer Center, University of Louisville, Louisville, KY 40292

TEICHER, BEVERLY. Dana-Farber Cancer Institute, Boston, MA 02115

VON HOFF, DANIEL D. Cancer Therapy and Research Center of South Texas, University of Texas Health Science Center at San Antonio, San Antonio, TX 78284

DE VRIES, ELISABETH G.E. Department of Medical Oncology, University Hospital Groningen, 9713 EZ Groningen, The Netherlands.

Preface

The importance of drug resistance in cancer chemotherapy cannot be over-stated. The 500,000 patients who die every year from cancer in the United States have, in most cases, been treated with chemotherapy. Many of these patients responded initially to chemotherapy, but death resulted from the development of drug-resistant tumors. In the first volume in the series. Drug Resistance in Chemotherapy the results of comprehensive laboratory studies aimed at understanding the mechanisms for resistance to individual agents and to the development of broad cross-resistance were described. In the past 2 years there has been substantial progress in understanding the molecular biology associated with these mechanisms of drug resistance. For the first time we are starting to understand which mechanisms are playing an important role in human tumors, and even more importantly, clinical trials have recently been initiated in an effort to reverse specific forms of drug resistance. The purpose of this volume is to describe the new advances, both at the molecular level and in the clinic regarding mechanisms of drug resistance and potential ways this resistance can be circumvented. This volume is focused upon mechanisms of resistance associated with two major classes of anticancer drugs: alkylating agents (including cisplatin) and the natural products (e.g., adriamycin and vinblastine).

The first section of the book describes new insights into the genetic mechanisms associated with drug resistance. The next section reviews the molecular biology of P-glycoprotein, and this is followed by an examination of the role of topoisomerase I and II in drug resistance. The next section describes studies on determining the importance of (P-170) in the multidrug resistant phenotype in human tumors. The structure-function relation-ships of agents that can reverse multidrug resistance associated with P-170 are then analyzed. Then we examine the recent clinical studies that are attempting to pharmacologically manipulate drug resistance associated with P-170 expression. The last section deals with drug resistance associated with alkylating agents and platinum complexes. The role of DNA repair and protein and nonprotein sulfhydryl in the expression of resistance to alkylating agents and platinum complexes is also described. The last chapter explores the clinical implications of these laboratory observations and describes clinical trials aimed at reversing resistance to alkylating agents and cisplatin.

It has become apparent that multiple mechanisms of drug resistance are playing a role in the clinical manifestations of drug resistance. The development of effective clinical strategies aimed at reversing drug resistance is dependent upon ultimately analyzing individual tumors to determine which mechanism is responsible for the development of drug resistance. I hope this book will provide the reader with an increased understanding of the complexity that surrounds drug resistance in human cancer. The mechanisms of drug resistance are complex and in many cases are multifactorial. Consequently, clinical reversal of drug resistance may ultimately require intervention at several different sites in the tumor cell, ranging from blocking efflux plumps to inhibition of cytosolic detoxification enzymes to inhibition of DNA repair.

1. New mechanisms of gene amplification in drug resistance (the episome model)

Daniel D. Von Hoff

Introduction

One of the greatest problems in clinical oncology today is the resistance of patients' tumors to conventional cancer chemotherapeutic agents. As is noted in the chapters in this volume, there are probably multiple mechanisms for the development of that resistance. In this chapter, new findings on one possible mechanism for drug resistance, namely, gene amplification, are presented.

Gene amplification (GA) is defined as a mechanism whereby cells can generate multiple copies of discrete regions of their genome. Gene amplification is one mechanism by which a cell can accumulate large amounts of a specific protein or RNA. The amplified genes are usually located either within expanded chromosomal regions, referred to as *homogeneously staining regions* (HSRs) or *abnormally banded regions* (ABRs), or in extrachromosomal elements called *minutes* or *double minutes*. There are now about 20 known examples of continuous cell lines in which amplification of a specific gene is known to be responsible for resistance to a specific drug [1]. There is also some evidence that DNA amplification can be responsible for drug resistance in tumors taken directly from patients. Amplification of the gene for dihydrofolate reductase (DHFR), the target enzyme for methotrexate, has been noted in ovarian cancer [2], small-cell lung cancer [3], and acute leukemia cells [4,5] from patients who have been treated with methotrexate. More recently, amplification of the multidrug resistance (*mdr*) gene (resistance to vinblastine and other agents) has also been described in sarcomas and other tumors [6,7]. Finally, amplification of the thymidylate synthase gene (resistance to 5 FU) has been described in a patient's rectal cancer specimen [8]. It must be stressed, however, that despite the numerous examples of GA in tumors taken directly from patients, the precise incidence of GA in a variety of human tumors has never been investigated. Therefore, it is unknown at this time just how important GA is as a mechanism for resistance in primary human tumors.

Genes responsible for drug resistance are not the only ones to be amplified. It has now been found that cellular counterparts of viral oncogenes (termed *cellular oncogenes*) can be found in both cell lines and in primary

Robert F. Ozols (ed.), MOLECULAR AND CLINICAL ADVANCES IN ANTICANCER DRUG RESISTANCE. Copyright © 1991.
Kluwer Academic Publishers, Boston. All rights reserved. ISBN 0-7923-1212-0

human tumors. It is also now clear that the presence of amplified oncogenes in patient's tumors may be an important prognostic factor. High levels of amplification of N-myc, HER-2/neu, and c-myc have already been shown to correlate with poor prognosis for patients with neuroblastoma [9], breast cancer [10], ovarian cancer [11], and small-cell lung cancer [12], respectively. From the above information, it is clear that gene amplification has some importance in the resistance of and progression of human tumors.

In recent years there have been many fine reviews written on the types of GA [1,13–18]. The purpose of the present discussion is to introduce the reader to a new possible mechanism involved in gene amplification, namely, the formation of circular, extrachromosomal DNA intermediates or episomes.

Extrachromosomal DNA in lower organisms

It has been known for some time that bacteria develop resistance to antibiotics such as tetracyclines or kanamycins because they possess small extrachromosomal circular DNA molecules (plasmids 2000–4000 base pairs in size) that contain drug-resistance genes [19–21]. The fact that these drug-resistance genes are found on plasmids, as opposed to on the main chromosomal DNA (4×10^6 base pairs), is important since antibiotic resistance requires large amounts of enzymes for neutralization. Because they are located on plasmids, the resistance genes are present in much higher copy numbers than they could be if they were located on the bacterial chromosome. The large copy number of the resistance gene can translate into large amounts of enzymes necessary to neutralize specific antibiotics.

Extrachromosomal DNA has also been identified in a number of other diverse organisms, such as yeast (the 2μ plasmid) [22], slime mold (gene coding for ribosomal RNA) [23], pea plants (gene function unknown) [24, 25], Tetrahymena (genes for ribosomal RNA) [26], Leishmania (DHFR gene for resistance to methotrexate) [27,28], and in a variety of insects (genes for ribosomal RNA) [29], and amphibians (genes for ribosomal RNA) [30].

Some of the extrachromosomal molecules are referred to as episomal DNA. Episomes are plasmids that have the ability to move on or off the main chromosomal elements.

With such a diverse group of organisms possessing extrachromosomal DNA in these cells, it is quite likely extrachromosomal DNA is important in nature. The work described below indicates extrachromosomal DNA may be important as an intermediate in gene amplification.

Extrachromosomal DNA as an intermediate in GA in animal tumor cells

To understand the early stages of gene amplification, the Wahl group at the Salk Institute began introducing genes into random genomic locations using gene transfer methods. They inserted a Syrian hamster CAD gene [*CAD* is an acronym for the multifunctional protein containing carbamylphosphate synthetase, apartate transcarbamylase, and dihydroorotase — amplification of this gene is responsible for resistance to the antitumor agent PALA or N-(phosphonacetyl)-L-aspartic acid] into a CAD-deficient Chinese hamster ovary cell line [31]. Most of the colonies that survived PALA after the gene transfer possessed a chromosomal localization for the gene (an HSR). However, one clone derived from this study was resistant to PALA (so it carried the CAD gene in an amplified form), but there was not a chromosomal localization for the CAD genes (none were found on HSRs, ABRs, or in double minutes [32,33]. In working on this puzzle (gene amplification and drug resistance without a localization of the amplified drug resistance gene), we have found that the amplified CAD genes are located on *submicroscopic circular supercoiled pieces of extrachromosomal DNA (episomes)*, which are approximately 250 kbp in size [32]. The cell line containing the episomes with CAD genes has been designated the C5R500 Chinese hamster ovary cell line. This episome is far below the size that can be detected as a minute or double minute by light microscopy.

The techniques used to isolate and identify the episome deserve some comment, since they have made their identification straightforward. Two techniques first used include the alkaline lysate procedure and the Eckhardt gel procedure. The alkaline lysate procedure was originally used to isolate circular viral DNA and plasmid DNA from linear chromosomal DNA [32, 34]. Use of this method caused lysis of tumor cells at high pH (pH 12.45). The high pH also denatures linear duplex DNA, while strands of covalently closed circular material remain intertwined. Upon neutralization and phenol extraction at high salt concentration, single-stranded DNA partitions at the interphase, while covalently closed circular DNA (episomal DNA) remains in the aqueous phase. This alkaline lysate material is further analyzed by agarose gel electrophoresis. This technique has been used to analyze large bacterial plasmids. With that system, the position of migration is approximately correlated with the logarithm of the molecular weight of the covalently closed circular molecule.

Based on our prior experience with human tuman cell lines with known episomes, we have found that the episomes may be quite fragile and can be "nicked" during processing of the cells. One way to attempt to avoid the "nicking" is to avoid manipulation of the cells by using a second technique, called the Eckhardt gel technique. This gel system was developed to analyze large bacterial plasmids [35] and the episomal form of the Epstein-Barr virus [34]. This gel system employs one set of wells in front of another set of wells. The front wells contain whole tumor cells, while the back wells contain a lysing buffer. The key feature of this gel method is that there is less manipulation of the cells, because whole cells are gently lysed in the well of the gel by migration of the lysing buffer from the back well into the front well at low voltage (50 V, 3 hr). The voltage is then increased (150 V),

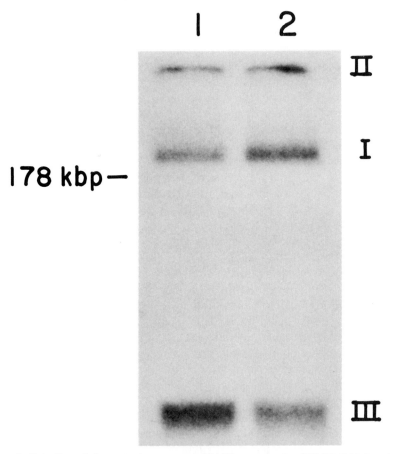

Figure 1. Detection of the extrachromosomal (CAD) gene in the C5R500 PALA-resistant CHO cell line. (See band next to Roman Numeral I.)

causing migration of circular DNA into the gel. The position of migration is correlated with the logarithm of the molecular weight of the covalently closed circular molecules [36]. The majority of the intact chromosomal DNA is retained at the well, and linear fragments of less than 120 kbp migrate near the xylene cyanol green front [33].

As an example of the above technique used to detect the 250 kbp episome in the PALA-resistant CHO cell line, please see Figure 1. The positive control that can be used in these experiments is the Raji cell line, which contains the EBV sequence, which is present in the Raji cells as a 178 kbp episome. The negative control in the experiment is a cell line in which the gene of interest is amplified but located on an HSR (a chromosomal location) in a cell line. This ensures that we do not have any "leak through" of an amplified sequence with a chromosomal location. Examples of these cell lines include the T_5S_{1-3} Chinese hamster ovary line, which includes 250 copies of the CAD gene on a chromosomal sequence. Based on past experience with such negative controls, we have *never* seen "leak through" of amplified chromosomal sequences into the alkaline lysate (episomal) material, even with such high copies of the amplified gene in the chromosomal sequence (250 copies).

As can be seen in Figure 1, there is ample evidence that the C5R500 cell line has submicroscopic circular supercoiled extrachromosomal DNA that is 250 kbp in size and contains amplified copies of the CAD gene.

We have documented that the CAD genes present in the episome are functional. Using the Brdu labelling Meselsohn Stahl technique [37], the CAD episomes replicate autonomously once per cell cylce in a semi-conservative manner [32,33]. Because the episomes were functional, we felt they were worthy of pursuit. Indeed, each episome must have an origin of replication. This origin of replication would be an ideal target for antineoplastic drug design. Determining the base pair sequence of that origin is an attainable goal if episomes could be demonstrated to be present in human tumors.

In addition to finding copies of the CAD gene amplified on episomes in CHO cells resistant to PALA, Wahl and colleagues have documented amplified copies of the adenosine deaninase gene, which codes for resistance to 2'-deoxycoformycin (2'-DCF) in mouse cells resistant to 2'-DCF [38].

Extrachromosomal DNA as an intermediate in GA in human tumor cells

Drug-resistance genes

The model described above by the Wahl group was a gene transfer model. One major question was whether there were other non-gene transfer model systems in which drug-resistance genes were located on circular extrachromosomal DNA (episomes). That question was addressed by Ruiz et al. by the use of a human tumor cell line resistant to vinblastine [39]. This cell line (the KB-VI line) is a squamous cell carcinoma line resistant to vinblastine based on the presence of the amplified *mdrl* gene [40]. To detect *mdr* gene-containing episomes in that line, we have utilized the relatively new technique of pulse field gel electrophoresis celled *filed inversion gel electrophoresis* (FIGE) [41–43]. Pulsed field gel electrophoresis can be used to separate large pieces of DNA as well as to migrate circular molecules into the gel. It is thought that conventional electrophoresis causes circular molecules to be arrested on the linear agarose polymer ("hoop-on-a-stick phenomenon"). The FIGE technique allows the circular molecules to migrate because the applied current has its polarity reversed every few seconds, which avoids the hang up of the circular DNA on the linear agarose polymer. FIGE can be used to resolve molecules below 1000 kbp in size. Along with the FIGE technique, whole KBVI cells were suspended in agarose blocks (designed to fit the size of the electrophoresis gel wells) [44], and DNA extraction was carried out in the agarose blocks (decreased shearing of the DNA allowing preservation of intact circular DNA molecule). Finally, the DNA in the blocks was irradiated with a ^{137}Cs source at a dose of 60 Gray (Gy) at a rate of 1.2 Gy/min prior to electrophoresis. This step linearized any circular molecules in the DNA from the KBV1 cells [45–47]. Using the above techniques (together termed the *gamma FIGE technique*), we were able to demonstrate that the KBV1 cells contained two species of *mdr*-containing circular molecules, 600 and 750 kbp in size. These molecules were also capable of autonomous semiconservative replication [39].

Using similar techniques (FIGE), Mauer et al. have documented that Hela cells resistant to methotrexate have copies of the dihydrofolate reductase gene located on extrachromosomal molecules 600–700 kbp in size [48]. The configuration of these extrachromosomal molecules they describe is uncertain, but from our review of the data presented in their paper, the molecules appear to be circular.

Finally, we have recently examined methotrexate-resistant human HEp2 squamous cells (known to contain amplified copies of the dihydrofolate reductase gene) for the presence of extrachromosomal copies of that gene. In addition to using the gamma FIGE technique described above, another technique, the CHEF technique (contour-clamped homogeneous electric field technique), has been used [49,50]. The CHEF technique is similar to the FIGE technique, except it allows resolution of molecules between 1000 and 9000 kbp in size. Using these techniques, we have documented that human tumor cell lines made resistant to methotrexate (by pressuring with methotrexate plus hydroxyurea and a phorbal ester) contain their amplified *dhfr* genes in autonomously replicating molecules ranging from 300 kbp (submicroscopic episomes) to over 4000 kbp (visible as double minutes) in size [46].

Oncogenes

In addition to drug-resistance genes being located on episomes, we have documented that the HL60 human promyelocytic leukemia cell line has amplified copies of the *c-myc* gene present on replicating episomes 250 kbp in size [51]. In addition, we have found copies of amplified *c-myc* in subclones of the Colo 320 DM human neuroendrocrine tumor cell line. These extrachromosomal molecules have ranged from 130 to 160 kbp in size.

Episomes can be precursors of double minutes

Carroll et al. have documented that upon passage of cells containing the CAD gene on episomes in higher concentrations of PALA, the submicroscopic episomes appear to multimerize and form microscopically

6

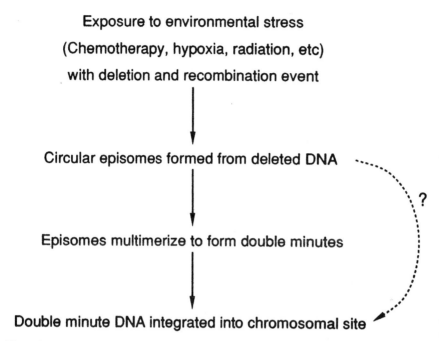

Exposure to environmental stress

(Chemotherapy, hypoxia, radiation, etc)

with deletion and recombination event

↓

Circular episomes formed from deleted DNA

↓

Episomes multimerize to form double minutes

↓

Double minute DNA integrated into chromosomal site

?

Figure 2. Proposed model for circular intermediates in gene amplification.

visible double minutes [52]. Vandevanter and Von Hoff have documented the same scenario for the methotrexate-resistant HEp-2 cell line. A selection for the larger (>1000 kbp size) molecule took place when the cells were carried in higher concentrations of methotrexate [46].

We have also recently documented that HL60 cells carried for increasing passage in cultures have their amplified copies of *c-myc* transferred from an episomal site to a site on double-minute chromosomes. With further passage in culture these *c-myc* copies become localized to a site within the chromosome [53]. These studies provide evidence that in human tumor cell lines there may be a progression from a submicroscopic extra-chromosomal site of oncogene amplification (episome) to a microscopically visible extrachromosomal site of amplification (the double minute) to an intrachromosomal site of amplification [53].

Proposed model for episomes or intermediate in GA

Recently, Wahl has proposed a model for GA taking into consideration the episome information reviewed above (Figure 2) [38]. In that model, a tumor cell, exposed to some environmental stress, such as hypoxia or a chemotherapeutic agent, has inhibition of replication or some other per-turbation of a chromosome structure (deletion and recombination event). The product of that perturbation is a circular extrachromosomal molecule

7

or episome. These episomes have the ability to replicate. If the selective pressure continues (e.g., methotrexate is present), the cells containing the episomes with the drug-resistance gene (e.g., dihydrofolate reductase) will have a greater advantage. With additional time in selective pressure, the episomes can multimerize to form double minutes. With additional time, the episomal DNA or double-minute DNA can integrate into a chromosomal site. This is certainly a highly simplified working model, but one that forms the basis for future experiments.

Possible way to exploit extrachromosomal location of drug-resistance genes

It is important to note that when the drug-resistance genes (or oncogenes) are present in an extrachromosomal compartment (on episomes or a double minutes), they are not in structures with centromeres, and hence randomly segregate at each mitosis, and consequently are vulnerable to loss from the cell population over time. On the other hand, if the amplified sequences are located on the chromosome on expanded chromosomal regions (HSRs) (which have centromeres), they segregate normally during mitosis and probably cannot be lost. The ability to eliminate the drug-resistance genes from resistant cells when the genes are located on an extrachromosomal site provides some chance for a therapeutic strategy.

It has long been known that one can eliminate antibiotic-resistance-gene containing plasmids from bacteria. By use of bacterial plasmid inhibitors, such as nalidixic acid, oxolinic acid, coumermycin A, or novobiocin, one can "cure" drug-resistance episomes in *E. coli* [54,55]. DNA intercalating agents, such as acridine orange, acriflavine, chloroquine, and ethidium bromide, are also capable of eliminating certain plasmids from bacterial hosts [56–60]. We have used a similar strategy to attempt to eliminate drug-resistance genes from both CHO and human tumor cell lines. To date, we have preliminary evidence that the ribonucleotide reductase inhibitor hydroxyurea can decrease drug-resistance gene copy numbers from both CHO (CAD gene) and human tumor (KBVI) cell lines [61]. Additional work on timing of exposures etc. is needed before practical applications of the data can be proposed. The other missing link in this approach is work to document that tumors taken from patients resistant to antineoplastics actually contain episomes with drug-resistance genes on them. That work is also ongoing.

Acknowledgments

This work was supported through a grant from the National Foundation for Cancer Research and through a Bristol Myers Drug Resistance Grant. A special thanks to Julia Perkins for her expert assistance in the preparation of this manuscript.

8

References

1. Stark, G.R. DNA amplification in drug resistant cells and in tumors. Cancer Surv. 5:1–23, 1986.
2. Trent, J., Buick, R.N., Olson, S., Horns, R.C., and Schimke, R.T. Cytologic evidence for gene amplification in methotrexate resistant cells obtained from patients with ovarian adenocarcinomas. J. Clin. Oncol. 2:8–15, 1984.
3. Curt, G.A., Carney, D.N., Cowan, K.H., Jolivet, J., Bailey, B.D., Drake, J., Kao-Shan, C.S., Minna, J., and Chabner, B. Unstable methotrexate resistance in human small cell carcinomas associated with double minute chromosomes. N. Engl. J. Med. 308:199–202, 1983.
4. Carman, M.D., Schornagel, J.H., Rivert, R., Srimatkandada, S., Portlock, A.S., and Duffy, T. Resistance to methotrexate due to gene amplification in a patient with acute leukemia. J. Clin. Oncol. 2:16–26, 1984.
5. Horns, R.C., Dower, W.J., and Schimke, R.T. Gene amplification in a leukemia patient treated with methotrexate. J. Clin. Oncol. 2:2–7, 1984.
6. Gerlach, J.H., Bell, D.R., Karakonsis, C.M., Slocum, H.K., Kartner, N, Rustum, Y.M., Ling, V., and Baker, R.M. P-glycoprotein in human carcinoma: evidence for multidrug resistance. J. Clin. Oncol. 5:1452–1460, 1987.
7. Bell, D.R., Gerlach, J.R., Kartner, N., Buick, R.N., and Ling, V. Detection of P-glycoprotein in ovarian cancer: a molecular marker associated with multidrug resistance. J. Clin. Oncol. 3:311–315, 1985.
8. Clark, J.L., Reizer, S.H., Mittelman, A., and Berger, F.G. Thymidylate synthase gene amplification in a colon tumor resistant to fluoropyrimidine chemotherapy. Cancer Treat. Rep. 71:261–265, 1987.
9. Seeger, R., Brodeur, G.M., Sather, H., Dalton, A., Siegel, S., Wong, K.Y., and Hammond, D. Association of multiple copies of the N-*myc* oncogene with rapid regression of neuroblastomas. N. Engl. J. Med. 313:1111–1116, 1985.
10. Slamon, D.J., Clark, G.M., Wong, S.F., Levin, W.J., Ullrich, A., and McGuire, W.L. Human breast cancer: correlation of relapse and survival with amplification of the HER-2/*neu* oncogene. Science 235:177–180, 1987.
11. Slamon, D.J., Godolphin, W., Jones, L.A., Holt, J.A., Wong, S.G., Keith, D.E., Levin, W.J., Stuart, S.G., Udove, J., Ullrich, A., and Press, M.F. Studies of the HER-2/*neu* proto-oncogene in human breast and ovarian cancer. Science 244:707–712, 1989.
12. Johnson, B.E., Battery, J., Linnoila, I., Becker, K.L., Makuch, R.W., and Snider, R.H. Changes in the phenotype of human small cell lung cancer cell lines after transfection and expression of the c-myc proto-oncogene. J. Clin. Invest. 78:525–532, 1986.
13. Stark, G. and Wahl, G.M. Gene amplification. Annu. Rev. Biochem. 53:447–491, 1984.
14. Schimke, R.T. Gene amplification drug resistance, and cancer. Cancer Res. 44:1735–1742, 1984.
15. Schimke, R.T. Gene amplification in cultured cells. Cell 37:705–713, 1984.
16. Alitalo, K., and Schwab, M. Oncogene amplification in tumor cells. Adv. Cancer Res. 47:235–281, 1980.
17. Schimke, R.T. Gene amplification in cultured cells. J. Biol. Chem. 263:5989–5992, 1988.
18. Stark, G.R., Debatisse, M., Giulotto, F., and Wahl, G.M. Recent progress in understanding mechanisms of mammalian DNA amplification. Cell 57:901–908, 1989.
19. Watanable, T. Infectious heredity of multiple drug resistance in bacteria. Bact Rev. 27:87–115, 1963.
20. Novick, R.P. Extrachromosomal inheritance in bacteria. Bacteriol. Rev. 33:210–235, 1969.
21. Eberhard, W.G. Why do bacterial plasmids carry some genes and not others? Plasmid 21:167–174, 1989.
22. Jayaram, J., Li, Y.-Y., and Broach, J.R. The yeast plasmid 2μ circle encodes components required for its high copy propagation. Cell 34:95–104, 1983.

9

23. Ferris, P.J., Vogt, V.M., and Truitt, C.I. Inheritance of extrachomosomal rDNA in *Physarum Polycephalum* Mol. Cell Biol. 3:635–642, 1983.
24. Van'T Hof, T. and Bjerknes, C.A. Cells of pea (*Pisum sativum*) that differentiate from G2 phase have extrachomosomal DNA. Mol. Cell. Biol. 2:339–345, 1982.
25. Van'T Hof, T., Bjerknes, C.A., and Delihas, N.C. Excision and replication of extrachromosomal DNA of pea (*Pisum sativum*). Mol. Cell. Biol. 2:172–181, 1983.
26. Cech, T.R. and Brehm, S.I. Replication of the extrachromosomal ribosomal RNA genes of *Tetrahymena thermophilia*. Nucleic Acids Res. 9:3531–3543, 1981.
27. Garvey, E.P. and Santi, D.V. Stable amplified DNA in drug-resistance *Leishmania* exists as extrachromosomal circles. Science 253:535–540, 1986.
28. Beverly, S.M., Coderre, J.A., Santi, D.V., and Schimke, R.T. Unstable DNA amplification in methotrexate-resistant Leishmania consist of extrachromosomal circles which relocalize during stabilization. Cell 78:431–434, 1984.
29. Gall, J.G. the genes for ribosomal RNA during oogenesis. Genetics 61(Suppl.):121–132, 1969.
30. McGregor, H.C. and Kezer, T. The chromosomal localization of a heavy satellite in the testis of *Plethodon c. cinereus*. Chromosoma. 33:167–182, 1971.
31. Wahl, G.M., de Saint Vince, R, and De Rose, M.L. Effect of chromosomal position on amplification of transfected genes in animal cells. Nature 307:516–520, 1984.
32. Carroll, S.M., Gaudray, P., De Rose, M.L., Emery, J.F., Meinkoth, J.L., Nakkim, E., Subler, M., Von Hoff, D.D., and Wahl, G.M. Characterization of an episome produced in hamster cells that amplify a transfected CAD gene at high frequency: functional evidence for a mammalian replication origin. Mol. Cell. Biol. 7:1740–1750, 1987.
33. Wahl, G.M., Carroll, S.M., Gaudray, P., De Rose, M.L., Emery, J., and Von Hoff, D.D. High frequency amplification of a transfected gene via excision of an autonomously replicating episomes. In: Accomplishment in Oncology: The Role of DNA Amplification in Carcinogenesis, Fortner (ed). J.B. Lippincott, Philadelphia, pp 45–57, 1987.
34. Gardella, T., Medveczky, P., Sairenji, T., and Mulder, C. Detection of circular and linear herpes wirus DNA molecules in mammalian cells by gel electrophoresis. J. Virol. 50: 248–254, 1984.
35. Eckhardt, T. A rapid method for identification of plasmid deoxyribonucleic acid in bacteria. Plasmid 1:584–588, 1978.
36. Cosse, F., Boucher, C., Julliot, J.S., Michel, M., and Denarie J. Identification and characterization of large plasmids in *Rhizobium meliloti* using gel agarose electrophoresis. J. Gen. Microbiol. 113:229–242, 1979.
37. Meselson, M. and Stahl, F.W. The replication of DNA in *E. coli*. Proc. Natl. Acad. Sci. USA 44:671–687, 1957.
38. Wahl, G.M. The importance of circular DNA in mammalian gene amplification. Cancer Res. 49:1333–1340, 1989.
39. Ruiz, J.C., Choi, K., Von Hoff, D.D., Rominson, I.B., and Wahl, G.M. Autonomously replicating episomes contain *mdr* 1 genes in a multidrug resistant human cell line. Mol. Cell. Biol. 9:109–115, 1989.
40. Fojo, A., Akiyama, S., Gottesman, M.M., and Pastan, I. Reduced drug accumulation in multiple drug-resistant human KB carcinoma cell lines. Cancer Res. 45:3002–3007, 1985.
41. Cantor, C.R., Smith, C.L., and Mathew, M.K. Pulse-field get electrophoresis of very large DNA molecules. Annu. Rev. Biophys. Chem. 17:287–304, 1988.
42. Levene, S.D. and Zimm, B.H. Separations of open-circular DNA using pulsed field electrophoresis. Proc. Natl. Acad. Sci. USA 84:4054–4057, 1987.
43. Carle, G.F., Franke, M., and Olsen, M.V. Electrophoretic separations of large DNA molecules by periodic inversion of the electric field. Science 232:65–68, 1986.
44. VanDevanter, D.R., Trammell, T.T.M., and Von Hoff, D.D. Simple construction of rubberbased agarose block molds for pulsed-field electrophoresis. BioTechniques 7:143–144, 1989.

10

45. Van der Bliek, A.M., Lincke, C.R., and Burst, P. Circular DNA of 3 T6R50 double minute chromosomes. Nucleic Acids Res. 16:4841–4851, 1988.
46. Von Hoff, D.D., Waddelow, T., Forseth, B., Davidson, K., Scott, J., Wahl, G. Loss of drug resistance gene-containing episomes from tumor cells is accelerated by hydroxyurea. Cancer Res. Accepted with revisions 1991.
47. VanDevanter, D.R., and Von Hoff, D.D. Acid depurination inhibits DNA transfer from agarose field inversion gels (FIGE). Applied and Theoretical Electrophoresis 1:159–192, 1990.
48. Mauer, B.J., Lai, E., Hamkalo, B.A., Hood, L., and Attardi, C. Novel submicroscopic extrachromosomal elements containing genes in human cells. Nature 327:434–437, 1987.
49. Von Hoff, D.D. Extrachromosomal circular DNA (episomes) formation as new mechanism for drug resistance and tumor progression (abst.). Invest. New Drugs 7:439, 1989.
50. Larson, J.J., Nicholson, A.W., and Siegel, A. Field inversion of large DNA fragments using an inexpensive unit. BioTechniques 5:228–232, 1989.
51. Von Hoff, D.D., Needham-VanDevanter, D.R., Yucel, T., Windle, B.E., and Wahl, G.M. Amplified human myc oncogenes localized to replicating submicroscopic circular DNA molecules. Proc. Natl. Acad. Sci. USA 85:4004–4008, 1988.
52. Carroll, S.M., DeRose, M.T., Gaudray, P., Moore, C.M., Needham-VanDeVanter, D.R., Von Hoff, D.D., and Wahl, G.M. Double minute chromosomes can be produced from precursors derived from a chromosomal deletion, Mol. Cell. Biol. 8:1525–1533, 1988.
53. Von Hoff, D.D., Forseth, B.J., Clare, N., Hansen, K.L., and VanDeVanter, D.R. Double minutes arise from circular extrachromosomal DNA intermediate which integrate into chromosomal sites in human HL60 leukemia cells. J Clin. Invest., 85:1887–1895, 1990.
54. Sugino, A., Peeables, C.L., Kreuzer, K.N., and Cozzarelli, N.R. Mechanism of action of nalidixic acid purification of *Escherichia coli* nala gene product and its relationship to DNA gyrase and a novel nick-closing enzyme. Proc. Natl. Acad. Sci. USA 74:4767–4771, 1977.
55. Gallagher, M., Weinberg, R., and Simpson, M.V. Effect of the DNA gyrase inhibitors novobiocin, nalidixic acid, and oxolinic acid, an oxidative phosphorylation. J. Biol. Chem. 261:8604–8607, 1986.
56. Bastarrachea, F. and Willetts, N.J. The elimination by acridine range of F30 from recombination deficient strains of *Escherichia coli* k12. Genetics. 59:153–166, 1968.
57. Hirota, Y., and Iijima, T. Acriflavine as an effective agent for eliminating F-factor in *Escherichia coli* K12. Nature 180:655–656, 1977.
58. Hahn, F.E. and Ciak, J. Elimination of resistance determinants from R-factor R_1 by intercalative compound. Antimicrob. Agents Chemother. 9:72–80, 1976.
59. Bouanchaud, D.H., Scavizzi, M.R., and Chabbert, Y.A. Elimination by ethidium bromide of antibiotic resistance in enterobacteria and staphylococci. J. Gen. Microbiol. 54:417–425, 1969.
60. Wolfson, J.S., Hooper, D.C., Swartz, M.N., and McHugh, G.L. Antagonism of the β subunit of DNA gyrase eliminates plasmids pβR 322 and pMG110 from *Escherichia coli*. J. Bacteriol. 152:330–344, 1982.
61. Von Hoff, D.D., VanDevanter, D., Forseth, B., Davidson, K., Waddelow, T., and Wahl, G. Hydroxyurea can decrease drug resistance gene copy numbers in tumor cell lines (abst.). Proc. Am. Assoc. Cancer Res., 31:378, 1990.

11

2. DNA-damage inducible genes

Matilda A. Papathanasiou and Albert J. Fornace, Jr.

Introduction

Most organisms can respond to changes in the environment by the induction of a variety of different genes. For example, exposure to elevated temperature, heat shock, leads to the increased transcription (induction) of a number of genes whose protein products, the heat-shock proteins (hsp*), may increase the cellular resistance to heat shock. Another example is the cellular exposure to toxic metal salts, such as cadmium, that leads to the induction of genes whose protein products, like metallothionein (MT), have a protective effect by binding these metal salts. As will be discussed throughout this chapter, exposure of cells to DNA-damaging agents can lead to the induction of a variety of genes. In a manner analogous to other stress responses, the products of DNA-damage-inducible (DDI) genes might be expected to have protective roles against genotoxic stress. This is clearly the case for bacteria, and a brief review of DDI genes in prokaryotes has been included for this reason. In eukaryotes, our understanding of DDI genes is less complete than in bacteria, but some evidence has already been found, particularly in yeast, that some DDI genes encode DNA repair functions. In mammalian cells, few DNA repair genes have been identified; thus, isolation of genes on the basis of DNA-damage inducibility offers an approach to identify genes involved in DNA damage processing.

In addition, the study of DDI genes may provide insight into how mammalian cells respond to genotoxic stress and lead to the elucidation of regulatory pathways that are activated by such stresses. The purpose of this chapter is to review our current understanding of DDI genes, with emphasis on those in mammalian cells; in particular, what genes have been found to

Abbreviations: ataxia telangiectasia (AT), bovine papilloma virus (BPV), Chinese hamster ovary (CHO), cis-Pt(II) diamminedichloride (DDP), DNA-damage inducible (DDI), extracellular protein synthesis-inducing factor (EPIF), heat-shock promoter elements (HSE), heat-shock protein (hsp), metallothionein (MT), methylmethane sulfonate (MMS), mitomycin C (MMC), N-acetoxy-2-acetylaminofluorene (AAAF), N-methyl-N'-nitro-N-nitrosoguanidine (MNNG), NAD(P)H:menadione oxidoreductase (Nmo-1), nitrogen mustard (HN2), 12-O-tetradecanoyl-phorbol-13-acetate (TPA), 3,7,8-tetrachlorodibenza-p-dioxin (TCDD), protein kinase C (PKC).

Robert F. Ozols (ed.), MOLECULAR AND CLINICAL ADVANCES IN ANTICANCER DRUG RESISTANCE. Copyright © 1991.
Kluwer Academic Publishers, Boston. All rights reserved. ISBN 0-7923-1212-0

be DDI in mammalian cells, what is known about their regulation, what are their functions, and is there evidence that such genes are involved in the cellular responses to chemotherapy agents? We will focus on cellular responses involving induction, i.e., changes in the transcription of particular genes. Although events such as gene amplification and mutation, which occur over much longer times, can be considered responses to genotoxic stress, they will not be addressed in this chapter.

DDI genes in simpler organisms, such as bacteria and yeast, and their regulation will also be discussed as models for how such responses may occur in mammalian cells. However, the responses to genotoxic stress in multicellular organisms might be expected to differ to some extent from simpler organisms and to be more complex. For example, effects such as the responses to tissue injury and apoptosis, programmed cell death [discussed in 1], are probably not relevant to single-cell organisms. When multicellular organisms are exposed to cytotoxic agents, whether they are DNA-damaging agents or not, the resultant cell injury and necrosis can lead to a variety of effects, such as inflammation, vascular injury, and hemorrhage; many of the cellular responses to such effects may have little to do with DNA-damage processing. Thus, in mammalian cells genotoxic stress might be expected to induce responses specific for DNA damage and more general stress responses to cell and tissue injury.

DDI genes in prokaryotes

The DDI response has been characterized best in *E. coli* [2] and involves at least three inducible systems of stress regulons (a regulon is a group of genes that is coordinately regulated): the *recA*/*lexA*-mediated SOS response, which is rapidly activated after exposure to many DNA-damaging agents, the adaptive response to alkylating agents, and the *oxyR*-mediated response to oxidative stress. In the case of the SOS response [2], approximately 20 different genes are coordinately induced after DNA damage. Evidence indicates that the signal for activation of this pathway is single-stranded DNA, produced by DNA damage or stalls in replication, and/or possibly the damaged DNA itself. This signal leads to activation of a specific proteinase function in the recA protein, which cleaves a repressor protein, lexA. The lexA protein binds to the regulatory region of SOS genes and, upon its removal by activated recA protein, transcription of these genes is increased. Many of the SOS genes code for DNA damage repair enzymes and factors important in recombination and mutagenesis. For example, the *uvr* genes code for the ABC excinuclease enzyme complex in *E. coli*. These enzymes work in unison as part of the nucleotide excision repair pathway to, first, recognize bulky damages in DNA, then to nick the DNA strand on both sides of the damage, and finally to remove the whole damaged region. Many chemotherapy agents produce such bulky lesions in DNA, particularly

14

interstrand cross-links, and nucleotide excision repair is involved in their removal. The functions of some other SOS genes are unknown; at least one, the *sulA* gene, codes for growth arrest. Thus, although *sulA* is not a DNA repair gene itself, a plausible reason why it is an SOS response gene is that by arresting growth and DNA synthesis, it allows the cell time to repair the damage prior to DNA replication and mitosis. Constitutive expression or overexpression of the SOS response can be deleterious to the cell.

An important physiologic role for the SOS response is to protect cells from the lethal consequences of DNA damage. Indeed, once the SOS response has been activated, if cells are challenged for a second time with a DNA-damaging agent, cell survival is markedly increased. A second DDI response in bacteria is the adaptive response to alkylating agents. If *E. coli* are treated with low doses of alkylating agents and then challenged with a larger dose, there is a marked protective effect by induction of this stress regulon, which codes for genes involved in the repair of base damage, such as base-excision repair mechanisms. Base-excision repair involves the removal of the damaged base itself with creation of an apurinic or apyrimidinic site. The *oxyR* response to oxidative stress is induced by a variety of different types of oxidative stress, such as H_2O_2. One target for oxidizing agents and free radicals is DNA. Thus, in *E. coli*, induction of the three regulons, briefly summarized here, results in responses to DNA damage that have protective effects for the cells.

Although the genes for each of the three DDI stress responses are distinct, each response is not always elicited individually; there can be some overlap between the DDI regulons, such as induction of more than one regulon by a single agent. For example, H_2O_2 is an oxidizing agent and a very effective trigger for the *oxyR* response, but it is also a DNA-damaging agent and will induce the SOS response [3]. Thus the same agent can activate more than one regulon. Additionally, alkylating agents at low doses induce the adaptive response, but they will also induce the SOS response, particularly at higher doses. Finally, these three DDI regulons are not isolated from other regulons that are inducible by other types of stress, such as the *htpR*-mediated heat-shock response and responses to starvation, heavy metals, or other adverse stimuli. In *E. coli* and *Salmonella typhimurium*, at least two genes of the *htpR* heat-shock regulon are also induced by DNA-damaging agents [3,4]. Thus a variety of genes, which are members of different regulons, may respond to genotoxic stresses. In some cases, this may be a specific response, such as induction of a DNA repair enzyme by DNA damage, while in others the induction may represent a more general stress response to cell injury. DNA-damaging agents have a variety of effects on the cell; they can produce both oxidative stresses and classic DNA damage. In addition, they may hit other important targets in the cell, such as membranes and proteins; thus a single agent can activate several different regulatory pathways that are all part of a complex network providing protection to the cells from various types of injuries.

DDI genes in smaller eukaryotes

DDI genes in yeast

The search for SOS-like responses in most eukaryotic cells has been limited, since few DNA repair genes have been isolated. Recently, an increasing number of such genes, some of which are inducible, have been isolated from the yeast *Saccharomyces cerevisiae*, using some of the many DNA repair mutants available in this organism [reviewed in 5]. The yeast DNA repair genes, which are designated the *RAD* genes, can be divided into different epistasis groups based on the sensitivity of single and double mutants to killing by DNA-damaging agents. The major epistasis groups are the *RAD3* group, which contains many genes involved in nucleotide excision repair; the *RAD52* group, which contains genes involved in recombinational repair processes; and the *RAD6* group, which contains a diverse group of genes, some of which are involved in mutagenic processes, while at least one, *RAD9*, encodes a growth arrest function. Division of the *RAD* genes into these general groups has served as a useful guide for how the products of these genes may interact in different DNA damage responses. Interestingly, members of all three epistasis groups have been reported to be DDI, including the *RAD1, RAD2, RAD6, RAD51, RAD52*, and *RAD54* genes [5]. A good example of a DDI response, which shares many of the characteristics of the *E. coli* SOS genes, is the *RAD2* nucleotide excision repair gene; these similarities include a role in DNA repair, i.e., incision at the site of damage, low-abundance mRNA, rapid induction by DNA damage, and induction of only 2- to 10-fold. The genes of certain other enzymes that are involved in DNA replication and repair, such as DNA ligase [6], DNA polymerase I [7], and ribonucleotide reductase [8], are also DDI. Cellular phenomena, such as induction of a recombinogenic function by DNA-damaging agents in yeast [9], are suggestive of SOS-like functions. However, the cellular responses to DNA-damaging agents in yeast differ in some respects from the SOS response and will probably prove to be more complex. For example, loss of inducibility of *RAD54* gene was found not to affect several cellular parameters, such as relative lethality after treatment with X-rays or alkylating agents [10].

In addition to the *RAD* genes, a variety of yeast genes of unknown function have been identified on the basis of DNA-damage inducibility. By differential hybridization screening, McClanahan and McEntee [11] isolated cDNA clones for four genes whose transcripts increased after DNA damage; these genes were designated *DDR* for "DNA damage responsive." The regulation of the *DDR* genes was found to be altered in different *rad* mutants, but not in a coordinate fashion for all four genes; these findings also support the proposition that DDI responses in yeast are complex and do not support a simple model for induction for the DDR genes [12]. The DIN (for "damage inducible") genes were also isolated on the basis of

16

DNA-damage inducibility and consist of six different DDI genes of unknown function [13]. Ruby and Szostak [13] estimated that there may be 80 or more DDI genes in yeast; this represents nearly 1% of the total genes in this organism. Thus, these observations indicate that the cellular responses to genotoxic stress in this eukaryote are complex and involve a substantial portion of the yeast genome.

As in bacteria, some yeast DDI genes are induced by other types of stress, which indicates that they may represent a more general stress response(s) to cellular injury or have different specific roles in different stress responses. For example, several of the DDR genes have been found to be induced by an unrelated type of stress, heat shock [14]. The yeast polyubiquitin gene is also inducible by either heat shock or exposure to DNA-damaging agents. As its name implies, ubiquitin probably has a variety of functions in eukaryotic cells, including a role in the removal of damaged proteins, which would be produced by stresses such as heat shock [discussed in 15]. The recent finding that the RAD6 gene encodes a ubiquitin-conjugating enzyme suggests that ubiquitin may play another role in the cellular response to DNA damage [16]. From this discussion of DDI genes in yeast, one can see that the responses to genotoxic stress in eukaryotes can be complex and may include both specific responses to DNA damage and more general stress responses. Considering that many genes have been fairly conserved throughout eukaryotic evolution, a similar situation might be expected in mammalian cells.

DDI genes in insect cells

While a comprehensive discussion of DNA-damage responses in insect cells is beyond the scope of this chapter, several points with relevance to DDI genes have been included. In *Drosophila*, several genes have been identified on the basis of being DDI; one of these genes was induced by either ultraviolet (UV) radiation or heat shock [17]. DDI responses have also been studied in *Drosophila* at the protein level using two-dimensional gel electrophoresis. Compared to mammalian cells, the *Drosophila* genome is less complex, and a larger fraction of the protein products of these genes can be resolved by two-dimensional gels. Interestingly, a large number of proteins were found to increase in abundance after DNA damage [18]. The most effective inducing agent was the alkylating agent methylmethane sulfonate (MMS), which induced 25 proteins. A complex pattern of induction was found for different DNA-damaging agents; e.g., some were induced by MMS and UV radiation, while others were induced by only one of these agents. Several of these proteins were also induced by heat shock. The tumor promoter and protein kinase C inducer 12-O-tetradecanoyl-phorbol-13-acetate (TPA) was a weak inducing agent in this system, and many proteins were not induced by this agent. These results are somewhat reminiscent of findings in bacteria and yeast, and indicate that the cellular responses to DNA damage are complex, involving many genes, and that they include both DNA-damage-specific stress responses and more general stress responses.

An interesting finding in insect cells is that there is indirect evidence for an X-ray stress response that provides substantial protection from cell killing by this agent [19]. A particular lepidopteran cell line has been found to be markedly resistant to X-rays (e.g., the D_{10} is 200 Gy or 20 krads). Split dose experiments suggest that the first dose stimulated a repair system not present or present at lower levels in unirradiated cells. If cells were treated with agents that inhibit protein or RNA synthesis, this protective response was blocked. These results suggest that ionizing radiation induces certain genes and that the protein products of these genes reduce the toxicity of this DNA-damaging agent.

Evidence for SOS-like responses in mammalian and other higher eukaryotic cells

A variety of experiments, modeled after studies of the SOS response in bacteria, provide indirect evidence that a similar response(s) may also exist in mammalian cells. For example, it is commonly known that exposure of cells containing latent viruses to DNA-damaging agents can activate lytic infection, which is analogous to the prophage (bacterial virus) induction in bacteria [20]. A variety of cell survival studies, among which a classic example is certain split-dose emperiments, also show some similarities to the bacterial response. In these experiments cells are treated with two doses of DNA-damaging agents; the first one is usually a small dose, which is nontoxic and is used to induce SOS-like responses, while the second one is a larger dose that produces appreciable cytotoxicity. If a protective response is induced by the first exposure, cytotoxicity would be expected to be reduced with the second exposure. As a result, cell survival after a split-dose experiment is higher than survival from a single-dose experiment; this phenomenon has been found in a variety of mammalian cells [20]. However, the magnitude of this protection in mammalian cells is usually less than that seen in bacteria. In addition, the first dose can cause changes in cell-cycle distribution and other parameters that may influence cell survival. Another indication for DDI responses in mammalian cells is the inhibition of protein synthesis by cycloheximide, which has been shown to decrease cell survival of marsupial cells exposed to UV radiation [21]. Since the primary action of cycloheximide is inhibition of protein synthesis, one could infer from these experiments that cycloheximide inhibits the synthesis of proteins coded for by DDI genes. However, cycloheximide can have other effects including perturbation of cell-cycle progression or even changes in chromatin structure that could alter cellular lethality. At the protein level, the activity of several repair-related proteins has been found to be DDI. For example, in frog cells, enzymatic photorepair, which is a type of repair specific for pyrimidine

18

dimers produced by UV, is inducible only by UV radiation [22]. The activity for O^6-alkylguanine-DNA alkyltransferase, a protein involved in the repair of a certain type of DNA alkylation damage, has been found to be induced severalfold in rat liver after treatment with certain alkylating agents; however, a similar effect also occurred after treatments, such as partial hepatectomy, which indicates that this response is not specific for DNA damage [23].

Evidence for repair can also be inferred from studies using viruses to assay inducible repair phenomena. Viral host-cell reactivation experiments offer the advantage that the yield of infectious virus is evaluated rather than cytotoxicity. In these types of experiments, mammalian host cells are pretreated with various physical or chemical agents that cause DNA damage, and they are subsequently infected with viruses treated with DNA-damaging agents, such as UV radiation. The yield of repaired virus is measured by scoring the number of plaques that form on the tissue culture plate. The yield of infectious virus is higher when the host cells have been pretreated compared to the yield from the same cells untreated, suggesting that some inducible protective response had been elicited in the host cells and affected the repair of the virus [20]. Complications in the interpretation of host-cell reactivation experiments are many and include multiplicity reactivation effects and the fact that often times the effects seen are not pronounced. Some of these limitations have been overcome by using an expression vector-host cell reactivation assay to measure cellular DNA repair capacity [24]. In this case an expression vector, treated with UV, was introduced into monkey cells that had been pretreated with UV or mitomycin C (MMC) 24–48 hr previously, and the relative expression of a reporter gene in the plasmid DNA was measured (instead of viral survival). Higher expression was found in the pretreated cells compared with expression in untreated cells. When mutations were studied [25], the yield of mutations changed using a shuttle vector that was introduced into mammalian cells briefly and then was recovered and transfected into bacteria. Pretreatment of cells with DNA-damaging agents, or with conditioned medium from damaged cells, caused an enhancement of mutagenesis of the UV-damaged vector [25]. All the studies discussed here provide evidence that DNA repair capacity can be enhanced in cells pretreated with DNA-damaging agents and therefore suggest that mammalian cells have some means of recovering from DNA damage in a manner reminiscent of the bacterial response. Obviously, to understand such responses at the molecular level, the most direct approach is to identify DDI genes and then study both their function and regulation.

Mammalian DDI genes

If DDI responses in mammalian cells are similar to those in bacteria and smaller eukaryotes, such responses would be expected to be complex and involve many genes. There is increasing evidence that this is, in fact, the case for mammalian cells. Like simpler organisms, many of these DDI genes may represent responses to stresses more general than only DNA damage. As discussed in the Introduction, cell and tissue injury could also lead to the induction of a variety of stress-type genes that may not be specific for DNA damage. Many DDI genes that have been identified in mammalian cells probably represent such responses, based on the spectrum of agents that induce them. In addition, other genes have been identified that are more specifically induced by DNA-damaging agents. In the following discussion, various mammalian DDI genes have been grouped based on the pattern of inducing agents.

DDI genes induced by protein-kinase-mediated mechanisms

Induction of a number of DDI genes in human and other mammalian cells has been found to be mediated by one or more protein kinases [recently reviewed in 26]. Kinases, such as protein kinase C (PKC) and cAMP-dependent kinase, play central roles in the relay of information along signal pathways within the cell [27]. PKC requires Ca^{2+} and phospholipid for its activation, which can occur in the cell membrane after binding of hormones or growth factors to various receptors. PKC is also activated both in vitro and in vivo by the tumor promoter TPA; TPA dramatically increases the affinity of PKC for Ca^{2+} with activation of this enzyme and its translocation to the membrane. Activated PKC can phosphorylate a large number of cellular proteins and thus rapidly change their activity. The end result of many signal transduction pathways is the induction of specific genes. This induction is mediated by transcription factors that bind to the regulatory regions of the genes. Transcription factors, such as the c-fos component of the AP-1 transcription factor, can be phosphorylated. PKC and possibly other kinases obviously play a central role in multiple signal pathways, since TPA induces activation of a variety of transcription factors, such as both components (c-fos and c-jun) of AP-1, and others such as NFκB, and the p67 and p62 serum response factors [28]. While a comprehensive discussion of these important signal transduction pathways is beyond the scope of this review, several general comments can be made that may aid the reader in understanding the effect of DNA-damaging agents. First, not all of the components of these pathways and their interactions have been elucidated at the present time; this is an area of active investigation and the reader should be aware that our understanding of these processes is incomplete. Second, these pathways may often operate separately but can also converge, such as in the case of PKC (Figure 1), to form a complex network. Third, these pathways are probably involved in the regulation of many important cell processes, such as cell growth. Finally, many growth factors, hormones, their receptors, and oncogenes will certainly prove to be important components of these pathways.

Herrlich's group has pioneered the study of DDI genes that are induced

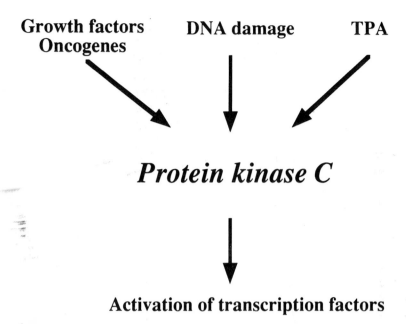

Growth factors   **DNA damage**   **TPA**
Oncogenes

Protein kinase C

Activation of transcription factors

Figure 1.

by PKC-mediated mechanisms [reviewed in 26]. Using two-dimensional gel electrophoresis with human fibroblasts, they first found that at least eight abundant proteins increased in abundance after UV irradiation of the cells [29]. This response was mediated by PKC or a similar protein kinase because TPA also induced the same proteins. Evidence was also found that this response could be elicited in untreated cells by an extracellular factor that was produced by the treated cells; this factor, named *extracellular protein synthesis-inducing factor* (EPIF), was activated by either DNA-damaging agents or TPA. cDNA clones for several of these DDI and TPA-inducible proteins were isolated, and included human MT IIA and collagenase [26]. Both at the protein and mRNA levels, these DDI genes were maximally induced 20–50 hr after treatment with DNA-damaging agents, while the time was somewhat shorter for TPA. The most effective doses of UV radiation for induction were $20 \, \text{J} \cdot \text{m}^{-2}$ or more; these doses characteristically produce high cytotoxicity (clonagenic survival <1%). Interestingly, these doses were reduced in UV-sensitive mutants. As seen in Table 1, a substantial number of DDI genes are induced by protein kinase-mediated mechanisms based on their inducibility by TPA. These genes code for proteins with diverse functions, which, in the case of proteins such as collagenase, may include responses to tissue injury. These results indicate

21

Table 1. Evidence for DNA damage inducible genes in mammalian cells

	Representative Agents	Comments	References
Genes/mRNA			
Human collagenase	UV, alk, TPA	Stress responses mediated by	52
Human MT IIA	UV, alk, TPA	the AP-1 transcription factor	53
Human plasminogen activator	UV, TPA		26,31
c-fos[a]	UV, alk, TPA, HS		30,54
c-jun	UV, TPA		54
Ornithine decarboxylase	UV, TPA		55
HIV-1	UV, alk, TPA		32,56
SV40 transcriptional enhancer	UV, alk, TPA		26,33
TIS	TPA, EGF, FGF	Induced by multiple pathways,	34
p53[b]	UV, NQO	tumor antigen and tumor supressor gene	57
Cystatin A	UV	keratinocytes	45
Keratin	UV, TPA	"	45
GAPDH	UV	"	45
spr I, *spr* II	UV, TPA, NQO	"	58
β-actin	Alk		59
Glutathione transferase	TPA	Response to oxidative stress	60
Heme oxygenase	UV, H_2O_2	"	61
Nmo-1	MMS, quinones	"	1
Ubiquitin	Alk, HS		15
MT I, MT II	UV, MMS	Coordinate rapid induction in hamster cells[c]	39
β-polymerase	Alk, H_2O_2	rapid induction in CHO cells	44
DDI genes Class I	UV, AAAF	"	46
Class II	UV, alk, H_2O_2	"	46
gadd genes (Class II subgroup)	UV, alk, H_2O_2, Growth arrest	Evidence for coordinate regulation	49
Proteins			
Class I MHC proteins	UV, alk		62
X-ray inducible	X-rays		51,63
EPIF	UV, alk, TPA	Mediates TPA response(s)	64

[a] Multiple mechanisms, both transcriptional and posttranscriptional, can account for increased expression of *c-fos*.
[b] Post-transcriptional.
[c] Chinese hamster V79 fibroblasts.
The abbreviations used are alk = alkylating agents; EGF = epidermal growth factor; EPIF = extracellular protein synthesis-inducing factor; FGF = fibroblast growth factor; *gadd* = growth arrest DNA damage-inducible; GAPDH = glyceraldehyde-3-phosphate dehydrogenase; MHC = major histocompatibility; MT = metallothionein; TIS = TPA inducible sequences.

that PKC (and possibly other kinases) play important roles in the cellular stress responses.

Our understanding of the mechanisms involved in the induction of DDI genes has been furthered by the findings of Herrlich's group and others that DNA damage activates certain transcription factors [26]. In the case of the collagenase gene, induction is mediated by interaction of the AP-1 transcription factor with a TPA-inducible enhancer in the promoter of this gene. What this means is that the AP-1 transcription factor is somehow activated by DNA damage and then binds to a control region in the collagenase gene with resultant increased transcription. The AP-1 transcription factor consists of the two proteins *c-fos* and *c-jun*; activation could be mediated by a variety of mechanisms, including phosphorylation. Activation of AP-1 involves protein kinase, since TPA will also induce it and protein kinase inhibitors will inhibit it. TPA or DNA damage lead to the activation of several different transcription factors [28]. In addition to AP-1, these agents will activate a NFκB transcription factor that binds to the HIV-1 enhancer (a control region in the human immunodeficiency virus); TPA or DNA-damaging agents also activate the serum response factors p67 and p62 that regulate the *c-fos* gene. As with AP-1, activation of these other transcription factors is mediated by PKC. However, the effect of TPA is not identical to that of DNA-damaging agents, e.g., only TPA causes translocation of PKC to the membrane. A reasonable interpretation of these observations is that DNA-damaging agents and TPA may involve different pathways that converge at PKC. Obviously, this story is incomplete and its elucidation will be exciting to follow.

Another factor that plays a central role(s) in the induction of DDI and TPA-inducible genes is the transcription factor and oncogene *c-fos*. As discussed above, this protein and *c-jun* form the AP-1 transcription factor that is activated by DNA damage and increases the transcription of the collagenase and other genes. Interestingly, both the *c-fos* and the *c-juns* genes are DDI (see Table 1). In both human and rodent cells, *c-fos* mRNA increased rapidly after treatment with a variety of DNA-damaging agents, TPA, or a different stress, heat shock [26,30]. Induction of *c-fos* by DNA-damaging agents or TPA is mediated by PKC, since induction is blocked by protein kinase inhibitors [26]. In the case of heat shock, induction is by both trancriptional and post-transcriptional mechanisms [30]. When cells were depleted of *c-fos*, the UV-induced induction of both collagenaes and HIV-1 were reduced [26]. This effect on collagenase would be expected, since it is induced via AP-1, however, the HIV-1 enhancer was induced via NFκB, indicating *c-fos* can affect other transcriptional factors. This result with HIV-1 suggests that *c-fos* may play a central role(s) in the PKC-mediated DDI response, in addition to its role in AP-1.

As shown in Table 1, a variety of DDI genes are induced by PKC-mediated mechanisms(s), based on their induction by TPA. For example, plasminogen activator, which might be expected to play a role in the response to tissue injury, has been found to be DDI in human cells [31]. Like collagenase and other genes studied by Herrlich's group, this induction appeared to be mediated by an extracellular factor that was produced by UV-irradiated cells. Several viral genes, such as HIV-1 [32] and SV40 [33], are also included in this group; as described earlier, one effect of the SOS response in bacteria is prophage (bacterial virus) induction. A variety of other genes, such as the TIS genes (for TPA inducible sequences) [34], have been isolated on the basis of TPA inducibility; these genes are also induced by growth factors and would be expected to be DDI. PKC may have importance in the cellular response to clinically important cytotoxic agents. In particular, TPA treatment was found to increase the resistance of human tumor cells to certain chemotherapy agents; this multidrug resistance was due to decreased accumulation of drug [35]. In rodent liver cells, DNA-damaging agents have been found to induce an increase in the mRNA level of the MDR-1 gene [36]; this effect may be cell-type specific, since we have found no evidence for induction of the same gene in Chinese ovary cells (CHO), even though it is expressed in these cells (unpublished data).

Metallothionein

The MT genes encode cysteine-rich small proteins that bind heavy metals and can protect against their toxic effects [37]. In addition to their role in metal homeostasis, other functions have been suggested for MTs on the basis of their induction by a variety of different stresses. For example, in vivo MT levels are also increased by glucocorticoids, interferon, surgical trauma, and tissue inflammation, as well as during certain developmental stages [37,38]. MT genes are induced by UV radiation in both human cells [26] and rodent cells [39], however, the kinetics of induction differed appreciably in the two cell types. In the case of human fibroblasts, MT IIa induction was similar to that of collagenase and was mediated by EPIF; maximum induction of only several fold occurred slowly and with relatively high doses, $>20 \, J \cdot m^{-2}$. In contrast, in a Chinese hamster lung fibroblast cell line designated V79, maximal induction of the two MT genes was rapid, within 4 hr, and occurred at a lower less toxic dose, $10 \, J \cdot m^{-2}$, where cell survival was greater than 10%. In contrast to human cells, induction of MT II mRNA in V79 cells was much stronger, up to 30-fold, and was similar in magnitude to that for heavy metals. This strong induction of MT in V79 cells was fairly specific for UV radiation, since no induction was seen after treatment with X-rays, H_2O_2, or heat shock, and induction of only several-fold occurred with MMS. MT genes contain multiple regulatory elements, e.g., the regulatory regions for metal, glucocorticoid, and the inflammatory response induction map to different 5' regions in the promoter of these genes [37]. Considering that the UV treatment, which produced maximal

24

Table 2. Evidence for increased expression of DDI genes in chemoresistant cell lines[a]

Gene(s)	Cell Line[b]	Drug Resistance	Reference
MT	2008 ovarian ca[c]	DDP	65
	COLO-316 ovarian ca	DDP	65
	HE_{100} epithelial	DDP	66
	$C11D_{100}$ mouse fibroblast	DDP	66
	A253 head and neck ca	DDP, ME,[d] CL[e]	41
	SCC25	DDP, ME, CL	41
	G3361 melanoma	DDP, ME, CL	41
	SW2 small cell	DDP, ME, CL	41
	SL6 large cell ca	DDP, ME, CL	41
	L1210/DDP murine leukemia	DDP, ME, CL	41
	$A2780^{CP}$ ovarian ca	DDP	d
	$A2780^{Me50}$ ovarian ca	ME	d
	$A2780^{CP}$ ovarian ca	DDP	d
	$A2780^{Me50}$ ovarian ca	ME	d
	PEO4 ovarian ca	DDP	d
ß-polymerase	P388 murine leukemia[e]	DDP, alk	67
	Raji-HN2	HN2	f
DDIA33	C13 hamster	MNNG	g
*gadd*45	PEO4 ovarian ca	DDP	d
*gadd*153	Raji-HN2	HN2	f

[a] RNA levels were compared to the respective parent cell line, or in the case of PEO4, a cell line derived from a biopsy prior to DDP treatment of the same patient.

[b] Cell lines were derived from human tumors unless otherwise specified.

[c] Abbreviations are ca = carcinoma; Me = melphalan; Cl = chlorambucil.

[d] Fornace, Hamilton, and Ozols, unpublished data.

[e] The activity of the ß-polymerase enzyme was found to be elevated.

[f] Fornace and Tan, unpublished data.

[g] Fornace and Goth-Goldstein, unpublished data.

induction in V79 cells, produced no induction in human fibroblasts [39], it would not be surprising if the EPIF-responsive region in the human genes differed from the regulatory region in the V79 MT genes, which was strongly and rapidly induced by UV.

Many authors have suggested that MT may protect against DNA-damaging agents [37]. MT is sulfhydryl-rich and can function as a hydroxyl radical scavenger in vitro [40]. MT is both DDI and is overexpressed in certain chemotherapy-resistant human tumor cell lines (Table 2). Several groups [discussed in 26] have found that cells containing increased MT can be somewhat radioresistant in clonagenic cell survival assays. However, these results have been inconsistent, e.g., V79 cells and CHO cells (which do not express either MT) have the same sensitivity to many DNA-damaging agents, including UV radiation and X-rays (our unpublished data). Often these studies suffer from the fact that the cells used are not well matched or

Table 3. Induction of stress response genes as measured by increased mRNA

| | RNA Level with Given cDNA probe[a] | | | | | |
	β-Polymerase	Ubiquitin	TPA Inducible Genes	hsp70	DDIA18 (Class I)	gadd (Class II)
Heat shock[b]	−	+	+/−[c]	+	−	−
MMS	+	+	+	−	−	+
MNNG	+	−	+	−	−	+
H$_2$O$_2$	+	−	+	−	−	+
UV radiation	−	−	+	−	+	+

[a] The relative abundance of mRNA from treated samples compared to untreated CHO cells was determined by dot blot hybridization; "+" indicates significant induction and "−" indicates no appreciable induction. Data are taken from refs. 15, 28, 30, 44, 46.

[b] CHO cells were harvested 4 hr after the start of treatment for all samples. Cell treatments were heat shock, 9 min at 45.5°; MMS, 100 μg/ml for 4 hr; MNNG, 30 μM for 4 hr; H$_2$O$_2$, 400 μM for 1 hr; UV radiation, 14 J · m^{-2}.

[c] c-fos was strongly induced by heat shock in both human and CHO cells, but some other TPA-inducible genes were not [26,30].

that MT is induced by heavy metals, such as Cd^{2+}, which may have other effects on the cell. For these reasons, studies have been conducted with cell lines isogenic, except for the presence or absence of a MT gene in a bovine papilloma virus (BPV) expression vector [41–43]. With this approach, one group has reported that overexpression of MT can provide some protection to alkylating agents or cis-Pt (II) diamminedichloride (DDP) using a non-clonagenic survival assay [41]. However, using clonagenic survival we have found that protection from DNA-damaging agents (X-rays, UV, HN$_2$, or H$_2$O$_2$) was not convincing in the same BPV-MT and additional BPV-MT lines, with the exception of a small protective effect for near UV radiation [41]. These results would appear to rule out a general radical scavenging for MT, since no protection was seen for X-rays or H$_2$O$_2$. With a similar BPV vector, Herrlich's group has also found that increased expression of MT provided no protection, as measured by clonagenic survival, from X-rays; however, they did find protection from MNNG cytotoxicity [26]. In similar experiments, increased MT expression did not increase DDP clonagenic survival [43]. If MT does protect against certain types of DNA-damaging agents, then this protection may be cell-type specific due to the magnitude of MT induction, varying levels of non-MT sulfhydryls, and other possible protective mechanisms.

Ubiquitin

As is the case for yeast, the mammalian ubiquitin genes are stress inducible and may play a role(s) in the cellular responses to DNA-damaging agents

[15]. This highly conserved protein has a variety of important roles in the cell, including a role in the removal of abnormal or damaged proteins and in yeast a role in DNA repair (see DDI genes in yeast). In eukaryotes, the major source for ubiquitin is the polyubiquitin gene(s). Both polyubiquitin genes are induced by heat shock, and ubiquitin is one of the most abundant heat-shock proteins (hsp) in human and rodent cells [14]. Since the comparable polyubiquitin genes in both yeast and chicken cells are heat-shock inducible and contain heat-shock promoter elements (HSE) [discussed in 15], ubiquitin is probably a hsp in all or most eukaryotes. In addition to HSE, mammalian polyubiquitin genes also probably contain one or more additional stress-inducible elements in their promoters, since ubiquitin mRNA is rapidly induced by such agents as MMS, DDP, or HN_2 under conditions where the other hsp mRNA are not [15]. In contrast, other hsp transcripts only increased slowly with very high and toxic doses of MMS and were not strongly induced. The induction of ubiquitin in mammalian cells by alkylating agents may not represent a specific stress response for DNA damage. As seen in Table 3, MMS was an effective inducing agent, while MNNG was not; both these agents produce similar levels of total DNA alkylation, but MMS produces an order of magnitude more protein alkylation. Thus, the signal for ubiquitin induction may be damage to cellular proteins rather than DNA.

β-polymerase

In contrast to the mammalian DDI genes already discussed, the induction of the β-polymerase gene may represent a stress response more specific for DNA damage [44]. β-polymerase is the first mammalian gene known to be involved in DNA repair that is also DDI. The product of the β-polymerase gene can fill in the gaps created in DNA after damaged residues have been excised. β-polymerase is probably the polymerase responsible for the repair replication step of base-excision repair, which is sometimes called short-patch repair. β-polymerase mRNA was found to be specifically induced in CHO cells by alkylating agents and similar agents producing base damage that is repaired by base-excision repair mechanisms (see Table 3). It was not induced by UV radiation, heat shock, or other types of stresses. It is particularly interesting to note that in the case of alkylating agents, MMS and MNNG induced a similar increase in β-polymerase mRNA at doses producing equivalent DNA alkylation [15,30,44], even though alkylation to other cellular targets, in particular proteins, was 10 times greater for MMS. β-polymerase inducibility by alkylating agents has been confirmed with expression vectors made by linking the promoter of the human β-polymerase gene to a reporter gene (CAT — chloramphenicol acetyl transferase). The promoter of the β-polymerase gene has been recently found to contain a DDI element, a palindromic sequence 5' to the transcription start site, that is induced by MNNG treatment [P.S. Kedar, et al., submitted for publication].

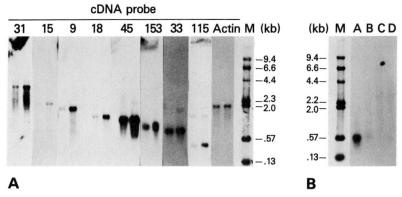

Figure 2. Blots of RNA from unirradiated and UV-irradiated Chinese hamster cells. *A*: Equal amounts of polyA RNA from untreated (left lane of each pair) and irradiated (right lane) CHO cells were size-separated and hybridized with labelled cDNA probes (DDIA prefix has been omitted). *B*: RNA from V79 cells (lanes A and B) or CHO cell (lane C and D) were hybridized with labelled metallothionein II probe. The UV dose was $14 \, \text{J} \cdot \text{m}^{-2}$ in panel A and lane C of panel B, and $17 \, \text{J} \cdot \text{m}^{-2}$ for lane A of panel B. Size markers, designated M, consisted of labelled single-stranded DNA.

These and other findings indicate that the induction of this gene by DNA-damaging agents is not mediated by the AP1 transcription factor but by another factor(s) that is activated by certain DNA-damaging agents. The β-polymerase gene has several properties in common with many bacterial and yeast DNA-repair genes: rapid induction of 2- to 10-fold, low abundance transcripts, and induction specific for DNA damage. These results for the β-polymerase gene indicate that specific DDI responses exist in mammalian cells.

DDI genes isolated by hybridization subtraction

The induction of DDI genes may represent stress responses that are specific for DNA damage or more general responses to cell injury and cell lethality. As discussed above, both β-polymerase and many bacterial and yeast DNA-repair genes share several properties not found for many other mammalian DDI genes. For example, the transcripts for many of the TPA-inducible genes were induced (increased in abundance) only slowly by DNA damage at high toxic doses. The UV-induction of several abundant transcripts in human keratinocytes was similar [45]; optimal induction was found 12 hr or more after high UV doses, $35-50 \, \text{J} \cdot \text{m}^{-2}$, and some were induced by TPA. In order to identify genes whose induction may be similar to that of bacterial and yeast DNA repair genes, a hybridization subtraction approach was developed to isolate cDNA clones encoding low-abundance transcripts that

28

Table 4. Induction of DNA-damage-inducible transcripts by various agents in CHO cells

---

Class I: A18[a], A26, A50, A70, A88, A109, A115, A143, A144, A162
    Induced 2- to 6-fold by UV radiation
    Also induced by the UV-mimetic agent AAAF[b] (for cDNA clones tested)
    Not induced by MMS, H_2O_2, heat shock, TPA, or growth arrest
Class IIa: A7, A8, A9, A15, A29, A31, A33, A77, A94, A99
    Induced 2- to 6-fold by UV radiation and 2- to 10-fold by MMS
    Many also induced by H_2O_2 and other agents that produce high levels of DNA base
      damage
    Not induced by heat shock (except for A15), TPA (except for A31 and A99), growth arrest
      (except for A7 and A33), adriamycin, or X-rays
Class IIb: A34, A45, A153
    Similar to Class IIa except for >10-fold induction by MMS
    Induced by growth arrest

---

[a] Numbers indicate individual cDNA clones from the CHO library [46].
[b] Cells were harvested 4 hr after the start of treatment; *N*-acetoxy-2-acetylaminofluorence
(AAAF).

are rapidly induced twofold or more by DNA-damaging agents [46]. CHO cells were UV-irradiated with a dose, $14 \, J \cdot m^{-2}$, where cellular DNA would be expected to be the major target, and then harvested only several hours later. As seen in Figure 2 and Table 4, this approach was effective in isolating a large number of cDNA clones encoding low-abundance DDI transcripts. Such a large number was not unexpected, considering that there are probably 80 or more DDI genes in yeast [13], which has less than one-tenth as many genes in their entire genome.

The cDNA clones of Table 4 were divided into two general classes based on the spectrum of inducing agents. The Class I clones were found to encode transcripts that were only induced by UV radiation and the UV-mimetic agent AAAF; both these agents produce high levels of base damage, which is repaired by nucleotide excision repair. No induction was found by a variety of other agents. One of these clones, DDIA18, was found to encode a nucleic acid single-stranded binding protein that is very highly conserved in rodent and human cells [46]. Class II transcripts were found to be induced by MMS. Most were induced also by other base-damaging agents, such as H_2O_2, HN2, melphalan, DDP, etc. Interestingly, the patterns of induction for the DDI transcripts of Table 4 were reminiscent of the responses in *Drosophila*, as measured by two-dimensional gel protein gel electrophoresis (see DDI genes in insect cells). In contrast to many other mammalian DDI genes, most of those in Table 4 were induced more rapidly, were induced at lower UV doses, and were not induced by TPA. Most were also not induced by heat shock. Based on these results, the induction of many of these DDI transcripts appear to represent specific stress responses to DNA damage.

29

Growth arrest- and DNA-damage-inducible (gadd) *genes*

DNA damage delays progression through the cell cycle and entry into mitosis. In many cases such delays probably represent active processes and not simply the deleterious effects of the damage. For example, in *E. coli* a role in the inhibition of cell growth is played by the *sulA* gene, a member of the SOS regulon that is induced by DNA damage [2]. In yeast the *RAD9* gene product is responsible for the arrest of cells after DNA damage in the G_2 phase of the cell cycle, and this response is absent in the radiosensitive *rad9* mutant [47]. In addition, the transient inhibition of DNA synthesis seen after DNA damage is decreased or absent in certain DNA-damage-sensitive mutants identified in human, rodent, *Drosophila*, slime mold, and fungal cells [48]. We have recently found that several of our DDI genes may play a role in such processes [49]. Five of the Class II clones in Table 4 (two of the Class IIa and all three Class IIb), designated *gadd*, were found to encode transcripts that were induced after growth arrest, such as medium depletion or serum reduction. Two of these clones, A45 and A153 (now designated *gadd45* and *gadd153*), hybridized well at high stringency to RNA from mouse, rat, and human cells; in all cases, the same pattern of induction by DNA-damaging agents or growth arrest signals was found. A variety of experiments indicate that these genes are coordinately induced and represent members of the same regulon that is activated by DNA damage or other growth arrest signals [49]; moreover, this regulon may be involved in negative growth control.

Oxidative stress response

As discussed earlier for the *oxyR* and SOS regulons in *E. coli*, many oxidizing agents can damage DNA, and cellular responses to oxidative stress and DNA-damaging often overlap. There is increasing evidence that this is also the case for mammalian cells. For example, the oxidizing agent, H_2O_2, was an effective inducing agent for many of the MMS-inducible transcripts of Table 4. At the doses used, both these agents produced substantial levels of base damage in the cellular DNA. As listed in Table 1, some genes whose products are involved in detoxifying oxidizing agents have been found to be inducible by DNA-damaging agents or TPA.

The NAD(P)H:menadione oxidoreductase (*Nmo-1*) gene has several properties that might be relevant to DDI genes [1]. This gene is a member of the aromatic hydrocarbon [*Ah*] receptor gene battery that is involved in the metabolism of drugs and carcinogens, such as benzo[a]pyrene. Drug-metabolizing enzymes are clinically divided into Phase I (monooxygenation) and Phase II (conjugation) reactions. Two of the [*Ah*] battery genes encode Phase I P450 enzymes, and the other four [*Ah*] genes code for *Nmo-1* and three other Phase II enzymes. The *Nmo-1* gene product detoxifies quinones by a two-electron reduction, resulting in hydroquinones that are readily

Table 5. Summary of the responses of three sets of stress-response genes

	$TCDD^a$ Treatment	c^{14Cos}/c^{14Cos} Mouse	MMS Treatment
[*Ah*] battery Phase I genes	+	−	−
[*Ah*] battery Phase II genes	+	+	+
gadd genes	−	+	+

[a] 2,3,7,8-tetrachlorodibenzo-*p*-dioxin (TCDD) activates both Phase I and Phase II [*Ah*] battery genes via binding to the *Ah* receptor in liver cells.

conjugated and excreted from the cell. Since quinones cause extensive DNA and protein alkylation, higher Nmo-1 activity would by advantageous to the cell. Interestingly, the *Nmo-1* and other phase II genes of the [*Ah*] gene battery are overexpressed in the c^{14Cos}/c^{14Cos} mouse mutant, which has a 1.1 cM deletion on chromosome 7; this region apparently contains one or more regulatory genes that modulate the expression of genes that are on other chromosomes [discussed in 1]. In addition to the *Nmo-1* gene, the *gadd* genes are also overexpressed in this mutant, while none of the other DDI genes were [49]. A further similarity between the *Nmo-1* and *gadd* genes was the finding that *Nmo-1* mRNA is induced in Hepa-1 liver cells by MMS [1]. The responses of these genes are summarized in Table 5. The increased expression of the *Nmo-1* gene and the *gadd* genes in the deletion mutant would suggest that a gene on chromosome 7 might encode one or more *trans*-acting factors that would be negative effectors of the *Nmo-1* and the *gadd* genes. Induction of these genes may thus be mediated by removal of this repressor. Interestingly, the SOS response is also mediated by removal of the *lexA* repressor. In addition, the *sulA* SOS gene encodes a growth arrest function.

A role for DDI genes in chemotherapy resistance?

As discussed elsewhere in this volume, there appear to be multiple mechanisms for chemoresistance in tumor cells, including alterations in drug uptake and efflux, metabolism, binding to DNA, and DNA repair. Since in both bacteria and eukaryotes many stress-response genes code for proteins that protect the cell from the particular stress, it would be reasonable to assume that some mammalian DDI genes may do the same for DNA damage. Even though the functions of many of DDI genes are uncertain at the present time, increased expression of a DDI gene in a particular chemoresistant tumor cell lines would imply a possible role in its resistance. In Table 2, we have shown results for a variety of drug-resistant cell lines that are resistant to base-bamaging agents, such as various alkylating agents or DDP, and do not have the *mdr-1* phenotype. As seen in this table, which includes preliminary unpublished results with several of our DDI clones, there is clearly evidence for increased expression of certain DDI genes, which warrants further study of the role of DDI genes in chemoresistance. Often chemoresistance appears multifactorial, even in the same cell line, and cannot easily be explained by a mutation or amplification of a single gene. However, if a regulatory factor that controls the expression of a regulon of stress-response genes was altered in a chemoresistant cell, then this single change could produce a variety of different effects.

Evidence for an x-ray-stress response

Most of this chapter has dealt with genes that are induced by UV radiation and other agents producing high levels of DNA base damage; however, the possibility exists that there may be genes induced by other types of genotoxic stress. For example, at biologically relevant doses x-radiation produces relatively little base damage, but it is an effective strand-breaking agent that probably results in chromosome breaks [50]. As summarized in Table 1, there is evidence at the protein level that certain genes can be induced by biologically relevant doses of x-rays in human cells. In one study [51], a correlation was observed between the magnitude of the induction of one protein and the ability of cells to recover from the potentially lethal effects of x-rays. The induction of some of these proteins appeared to be decreased in radiation-sensitive mutants, such as ataxia telangiectasis (AT) [51]. One effect of x-rays is the transient inhibition of DNA synthesis, which is reduced in AT cells. Since several of our DDI genes were associated with growth arrest, induction of these genes was recently studied in human cells. Interestingly, the *gadd45* gene was found to be clearly x-ray-inducible with doses as low as 2 Gy [68]. In AT cells, this gene was also rapidly inducible by x-rays or MMS, but the magnitude of the induction was substantially less than that in normal cells. These observations demonstrate that there is at least one x-ray-inducible gene in human cells, and indicate that an x-ray-stress response(s) exists in human cells.

Concluding remarks

The purpose of this chapter is to familiarize the reader with some of the aspects of DDI genes. Considering that nearly all of the known mammalian DDI genes have been identified in the last five years, our understanding of these genes, their regulation, and their function is in many respects incomplete and is certain to increase in the next several years. Several general comments can be made about these genes and their regulation. The first is that there are many DDI genes in mammalian cells. Approximately 1% of all the genes in yeast may be DDI [13]; 1% of the mammalian genome is 10^3 genes! A second important point is that the regulation of these genes is complex and probably involves multiple regulatory pathways in mammalian cells. For example, the results in Table 3 alone suggest that there are at least 5 DNA-damage stress responses (β-polymerase, ubiquitin, TPA-inducible genes, *DDIA18*, and the *gadd* genes), based on their patterns of induction by different damaging agents. For example, the TPA-inducible genes appear to represent a stress response different from that of the β-polymerase type of response, which was not induced by heat shock or UV, and was induced by single-base damaging agents. Some of these stress responses may be specific for DNA damage, while others probably represent more general stress responses to cell injury. A final point is that stress responses to different classes of DNA-damaging agents may involve both common and different genes. For example, β-polymerase was induced by alkylating agents in CHO cells, but not by UV radiation. This raises the possibility that new DDI genes might be identified using inducing agents other than UV radiation. Perhaps mammalian genes exist that are specifically induced by agents such x-rays, interestrand cross-linking agents, topoisomerase inhibitors, or other types of DNA-damaging agents.

References

1. Nebert, D.W., Peterson, D.D., and Fornace, A.J. Jr. Cellular responses to oxidative stress: the [*Ah*] gene battery as a paradigm. Environ. Health Persp., 88:13–25, 1990.
2. Walker, G.C. Mutagenesis and inducible responses to DNA damage in *E. coli*. Microbiol. Rev. 48:60–93, 1990.
3. VanBogelen, R.A., Kelley, P.M., and Neidhardt, F.C. Differential induction of heat shock, SOS, and oxidation stress regulons and accumulation of nucleotides in *E. coli*. J. Bacteriol. 169:26–32, 1987.
4. Morgan, R.W., Christman, M.F., Jacobson, F.S., Storz, G., and Ames, B.N. Hydrogen peroxide-inducible proteins in *Salmonella typhimurium* overlap with heat shock and other stress proteins. Proc. Natl. Acad. Sci. USA 83:8059–8063, 1986.
5. Friedberg, E.C. DNA repair in the yeast *Saccharomyces cerevisiae*. Microbiol. Rev. 52:70–102, 1988.
6. Johnson, A.L., Barker, D.G., and Johnson, L.H. Induction of yeast DNA ligase genes in exponential and stationary phase cultures in response to DNA damaging agents. Curr. Genet. 11:107, 1986.
7. Johnson, L.H., White, J.H.M., Johnson, A.L., Luccini, G., and Plevani, P. The yeast DNA polymerase I transcript is regulated in both mitotic cell cycle and in miosis and is also induced after DNA damage. Nucleic Acids Res. 15:5017, 1987.
8. Elledge, S.J. and Davis, R.W. Identification and isolation of the gene encoding the small subunit of ribonucleotide reductase from *S. cerevisiae*: a DNA damage-inducible gene required for mitotic viability. Mol. Cell. Biol. 7:2783–2793, 1987.
9. Cendari, E., Vellosi, R., Galli, A., and Bronzetti, G. Inducibility of gene conversion in *Saccharomyces cerevisiae* treated with MMS. Mut. Res. 174:271, 1986.
10. Cole G.M., and Mortimer R.K. Failure to induce a DNA repair gene, RAD54, in *Saccharomyces cerevisiae* does not affect DNA repair or reconbination phenotypes. Mol. Cell. Biol. 9:3314–3322, 1989.

11. McClanahan, T. and McEntee, K. Specific transcripts are elevated in *Saccharomyces cerevisiae* in response to DNA damage. Mol. Cell. Biol. 4:2356–2363, 1984.
12. Maga, J.A., McClanahan, and McEntee, K. Transcriptional regulation of DNA damage responsive (*DDR*) genes in different rad mutant strains of *Saccharomyces cerevisiae* MGG 205:276–284, 1986.
13. Ruby, S.W. and Szostak, J.W. Specific *Saccharomyces cerevisiae* genes are expressed in response to DNA-damaging agents. Mol. Cell. Biol. 5:75–84, 1985.
14. McClanahan, T. and McEntee, K. DNA damage and heat shock dually regulate genes in *Saccharomyces cerevisiae*. Mol. Cell. Biol. 6:90–96, 1986.
15. Fornace, A.J. Jr., Alamo, I. Jr., Hollander, M.C., and Lamoreaux, E. Ubiquitin RNA is a major stress-induced transcript in mammalian cells. Nucleic Acids Res. 17:1215–1230, 1989.
16. Jentsch, S., McGrath, J.P., and Varshavsky, A. The yeast DNA repair gene RAD6 encodes a ubiquitin-conjugating enzyme. Nature 329:131–134, 1987.
17. Vivino, A.A., Smoth, M.D., and Minton, K.W. A DNA damage responsive *Drosophila melanogaster* gene is also induced by heat shock. Mol. Cell. Biol. 6:4767–4769, 1986.
18. Akaboshi E. and Howard-Flanders P. Proteins induced by DNA-damaging agents in cultured Drosophila cells. Mut. Res. 227:1–6, 1989.
19. Koval, T.M. Enhanced recovery from ionizing radiation damage in a lepidoteran insect cell line. Radi. Res. 115:413–420, 1988.
20. Paoletti, C., et al. Inducible responses to DNA damages, CNRS symposium. Biochimie 64:541–848, 1982.
21. Hoy, C.A. and Rupert, C.S. Cycloheximide-sensitive recovery from 254 nm UV light damage in cultured marsupial cells. Mut. Res. 140:199–203, 1984.
22. Chao, C.C.-K. and Chao S.L. Federation of European Biochemical Societies, Elsevier Publishers, 1987.
23. Yarosh, D.B. The role of O6-methylguanine-DNA methyltransferase in cell survival, mutagenesis and carcinogenesis. Mut. Res. 145:1–16, 1985.
24. Protic, M., Roilides, E., Levine, A.S., and Dixon, K. Enhancement of DNA repair capacity of mammalian cells by carcinogen treatment. Somat. Cell Mol. Genet. 14: 351–357, 1988.
25. Roilides E., Minson, P.J., Levine A.S., and Dixon, K. Use of a simian virus 40-based shuttle vector to analyze enhanced mutagenesis in mitomycin C-treated monkey cells. Mol. Cell. Biol. 8:3943–3946, 1988.
26. Kaina, B., Stein, B., Schönthal, A., Rahmsdorf, J., Ponta, H., and Herrlich, P. An update of the mammalian UV response: gene regulation and induction of a protective. In: DNA repair mechanisms and their biological implications in mammalian cells efunction. Eds Lambert, M.W. and Laval, J. Plenum Press, New York, pp. 149–165, 1989.
27. Nishizuka, Y. Studies and perspectives of protein kinase C. Science 233:305–312, 1986.
28. Stein, B., Rahmsdorf, H.J., Steffen, A., Litfin, M., and Herrlich, P. UV-induced DNA damage is an intermediate step in UV-induced expression of human immunodeficiency virus type 1, collagenase, c-fos, and metallothionein. Mol. Cell. Biol. 9:5169–5181, 1989.
29. Schorpp, M., Mallick, U., Rahmsdorf, H.J., and Herrlich, P, UV-induced extracellular factor from human fibroblasts communicates the UV response to nonirradiated cells. Cell 37:861–868, 1984.
30. Hollander, M.C. and Fornace, A.J. Jr. Induction of *fos* RNA by DNA damaging agents. Cancer Res. 49:1687–1692, 1989.
31. Miskin, R. and Ben-Ishai, R. Induction of plasminogen activator by UV light in normal and xeroderma pigmentosum fibroblasts. Proc. Natl. Acad. Sci. USA 78:6236, 1981.
32. Valerie, K., Delers, A., Bruck, C., Thiriart, C., Rosenberg, H., Debouck, C., and Rosenberg, M. Activation of human immunodeficiency virus type 1 by DNA damage. Nature 333:78–81, 1988.
33. Imbra, R.J. and Karin, M. Phorbol ester induces the transcriptional stimulatory activity of the SV40 enhancer. Nature 32:555–557, 1986.

34. Lim, R.W., Varnum, B.C., O'Brian, T.G., and Herschman, H.R. Induction of tumor promotor-inducible genes in murine 3T3 cell lines and tetradecanoyl phorbol acetate-nonproliferative 3T3 variants can occur through protein kinase C-dependent and -independent pathways. Mol. Cell. Biol. 9:1790–1793, 1989.

35. Fine, R.L., Patel, J., and Chabner, B.A. Phorbol esters induce multidrug resistance in human breast cancer cells. Proc. Natl. Acad. Sci. USA 85: 582–586, 1988.

36. Burt R.K. and Thorgeirsson, S.S. Coinduction of MDR-1 multidrug-resistance and cytochrome P-450 genes in rat liver by xenobiotics. J. Natl. Cancer Inst. 80, 1383–1386, 1988.

37. Hamer, D.H. Metallothionein. Annu. Rev. Biochem. 55:913–951, 1986.

38. Matsubara, J., Tajima, Y., and Karasawa, M. Metallothionein induction as a potent means of radiation protection in mice. Radiat. Res. 111:267–275, 1987.

39. Fornace, A.J. Jr., Schalch, H., and Alamo, I. Jr. Coordinate induction of metallothionein I and II in rodent cells by UV-irradiation. Mol. Cell. Biol. 8:4716–4720, 1988.

40. Thornalley, P.J. and Vasak, M. Possible role for MT in protection against radiation-induced oxidative stress. Kinetics and mechanism of its reaction with superoxide and hydroxyl radicals. Biochem. Biophs. Acta 827:36–44, 1985.

41. Kelley, A.L., Basu, A., Teicher, B.A., Hacker, M.P., Hamer, D.H., and Lazo, J.S. Overexpression of metallothionein confers resistance to anticancer cells. Science 241:1813, 1988.

42. Fornace, A.J. Jr., Papathanasiou, M.A., Tarone, R.E., Wong, M., Mitchell, J., and Hamer, D.H. DNA-damage-inducible genes in mammalian cells. Prog. Clin. Biol. Res. 340A:315–25, 1990.

43. Schilder, R.J., Hall, L., Fojo, A.T., Monks, A., Handel, L.M., Fornace, A.J., Jr., Hamer, D.H., Young, R.C., Ozols, R.F., and Hamilton, T.C. Metallothionein gene expression and resistance to cisplatin in human ovarian cancer. Int. J. Cancer 45:416–422, 1990.

44. Fornace, A.J. Jr., Zmudzka, B.Z., Hollander, M.C., and Wilson, S.H. Induction of mammalian β-polymerase mRNA by DNA damaging agents in Chinese hamster ovary cells. Mol. Cell. Biol. 9:851–853, 1989.

45. Kartasova, T., Cornelissen, B.J., Belt, P., and Van de Putte, P. Effects of UV, 4-NQO and TPA on gene expression in cultured human epidermal keratinocytes. Nucleic Acid Res. 15:5945–5962, 1987.

46. Fornace, A.J. Jr., Alamo, I. Jr., and Hollander, M.C. DNA damage-inducible transcripts in mammalian cells. Proc. Natl. Acad. Sci. USA 85:8800–8804, 1988.

47. Weinert, T.A. and Hartwell, L.H. The RAD9 gene controls the cell cycle response to DNA damage in Saccharomyces cerevisiae. Science 241:317–322, 1988.

48. Lavin, M.F. and Schroeder, A.L. Damage-resistant DNA synthesis in eukaryotes. Mut. Res. 193:193–206, 1988.

49. Fornace, A.J. Jr., Nebert, D., Hollander, M.C., Papathanasiou, M., Fargnoli, J., and Holbrook, N. Mammalian genes coordinately regulated by growth arrest signals and DNA-damaging agents. Mol. Cell. Biol. 9:4196–4203, 1989.

50. Friedberg, E.C. DNA Repair. W.H. Freeman, New York, 1984.

51. Boothman, D.A., Bouvard, I., and Hughes, E.N. Identification and characterization of X-ray-induced proteins in human cells. Cancer Res. 49:2871–2878, 1989.

52. Angel, P., Baumann, I., Stein, B., Delious, H., Rahmsdorf, H.J., and Herrlich, P. 12-O-tetradecanoyl-phorbol-13-acetate induction of the human collagenase gene is mediated by an inducible enhancer element located in the 5'-flanking region. Mol. Cell. Biol. 7:2256, 1987.

53. Angel, P., Poting, A., Mallick, U., Rahmsdorf, H.J., and Herrlich, P. Induction of metallothionein and other MRNA species by carcinogens and tumor promoters in primary human fibroblasts. Mol. Cell. Biol. 6:1760–1766, 1986.

54. Schontal. A. Stein, B., Ponta, H., Rahmsdorf, H.J., and Herrlich, P. Nuclear protooncogenes determine the genetic program in response to external stimuli. Cold Spring

Harbor Symp. Quant. Biol. 53 (Pt 2):779–787, 1988.

55. Verma, A.K., Hsienh, J.T., and Pong, R.C. Mechanisms involved in ornithine decarboxylase induction by 12-O-tetradecanoylphorbol-13-acetate, a potent mouse skin tumor promoter and an activator of protein kinase C. Adv. Exp. Med. Biol. 250:273–290, 1988.

56. Kaufman, J.D., Valandra, G., Roderiguez, G., Bushar, G., Giri, C., and Norcross, A. Phorbol ester enhances human immunodeficiency virus-promoted gene expression and acts on a repeated 10-base-pair functinal enhancer element. Mol. Cell. Biol. 7:3759, 1987.

57. Maltzman, W. and Czyzyk, L. UV irradiation stimulates levels of p53 tumor antigen in nontransformed mouse cells. Mol. Cell. Biol. 4:1689, 1984.

58. Kartasova, T. and Van de Putte, P. Isolation, characterization and UV-stimulated expression of two families of genes encoding polypeptides of related structure in human epidermal keratinocytes. Mol. Cell. Biol. 8:2195–2203, 1988.

59. Kleinberger T., Flint, Y.B., Blank, M., Etkin, S., and Lavi, S. Carcinogen-induced trans activation of gene expression. Mol. Cell. Biol. 8:1366–1370, 1988.

60. Sakai, M., Okuda, A., and Muramatsu, M. Multiple regulatory elements and phorbol 12-O-tetradecanoate 13-acetate responsivness of the rat placental glutathione transferase gene. Proc. Natl. Acad. Sci. USA 85:9456–9460, 1988.

61. Keyse, S.M. and Tyrrel, R.M. Heme-oxygenase is the major 32-kDa stress protein induced in human skin fibroblasts by UV A radiation, hydrogen peroxide, and sodium arsenite. Proc. Natl. Acad. Sci. USA 86:99–103, 1989.

62. Lambert, M.E., Ronai, Z.A., Weinstein, I.B., and Garrels, J.I. Enhancement of major histocompatibility class I protein synthesis by DNA damage in cultured human fibroblasts and keratinocytes. Mol. Cell. Biol. 9:847–850, 1989.

63. Wolff, S. Are radiation-induced effects hormetic? Science 245:575, 1989.

64. Rotem, N., Axelrod, J.H., and Mishkin, R. Induction of urokinase-type plasminogen activator factor by UV light in human fetal fibroblasts is mediated through a UV-induced secreted protein. Mol. Cell. Biol. 7:622–631, 1987.

65. Andrews, P.A., Murphy, M.P., and Howell, S.B. Metallothionein-mediated cisplatin resistance in ovarian carcinoma cells. Cancer Chemother. Pharmacol. 19:149–154, 1987.

66. Bakka, A., Endresen, L., Johnsen, A.B.S., Edminson, P.D., and Rugstad, H.E. Resistance against cis-dichlorodiammineplatinum in cultured cells with a high content of metallothionein. Toxicol. Appl. Pharmacol. 61:215–226, 1981.

67. Kraker, A.J. and Moore, C.W. Elevated DNA polymerase beta activity in a cisdiamminedichloroplatinum(II) resistant P338 murine leukemia cell line. Cancer Lett. 38:307, 1988.

68. Papathanasiou, M.A., Kerr, N., Robbins, J.H., McBride, O.W., Alamo, I., Jr., Barrett, S.F., Hickson, I., and Fornace, A.J., Jr. Induction by ionizing radiation of the gadd45 gene in cultured human cells: lack of mediation by protein Kinase C. Molec. Cell. Biol. 11: 1009–1016, 1991.

3. Molecular biology of P-glycoprotein

Marilyn M. Cornwell

Introduction

Since the advent of chemotherapy it has been observed that certain types of cancer are rarely sensitive to treatment with chemotherapy. Other cancers that are initially responsive to treatment eventually become resistant to the treatment regimen being used and to some other drugs as well. Resistance to chemotherapy remains one of the fundamental barriers to curative treatment. The mechanisms by which tumor cells become drug resistant have been under intensive study. It is clear from the accumulated data that drug resistance is a complex phenomenon, including more than one mechanism. Resistance may be caused by a change in one, more than one, facet of drug interaction with a cell, from drug influx/efflux and drug metabolism to drug-target site interactions.

One of the most well-studied types of resistance is resistance to multiple structurally dissimilar hydrophobic chemotherapeutic agents, or MDR. This phenomenon has been modelled using rodent and human cells in culture [1–3]. The results of studies over the past two decades indicate that MDR is a complex phenotype that may involve the activities of several cellular proteins. The most well-understood mechanism, however, involves the plasma membrane multidrug transporter P-glycoprotein, which has been shown to mediate decreased cellular accumulation of certain hydrophobic drugs [reviewed in 4–6]. The evidence for the role of P-glycoprotein in multidrug resistance and the procedures used to clone the *mdr* genes have been recently reviewed [4–6]. This review focuses on the current knowledge of the structure and regulation of the genes that encode P-glycoproteins.

The *MDR* multigene family

The *MDR* genes are a family of related sequences that have extensive homology between species. In humans, two *MDR* genes have been identified, only one of which has been shown to be involved in the multidrug resistance phenotype. In rodents, three *MDR* genes have been identified,

Robert F. Ozols (ed.), MOLECULAR AND CLINICAL ADVANCES IN ANTICANCER DRUG RESISTANCE. Copyright © 1991.
Kluwer Academic Publishers, Boston. All rights reserved. ISBN 0-7923-1212-0

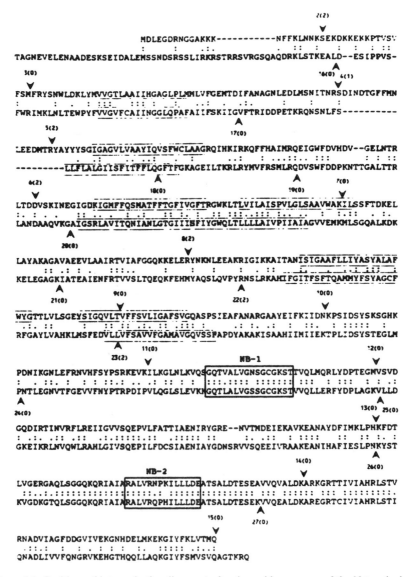

Figure 1A. Positions of introns in the alignment of amino acid sequences of the N-terminal and C-terminal halves of *MDR1*-encoded P-glycoprotein. Identical amino acid residues are indicated by colons; functionally similar residues (A,S,T; D,E; N,Q; R,K; I,L,M.V; F,Y,W) are indicated by dots. Potential transmembrane segments are enclosed in thin boxes. Potential nucleotide-binding sites (NB-1 and NB-2) are enclosed in thick boxes. Positions of introns are marked by arrows, intron numbers, and intron types (in parentheses). (From Chen et al. [13], permission.)

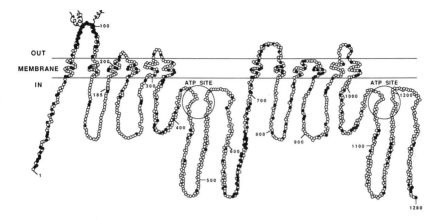

Figure 1B. Model of the human multidrug transporter. The filled circles represent amino acids that differ between human *MDR1* and mouse *mdr1*, the most divergent human and mouse sequences that are still functional in conferring drug resistance. The ATP-binding sites are circled. Putative N-linked carbohydrates are shown as curly lines. The mutation that is associated with preferential colchicine resistance, glycine to valine at position 185, is shown as a cross-hatched square. (From Kane et al. [14], with permission.)

two of which play a role in multidrug resistance. Related sequences have been identified in several other species in which genetic evidence suggests that the genes encode proteins with critical transport function.

The human MDR *genes*

The two human *MDR* genes, *MDR1* [7] and *MDR2* [8], are located within 330 bp of each other on chromosome 7 band q21.1 [9,10], coincident with the location of the cystic fibrosis gene and *met* protooncogene [10]. Comparison of their coding sequences indicates that *MDR1* and *MDR2* are 85% homologous, although only *MDR1* is involved in multidrug resistance [11, 12]. Recent studies of the human *MDR1* genomic structure indicates that the gene has 27 exons (Figure 1A) [13]. Both *MDR1* and *MDR2* encode approximately 1280 amino acids, with 12 transemembrane domains and two nucleotide binding domains [14,15] (Figure 1B). Although the encoded protein has two very similar halves, the exon/intron organization of the each half is more similar between the *MDR* genes of different species than the exon/intron structure of the halves within the same gene [13]. From the elegant analysis of the exon/intron structure, it has been hypothesized that the *MDR1* gene arose through fusion of two similar primordial genes, rather than by duplication of a single gene [13]. A model of the origin of P-glycoprotein from two primordial genes is presented in Figure 2 [13].

Evidence that increased expression of the *MDR1* gene causes multidrug resistance [4–6] includes 1) increased expression and amplification of

39

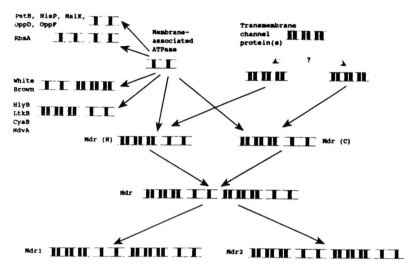

Figure 2. Proposed scheme for the evolution of *mdr* (P-glycoprotein) genes. Box with shaded bars, nucleotide-binding domain; box with black bars, membrane-bound domain. (From Chen et al. [13], with permission.)

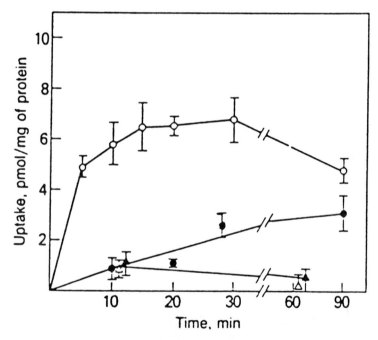

Figure 3. Time course of ATP-dependent vinblastine uptake in vesicles from drug-sensitive and drug-resistant KB cells. ³H-vinblastine accumulation was measured in membrane vesicles from drug-resistant cells (○, ●) and drug-sensitive cells (△, ▲), as described by Horio et al. [23], in the presence of ATP (○, △) or AMP (●, ▲). (From Horio et al. [43], with permission.)

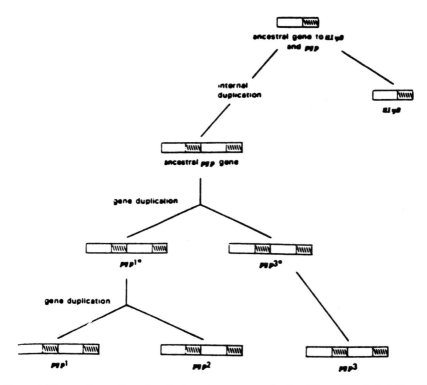

Figure 4. Proposed genealogy for the hamster *pgp* gene family. (From Ng et al. [29], with permission.)

MDR1 in multidrug resistance cells [16–19], 2) ATP and drug binding by P-glycoprotein [20–22], 3) ATP-dependent drug transport in isolated membrane vesicles from drug-resistant cells (Figure 3) [23], 4) localization of P-glycoprotein in the plasma mambrane [24], and 5) transfer of the multidrug resistance phenotype to sensitive cells by transfected *MDR1* cDNA [11]. In contrast, *MDR2* does not appear to be involved in the multidrug resistance, since attempts to confer the phenotype by transfection of the *MDR2* cDNA have failed thus far [25].

The rodent mdr *genes*

The three mouse and hamster *mdr* genes encode proteins similar in structure to the human *MDR* genes [15,26–29]. The hamster genes map to chromosome 1q26 [30], and the mouse genes map to chromosome 5 [31]. All the rodent genes are on the same chromosome, as are the human genes [32,33]. Analysis of the exon/intron structure of the mouse [33] and hamster [29] genes, along with comparison of amino acid sequence, suggests that the rodent genes resulted from a duplication event sometime after primates and

41

Table 1. Proposed classification of mammalian *mdr* sequences[a]

Source	*mdr* Gene Class	Other Designation	References
Human	*mdr1*	*MDR1*	7,82
	mdr2	*MDR2*	7,8,61
Rodent	*mdr1a*	*pgp1, mdr3*	26,27,64
	mdr1b	*pgp2, mdr1*	25–27,34
	mdr2	*pgp3, mdr2*	26,34

[a] Adapted from Hsu et al. [26].

rodents diverged. A model for the evolution of hamster *mdr* genes is shown in Figure 4 [29]. Mouse *mdr1a* and *mdr1b* (also called *mdr3* and *mdr1*, respectively) and their hamster homologs, *pgp1* and *pgp2*, encode proteins that are similar in amino acid sequence to human *MDR1* [26,27], and these rodent genes confer drug resistance. Within the *MDR1*-related genes, mouse *mdr1a* (*pgp1*) appears to be more like *MDR1* than mouse *mdr1b* (*pgp2*) [27,28]. Mouse *mdr2* and hamster *pgp3* are more related to human *MDR2*, and, like the human gene, neither *mdr2* nor *pgp3* has been shown to confer drug resistance [8,25,34]. The relationship of human and rodent *MDR* genes is outlined in Table 1 [27].

In general, the functional characterization of the rodent gene products has shown that 1) the *MDR1*-related sequences encode drug transport proteins [27] and 2) transfection of the corresponding cDNAs confers the full multidrug resistance phenotype [35].

MDR-*related sequences in other species*

Recent evidence suggests that *mdr*-like sequences exist in many species. In prokaryotes, certain subunits of several cellular export and import systems share sequence and structural homology with the P-glycoprotein ATP-binding region [15,26,36]. The strongest homologies are with *hylB*, the ATP-binding hemolysin export protein in *E. coli* [37]; NDVA, a glucan export protein in *Rhizobium meliloti* [38]; *lktB*, a toxin secretion component analogous to *hylB* in *Pasteruella haemolytica* [39]; and *cyaB*, involved in adenylate cyclase secretion in *Bordetella pertussis* [40]. Homologies exist between the ATP-binding regions of P-glycoprotein and the bacterial transport proteins hisP, malK, pstB, rbsA, oppD, and oppF [reviewed 36], as well as ftsE in *E. coli*, a protein involved in cell division [41] and nodI in *Rhizobium*, a protein involved in nodulation [42]. In these systems the homology to P-glycoprotein exists only in the ATP-binding subunit, not in the substrate-binding or integral membrane subunits [36,43]. The proposed relationship between the prokaryotic genes and the mammalian genes is shown in Figure 2 [13].

Several eukaryotic proteins thought to be involved in cellular transport are similar to P-glycoprotein. A homolog of *mdr*, *pfmdr*, has been cloned

42

and sequenced from the malaria parasite *Plasmodium falciparum* [44,45]. The *pfmdr* gene is amplified and transcript levels are increased in some strains of chloroquine-resistant *P. falciparum*. In yeast, the STE-6 gene is about 60% homologous at the amino acid level to human *mdr1*, and genetic evidence suggests that it encodes a protein involved in transport of the mating type factor **a**. The predicted structure of STE6 is virtually identical to P-glycoprotein [46,47]. In *Drosophila*, two genes involved in eye pigmentation, white and brown, encode proteins thought to be transporters of eye pigments [48,49]. Each contains an amino-terminal nucleotide binding site and hydrophobic regions in the carboxy-terminal third of the protein [50–52].

Regulation of *MDR* gene expression

Because increased *MDR1* gene expression has important implications for the treatment of human tumors, the regulation of *MDR1* gene expression is under intensive study. The expression of *MDR1* in human tumors is reviewed by Goldstein et al. in this series (Goldstein et al. Chapter 5).

Chromosomal aberrations

Pioneering work by Biedler and coworkers and Ling and coworkers showed that multidrug resistance was consistent with an amplification phenomenon [reviewed in 6]. First, multidrug-resistance revertants could be selected by simply growing the cells in the absence of drug for several weeks [6,53]. Secondly, multidrug-resistant cells in culture were shown to have amplified DNA in the form of HSRs (homogeneously staining regions) and/or double minute chromosomes [54]. Multidrug-resistance revertants were found to have lost these DNA abnormalities [55]. Subsequent work showed that the amplified sequences contained the P-glycoprotein (*mdr*) genes [7].

The P-glycoprotein amplicon contains five gene classes [12,32,56], and the organization of these genes within the amplicon is conserved among human, mouse, and hamster [12,57]. The product of one of the non-*MDR* genes has been identified as a cytosolic calcium-binding protein, homologous to calpain [32]. It is not known what role, if any, the non-*MDR* gene products from this amplicon play in the MDR phenotype.

Expression in normal tissues

The expression of the P-glycoprotein genes has been studied using molecular probes, as well as specific antibodies (summarized in Table 2). These studies have shown that a single species of mRNA of about 4.5 kb is expressed at high levels in human adrenal, kidney, colon, and liver, at intermediate levels in jejunum, pancreas, and brain, and at low levels in most other tissues [24,58–

Table 2. *mdr* gene expression in normal tissues

Organ	MDR1[a]	MDR2[b]	mdr1a[c]	mdr1b	mdr2	References
Adrenal	+++++	+	−	++++	++	58,61,64
Uterus			−	+	−	58
Pregnant uterus			−	+++++	−	58
Placenta			−	+++	−	58
Kidney	+++	++	+	++	−	58,64
Colon	++	−	+++	−	−	58,61,64
Liver	+++	+++	+	+	++	58,61,64
Jejunum	++					58
Rectum	++					58
Brain	++		+	++	−	58,64
Prostate	+					58
Skin	+					58
Muscle	+	−	+	+	++	58,61,64
Heart	+		++	++	++	58,64
Lung	+	−	++	+	++	58,61,64
Spleen	+	+	+	+	++	58,61,64
Bone marrow	+					58
Stomach	+	−	−	−	++	58,61,64
Esophagus	+	−				58,61
Ovary	+					58
Spinal cord	+		++	−	−	58,61,64
Testes			++	−	−	64
Bladder	+	−				58,61

MDR1 levels are quantitated by desitometry of slot blots, as described by Fojo et al. [58]. *MDR2* was detected by PCR amplification, as described by Chin et al. [61]. Rodent *mdr* gene expression was quantitated from Northern blots, as described by Croop et al. [64]. −, no detectable signal. A blank space signifies no data available.

61]. In those tissues where the gene is expressed at high levels, P-glycoprotein is localized to specific regions, primarily on the lumenal surfaces of secretory epithelium, such as bile canaliculi in the liver and proximal tubules of the kidney [24].

Recent studies have shown that human *MDR2* is coexpressed with *MDR1* in liver, kidney, adrenal, and spleen, but is not expressed in colon, lung, stomach, esophagus, breast, muscle, and bladder [8,62]. van der Bliek et al. have shown that in human liver *MDR2* transcripts are differentially spliced at the 3' end to form three splicing variants [8]. Differential expression of these transcripts has not been demonstrated, and the functional significance of these transcripts is not yet understood.

A somewhat different pattern of *mdr* expression has been observed in rodent tissues (Table 2). The three rodent genes are show a distinct pattern of tissue-specific gene expression [63–65]. The mouse *mdr1a* (or *mdr3*, *pgp1*) is expressed at high levels in intestine, lung, brain, heart, and testes, and at detectable levels in kidney, liver, muscle, spleen, and stomach [65]. The mouse *mdr1b* gene (*mdr1*, *pgp2*) is expressed at very high levels in adrenal, placenta, and the secretory epithelium of the gravid uterus; at high levels in heart and kidney; and at detectable levels in uterus, liver, muscle, spleen, brain, and lung [65,66]. No expression of *mdr1b* was detectable in intestine, spinal cord, testes, or stomach [65]. Expression of *mdr2* (*pgp3* was high in adrenal, liver muscle, spleen, and heart, but at undetectable levels in all other tissues [65].

The distinct pattern of *mdr* gene expression in normal tissues and the similarity between P-glycoproteins suggest that each of these gene products is involved in normal transport functions. It has been suggested that the bile canaliculi, kidney proximal tubule, and GI localization of the human gene products is consistent with the excretion of ingested toxic substances or unknown cellular metabolites [67]. The *MDR1* gene product in liver bile canalicular membranes has been shown to transport a variety of chemo-therapeutic agents in an ATP-dependent manner [68], indicating that the protein in unselected cells can use the same substrates as the P-glycoprotein in multidrug-resistant cells. High levels of *MDR1* expression in the adrenal suggests that steroids or other adrenocortical products may be transported by P-glycoprotein.

The localization and increased expression of P-glycoprotein in the endo-metrium of the gravid uterus in mouse (*mdr1b*) suggests that endogenous steroids may be a substrate for P-glycoprotein [66]. Progesterone has been shown to specifically interact with P-glycoprotein in multidrug-resistant cells and to increase the sensitivity of multidrug-resistant cells to vinblastine [69]. It is not yet known whether the human gene is expressed in the pregnant human uterus. It is possible that expression of the mouse *mdr1b* gene in the rodent uterus may not have a human counterpart.

Control of gene expression

Although increased expression of the *MDR* genes was originally associated with amplification of *MDR* DNA, it is clear from recent studies that *MDR* mRNA levels are regulated more specifically. First, increased steady-state levels of *MDR* mRNA can account for increased resistance in the absence of *MDR* gene amplification [19,70]. Second, high levels of expression in a relatively small number of normal tissues occurs in the absence of gene amplification [59]. In addition, the examination of hundreds of human tumor specimens has shown that increased *MDR1* mRNA is observed without *MDR1* gene amplification [59; see Goldstein et al., Chapter 5). Finally, recent studies have shown that *MDR1* is regulated by transcriptional, as well as post-transcriptional, controls.

Transcriptional control of the *MDR* gene has been indicated by induction by heat-shock and sodium-arsenite treatment of human renal adenocar-cinoma cells [71] and by retinoic-acid treatment of human neuroblastoma cells [72]. In the studies of heat-shock and sodium-arsenite inducibility, new RNA synthesis was required for induction [71], although increased tran-scription by nuclear run-on was not demonstrated. In addition, a post-

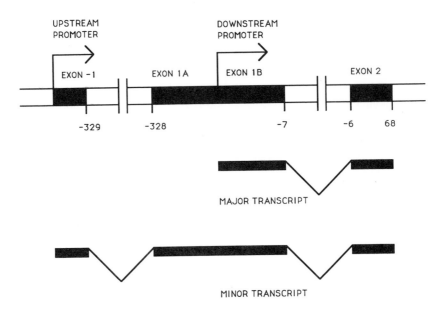

Figure 5. Diagram of transcription initiation in the *MDR1* gene. Numbers correspond to the cDNA residues at the exon-intron borders. The ATG initiation codon is at the beginning of exon 2. (Adapted from Chin et al. [62] and printed with permission.)

transcriptional component of *MDR1* regulation was indicated by the increased half-life of *MDR1* mRNA after sodium-arsenite treatment [71].

Evidence that the *MDR1* gene is regulated post-transcriptionally comes from studies done by treating rats with cytotoxic drugs or partial hepatectomy [reviewed in 67]. Damage to the rat liver by these treatments results in large increases in *MDR1* RNA levels [73]. In addition, treatment of rats with such agents as aflatoxin B1, isosafrole, phenothiazine, and TCDD, which induce drug catabolizing enzymes, such as P450 isoform **d**, results in increases in *MDR1* mRNA [74]. The mechanism of this regulation is not known, but new transcription is not seen in nuclear run-on assays [75].

Attempts to understand the regulation of *MDR1* expression have been hampered by the low level of expression in most cell lines. In the studies discussed above, the induction by heat-shock and arsenite treatment occurs in only one of almost 50 cell lines examined [71]. In addition, it is unclear at this time whether the post-transcriptional control observed is restricted to the rat liver system or whether it plays a major role in *MDR1* expression in human cells.

Analysis of RNAs from human multidrug-resistant cells has shown that two distinct promoter elements drive *MDR1* transcription [76,77] (Figure 5). P1 promoter activity is located within the first kilobase of sequences 5' to the transcription initiation site [77]. The major transcription start sites are located 136 and 140 bases upstream of the +1 translation start site (Figure

5). In most cell lines, normal tissues, and tumor samples studies to date, the P1 promoter initiates from these sites [77; Goldstein et al., Chapter 5]. Minor P1 transcription start sites located 156–80 bases upstream are present in RNAs from colchicine-selected MDR cell lines [76,77]. Transcripts initiating from the P2 promoter 500–600 bases upstream of the +1 ATG are found in colchicine-selected cell lines and in some human tumors [77,78]. These transcripts are somewhat unusual in that they contain P1 promoter sequences (exon 1a) (Figure 5) [62,77]. In some of these cell lines and tumors, P2 promoter activity accounts for 50–100% of *mdr1* transcription [76–78]. The significance of the P2 promoter activity is not yet clear, although it may be a function of drug treatment.

To study the regulation of *MDR1* expression, a genomic sequence containing P1 promoter activity was cloned [77]. P1 activity was demonstrated in transfection assays using a reporter gene [77]. Detection of promoter function required the presence of a viral enhancer, consistent with the low basal activity of the promoter observed in drug-sensitive cells [77]. Sequence analysis has shown the P1 promoter region contains a variety of consensus sequences for the binding of proteins known to be transcription factors (Figure 3). The P1 promoter is GC-rich, contains a "CCAAT"-box 200 bases upstream of the initiation site, but does not contain a canonical "TATA"-box within this region, although a TFIID consensus site is located about 350 bases upstream of the initiation site (Figure 6). Functional analysis of the *MDR1* promoters is far from complete. Many questions about the role of sequences within the P1 promoter still remain, especially with regards to tissue-specific expression of P-glycoprotein. The sequence and functional characterization of the P2 has not yet been reported, and whether there is any interaction between P1 and P2 remains to be determined.

A genomic DNA containing the mouse *mdr1* transcription initiation site has been sequenced, and a single initiation site has been identified by S1 nuclease mapping [33]. The mouse 5' flanking region, unlike the human sequence, contains a TATA-like sequence, a "GC" box, and a canonical CCAAT box [33]. It seems likely that regulatory mechanisms that differ between the mouse and human may be accounted for, at least in part, by what appear to be significant differences in regulatory sequences.

Molecular analysis of P-glycoprotein function

A concerted effort by a number of different laboratories to characterize to P-glycoprotein function at the molecular level has provided biochemical and genetic evidence that P-glycoprotein unidirectionally transports certain hydrophobic agents in an ATP-dependent manner [6]. The more difficult problem has been to define the transport activity of this protein mechanistically. There must be regions of the protein that are highly specific for substrate recognition, because although *MDR1* and *MDR2* are 85% homo-

CONSENSUS TRANSCRIPTION FACTOR BINDING SITES IN THE *MDR*1 DOWNSTREAM PROMOTER

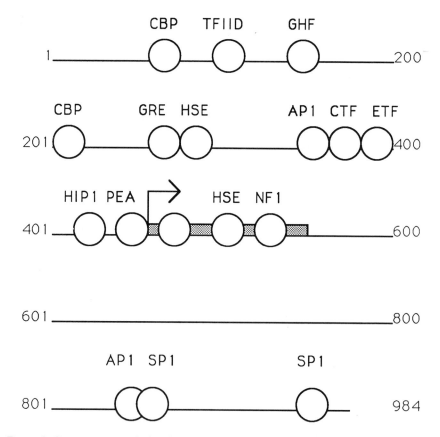

Figure 6. Consensus transcription factor binding sites in the *MDR1* downstream promoter. Sequences in the genomic promoter clone pMDR-P3 [77], 1–984 bp, are indicated by the solid line. Consensus binding sites are shown as a circle with the acronym for the factor or the sequence above. The arrow indicates the transcription initiation site, and the stippled box represents exon 1B [77].

logous, the *MDR2* gene product has not been shown to mediate multidrug resistance [24,34]. It is thought that the entire protein, including both ATP-binding regions, is functionally integrated, since neither half of the protein can function independently (Figure 7) [79]. Deletion analysis has shown that removal of 23 amino acids at the carboxy terminus of the protein-coding region reduces but does not eliminate the activity of the protein. However,

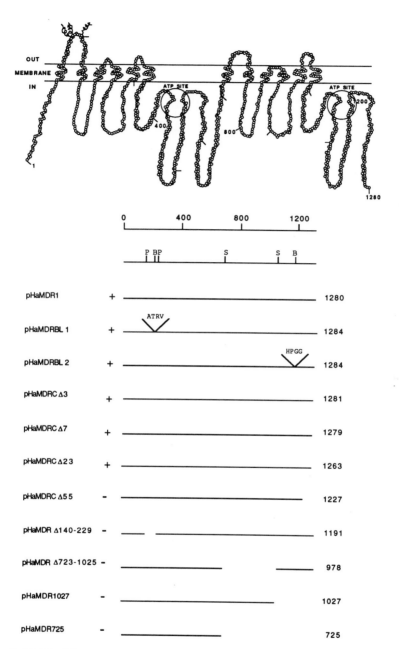

Figure 7. Model of human P-glycoprotein and linear representation of mutants. The ATP-binding sites are circled and putative N-linked sugars are shown as curly lines. The +− designation shown in the second column indicates whether or not drug resistance was conferred by the construct. On the frist line the amino acid position is shown, while on the second line a partial restriction map for the pertinent enzymes is given (P = *Pvu*II, B = *Bal*I, and S = *Stu*I). The four amino acid insertions for pHaMDRBL1 and pHaMDRBL2 are indicated above the line at the point of their insertion. For the mutants with the internal deletions, the line is disrupted in the area of the deletion. The final column indicates the number of amino acids expected for each mutant.

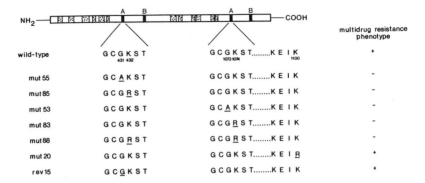

Figure 8. Effects of discrete mutations introduced at the nucleotide binding site of the *MDR1* protein on expression of multidrug resistance. *a*: Predicted structural domains of the *MDR1* protein. ■, A and B motifs of the nucleotide-binding site consensus sequence; □, putative transmembrane domains. *b*: Positions of the amino acid residues targeted by site-directed mutagenesis in the wild-type sequence and mutated residues (underlined) in the mutants. *c*: Ability (+) or inability (−) of the mutant cDNAs to confer multidrug resistance upon direct transfection into drug-sensitive cells [80]. (From [●●], with permission.)

deletion of 53 amino acids completely abolishes functional activity [79]. The same holds for deletion of 267 bp in the amino half (removing the first cytoplasmic loop to the fourth transmembrane domain) or 906 bp in the carboxy half (the sixth through twelfth transmembrane domains) [79] (Figure 7). Furthermore, mutational analysis of the ATP-binding regions has shown that the integrity of both these sites is required for P-glycoprotein function (Figure 8) [80]. The stoichiometries of drug binding, ATP hydrolysis, and transport, as well as the location of the drug-binding site(s), are not well defined. Recent studies using a photoactivatable drug in combination with proteolysis suggest that two distinct sites within P-glycoprotein are labelled by drug, indicating that either there are two drug-binding sites or that one site is composed of distinct regions within the two halves of the protein [81,82]. Similar experiments utilizing *MDR1-MDR2* chimeras or other structural mutants may provide additional insight into the structural requirements for drug-protein interactions.

Molecular characterization of the cDNAs from MDR cell lines has provided the first clues as to understanding the diverse substrate specificity of P-glycoprotein. Choi et al. observed that the P-glycoprotein in colchicine-selected human cells differed from that in vinblastine-selected or drug-sensitive cells at a single amino acid residue [83]. The "mutant" protein in colchicine-selected cells contains a valine at amino acid 185, while the "wild-type" sequence contains a glycine at that residue. To determine whether this subtle difference could account for preferential resistance to colchicine, the mutant gene was transfected into drug-sensitive cells. Transformants containing the mutant cDNA were relatively more resistant to colchicine than to adriamycin or vinblastine. Transformants containing the wild-type cDNA showed equivalent resistance to these agents [83]. Thus, amino acid 185, and the region containing this residue, may be involved in determining the substrate specificity of P-glycoprotein. This residue is within the region labelled with photoaffinity drug analogues [81,82]. It seems likely that discreet changes in protein sequence could account for variations in the pattern of cross-resistance observed in multidrug-resistant cell lines [4,53,84].

The three rodent gene products appear to also to confer differences in resistance. During stepwise vinblastine selection of the mouse J774.2 cell line, there is a switch from expression of *mdr1b* RNA (and a 140,000 Dal P-glycoprotein) to expression of *mdr1a* (and a 130,000 Dal P-glycoprotein) [27,85]. This switch might simply provide a selective advantage for cells expressing *mdr1a*. Alternatively, at high drug concentrations, cells may actively switch from *mdr1b* to *mdr1a* synthesis. Taken together with the tissue-specific expression of these two genes, the results are consistent with a differential function of their gene products in the mouse.

Summary

The molecular genetic characterization of MDR human, mouse, and hamster P-glycoprotein genes has identified several elements that may contribute to the diversity in multidrug-resistance phenotype associated with P-glycoprotein expression. First, spontaneous mutations within the *MDR* genes may alter the relative affinity of P-glycoprotein for certain drugs or alter the substrate specificity of the protein. Secondly, alternative splicing of *MDR* mRNA may result in isoforms with different substrate recognition or transport properties. Differential splicing has not thus far been demonstrated for human *MDR1* or mouse *mdr1a* and *mdr1b* genes. Finally, differential expression of *mdr* genes encoding P-glycoprotein isoforms with distinct properties appears to be a possible mechanism for generating diversity in MDR rodent cells.

References

1. Biedler, J.L. and Riehm, H. Cellular resistance to actinomycin D in Chinese hamster ovary cell in vitro: cross resistance, radiographic and cytogenetic studies. Cancer Res. 30:1174–1184, 1970.
2. Akiyama, S.-I., Fojo, A, Hanover, J.A., Pastan, I., and Gottesman, M.M Isolation and genetic characterization of human KB cell lines resistant to multiple drugs. Somat. Cell Mol. Genet. 11:117–126, 1985.
3. Howell, N., Belli, T.A, Zaczkiewics, L.T., and Belli, J.A. High level, unstable adriamycin resistance in a Chinese hamster mutant cell line with double minute chromosomes. Cancer Res. 44:4023–4030, 1984.
4. Croop, J.M., Gros, P., and Housman, D.E. Genetics of multidrug resistance. J. Clin. Invest. 81:1303–1309, 1988.

5. Gottesman, M.M. and Pastan, I. The multidrug transporter: a bouble edged sword. J. Biol. Chem. 263:12163–12166, 1988.
6. Endicott, J. and Ling, V. The biochemistry of P-glycoprotein-mediated multidrug resistance. An. Rev. Biochem. 58:137–171, 1989.
7. Roninson, I.B., Chen, J.E., Choi, K., Gros, P., Housman, D., Fojo, A., Shen, D., Gottesman, M.M., and Pastan, I. Isolation of human mdr DNA sequences amplified in multidrug-resistant KB carcinama cells. Proc. Natl. Acad. Sci. USA 83:4538–4542, 1986.
8. van der Bliek, A.M., Baas, F., de Lange, T., Kooiman, P.M., van der Veld-Koerts, T., and Borst, P. The human mdr3 gene encodes a novel P-glycoprotein homologue and gives rise to alternatively spliced mRNAs in liver. EMBO J. 6:3325–3331, 1987.
9. Callen, D.F., Baker, E., Simmers, R.N., Seshardri, R., and Roninson, I.B. Localization of the human multiple drug resistance gene, MDR1, to 7q21.1. Hum. Genet. 77:142–144, 1987.
10. Trent, J.M. and Witkowski, C.M. Clarification of the chromosomal assignment of the human P-glycoprotein/mdr1 gene: possible coincidence with the cystic fibrosis and c-met oncogene. Cancer Genet. Cytogenet 26:187–190, 1987.
11. Ueda, K., Cardarelli, C., Gottesman, M.M., and Pastan, I. Expression of a full-length cDNA for the human mdr1 gene confers resistance to colchicine, doxorubicin and vinblastine. Proc. Natl. Acad. Sci. USA 85:1595–1599, 1987.
12. van der Bliek, A.M., Baas, F., van der Veld-Koerts, T., Biedler, J.L., Meyers, M.B., Ozols, R.F., Hamilton, T.C., Joenje, H., and Borst, P. Genes amplified and overexpressed in human multidrug-resistant cell lines. Cancer Res. 48:5927–5932, 1988.
13. Chen, C., Clark, D., Ueda, K., Pastan, I., Gottesman, M.M., and Roninson, I.B. Genomic organization of the human multidrug resistance (MDR1) gene and origin of P-glycoproteins. J. Biol. Chem. 265:506–514, 1990.
14. Kane, S.E., Pastan, I., and Gottesman, M.M. Genetic basis of multidrug resistance of tumor cells. J. Bioenerg. Biomembr., 1990, in press.
15. Chen, C., Chin, J.E., Ueda, K., Clark, D.P., Pastan, I., Gottesman, M.M., and Roninson, I.B. Internal duplication and homology with bacterial transport proteins in the mdr1 (P-glycoprotein) gene from multidrug-resistant human cells. Cell 47:381–389, 1987.
16. Juliano, R.L. and Ling, V. A surface glycoprotein modulating drug permeability in Chinese hamster ovary cell mutants. Biochim. Biophys. Acta 455:152–162, 1976.
17. Riordan, J.R., Deuchars, K., Kartner, N., Alon, N., Trent, J., and Ling, V. Amplification of P-glycoprotein genes in multidrug-resistant mammalian cell lines. Nature 316:817–819, 1985.
18. Meyers, M.B., Spengler, B.A., Chang, T.D., Melera, P.W., and Biedler, J.L. Gene amplification-associated cytogenetic aberrations and protein changes in vincristine-resistant Chinese hamster, mouse, and human cells. J. Cell Biol. 100:588–596, 1985.
19. Shen, D., Fojo, A., Chin, J.E., Roninson, I.B., Richert, N., Pastan, I., and Gottesman, M.M. Human multidrug resistant cell lines: increased mdr1 expression can precede gene amplification. Science 232:643–645, 1986.
20. Cornwell, M.M., Safa, A.R., Felsted, R.L., Gottesman, M.M., and Pastan, I. Membrane vesicles from multidrug-resistant human cancer cells contain a specific 150–170 kDa protein detected by photaffinity labeling. Proc. Natl. Acad. Sci. USA 83:3847–3850, 1986.
21. Cornwell, M.M., Tsuruo, T., Gottesman, M.M., and Pastan, I. ATP-binding properties of P-glycoprotein from multidrug resistant KB cells FASEB J. 1:51–54, 1987.
22. Safa, A.R., Glover, G.J., Meyers, M.B., Biedler, J.L., and Felsted, R.L. Vinblastine photoaffinity labeling of high molecular weight surface membrane glycoprotein specific for multidrug resistant cells. J. Biol. Chem. 261:6137–6140, 1986.
23. Horio, M., Gottesman, M.M., and Pastan, I. ATP-dependent transport of vinblastine in vesicles from human multidrug-resistant cells. Proc. Natl. Acad. Sci. USA 85:3580–3584, 1988.
24. Thiebaut, F., Tsuruo, T., Hamada, H., Gottesman, M.M., Pastan, I., and Willingham,

52

M.C. Cellular localization of the multridrug-resistant gene product P-glycoprotein in normal human tissues. Proc. Natl. Acad. Sci. USA 84:7735–7738, 1987.

25. van der Bliek, A.M., Kooiman, P.M., Schneider, C., and Borst, P. Sequence of mdr3 encoding a human P-glycoprotein. Gene 71:401–411, 1988.

26. Gros, P., Croop, J., and Housman, D. Mammalian multidrug resistance gene: complete cDNA sequence indicates strong homology to bacterial transport proteins. Cell 47:409–411, 1986.

27. Hsu, S.I-H., Lothstein, L., and Horwitz, S.B. Differential overexpression of three mdr gene family members in multidrug-resistant J774.2 mouse cells. J. Biol. Chem. 264:12053–12062, 1989.

28. Endicott, J.A., Juranka, P.F., Sarangi, F., Gerlach, J.H., Deuchars, L.L., and Ling, V. Simultaneous expression of two P-glycoprotein genes in drug-sensitive Chinese hamster ovary cells. Mol. Cell. Biol. 7:4075–4081, 1987.

29. Ng, W.F., Sarangi, F., Zastawny, R.L., Veinot-Drebot, L., and Ling, V. Identification of members of the P-glycoprotein multigene family. Mol. Cell. Biol. 9:1224–1232, 1989.

30. Jongsma, A.P.M. Spengler, B.A., van der Bliek, A.M., Borst, P., and Biedler, J.L. Chromosomal localization of three genes coamplified in the multidrug-resistant CHRC5 Chinese hamster ovary cell line. Cancer Res. 47:2875–2878, 1987.

31. Martinsson, T. and Levan, G. Localization of the multidrug resistance-associated 170 kDa P-glycoprotein by in situ hybridization. Cytogenet. Cell Genet. 45:99–101, 1987.

32. van der Bliek, A.M., van der Velde-Koerts, T., Ling, V., and Borst, P. Overexpression and amplification of five genes in a multidrug resistant Chinese hamster ovary cell line. Mol. Cell. Biol. 6:1671–1678, 1986.

33. Raymond, M. and Gros, P. Mammalian multidrug-resistance gene: correlation of exon organization with structural domains and duplication of an ancestral gene. Proc. Natl. Acad. Sci. USA 86:6488–6492, 1989.

34. Gros, P., Raymond, M., Bell, J., and Housman, D. Cloning and characterization of a second member of the mouse mdr gene family. Mol. Cell. Biol. 8:2770–2778, 1988.

35. Gros, P., Ben Neriah, Y., Groop, J.M., and Housman, D.E. Isolation and expression of a cDNA (mdr1) that confers multidrug resistance. Nature 323:728–731, 1986.

36. Higgins, C.F., Hiles, I.D., Salmond, G.P.C., Gill, D.R., Downie, J.A., Evans, I.J., Holland, I.B., Gray, L., Buckel, S.D., Bell, A.W., and Hermodson, M.A. A family of related ATP-binding subunits coupled to many distinct biological processes in bacteria. Nature 323:448–450, 1986.

37. Felmlee, T., Pellett, S., and Welch, R.A. Nucleotide sequence of an *Escherichia coli* chromosomal hemolysin. J. Bact. 163:94–105, 1985.

38. Stanfield, S.W., Ielpi, L., O'Brchta, D., Helinski, D.R., and Ditta, G.S. The ndv gene product of *Rhizobium meliloti* is required for -(1 2) glucan production and has homology to the ATP-binding export protein Hy1B. J. Bacteriol. 170:3523–3530, 1988.

39. Strathdee, C.A. and Lo, R.Y.C. Cloning, nucleotide sequence, and characterization of genes encoding the secretion function of the *Pasteurella haemolytica* leukotoxin determinant. J. Bact. 171:916–928, 1989.

40. Glaser, P., Sakamoto, H., Bellalou, J., Ullmann, L, and Danchin, A. Secretion of cyclolysin, the calmodulin sensitive adenylate cyclase-haemolysin bifunctional protein of *Bordetella pertussis*. EMBO J. 7:3997–4004, 1988.

41. Gill, D.R., Hatfull, G.F., and Salmond, G.P.C. A new cell division operon in *Escherichia coli*. Mol. Gen. Genet. 205:134–145, 1986.

42. Evans, I.J. and Downie, J.A. The nodI gene product of *Rhizobium* leguminosarum is closely related to ATP-binding bacterial transport proteins: nucleotide sequence analysis of the nodI and nodJ genes. Gene 43:95–101, 1986.

43. Ames, G. Bacterial periplasmic transport systems: structure, mechanism, and evolution. Ann. Rev. Biochem. 55:397–425, 1986.

44. Wilson, C.M., Serrano, A.E., Wasley, A., Bogenschutz, M.P., Shankar, A.H., and Wirth,

D.F. Amplification of a gene related to mammalian mdr genes in a drug-resistant *Plasmodium falciparum*. Science 244:1184–1186, 1987.

45. Foote, S.J., Thompson, J.K., Cowman, A.F., and Kemp. D.J. Amplification of the multidrug resistance gene in some chloroquine-resistant isolates of *P. falciparum*. Cell 57:921–930, 1989.

46. McGrath, J.P. and Varshvsky, A. The yeast STE6 gene encodes a homologue of the mammalian multidrug resistance P-glycoprotein. Nature 340:400–404, 1989.

47. Kuchler, K., Sterne, R.E., and Thorner, J. EMBO J., in press, 1989.

48. Sullivan, D.T. and Sullivan, M.C. Transport defects as the physiological basis for eye color mutants of *Drosophila melanogaster*. Biochem. Genet. 13:603–613, 1975.

49. Sullivan, D.T., Bell, L.A., Paton, D.R, and Sullivan, M.C. Purine transport by malpighian tubules of pteridine-deficient eye color mutants of *Drosophila melanogaster*. Biochem. Genet. 17:565–573, 1979.

50. Dreesen, T.D., Johnson, D.H., and Henikoff, S. The brown protein of *Drosophila melanogaster* is similar to the white protein and to components of active transport complexes. Mol. Cell. Biol. 8:5206–5215, 1988.

51. O'Hare, K., Murphy, C., Levis, R., and Rubin, G.M. DNA sequence of the white locus of *Drosophila melanogaster*. J. Mol. Biol. 180:437–455, 1984.

52. Mount, S.M. Sequence similarity. Nature 325:48751, 1987.

53. Shen, D., Cardarelli, C., Hwang, J., Cornwell, M., Richert, N., Ishii, S., Pastan, I., and Gottesman, M.M. Multiple drug resistant human KB carcinoma cells independently selected for high-level resistance to colchicine, adriamycin, or vinblastine show changes in expression of specific proteins. J. Biol. Chem. 261:7762–7770, 1986.

54. Bradley, G., Juranka, P.F., and Ling, V. Mechanism of multidrug resistance. Biochim. Biophys. Acta 948:87–128, 1988.

55. Fojo, A.T., Whang-Peng, J., Gottesman, MN.M, and Pastan, I. Amplification of DNA sequences in human multidrug-resistant KB carcinoma cells. Proc. Natl. Acad. Sci. USA 82:7661–7664, 1985.

56. de Bruijn, M.H.L., van der Bliek, A.M., Biedler, J.L., and Borst, P. Differential amplification and disproportionate expression of five genes in three multidrug-resistant Chinese hamster lung cell lines. Mol. Cell. Biol. 6:4717–4722, 1986.

57. Stahl, F., Martinsson, T., Dahllof, B., and Levan, G. Amplification and overexpression of genes in SEWA murine multidrug-resistant cells and mapping of the P-glycoprotein genes to chromosome 5 in mouse. Hereditas 108:251–258, 1988.

58. Fojo, A.T., Shen, D., Mickley, L.A., Pastan, I., and Gottesman, M.M. Intrinsic drug resistance in human kidney cancer is associated with expression of a human multidrug resistance gene. J. Clin. Oncol. 5:1922–1927, 1987.

59. Fojo, A.T., Ueda, K., Slamon, D.J., Poplack, D.G., Gottesman, M.M., and Pastan I. Expression of a multidrug-resistance gene in human tumors and tissues. Proc. Natl. Acad. Sci. USA 84:265–269, 1987.

60. Sugawara, I., Kataoka, I., Morishita, Y., Hamada, H., Tsuruo, T., Itayama, S., and Mori, S. Tissue distriction of P-glycoprotein encoded by a multidrug resistant gene as revealed by a monoclonal antibody, MRK16. Cancer Res. 48:4611–4614, 1988.

61. Kakehi, Y., Kanamuaru, H., Yoshida, O., Ohkubo, H., Nakanishi, S., Gottesman, M.M., and Pastan, I. Measurement of multidrug resistance messenger RNA in urogenital cancers: elevated expression in renal cell carcinoma is associated with intrinsic drug resistance. J. Urol. 139:862–865, 1988.

62. Chin, J.E., Soffir, R., Noonan, K.E., Choi, K., and Roninson, I.B. Structure and expression of the human MDR (P-glycoprotein) gene family. Mol. Cell. Biol. 9:3808–3820, 1989.

63. Baas, F. and Borst, P. The tissue dependent expression of hamster P-glycoprotein genes. FEBS Lett. 229:329–332, 1988.

64. Mukhopadhyay, T., Batsakis, J.G., and Kuo, M.T. Expression of the mdr (P-glycoprotein) gene in Chinese hamster digestive tracts. J. Natl. Cancer Inst. 80:269–275, 1988.

54

65. Croop, J.M., Raymond, M., Haber, D., Devault, A., Arceci, R.J., Gros, P., and Housman, D.E. The three mouse multidrug resistance genes are expressed in a tissue-specific manner in normal mouse tissues. Mol. Cell. Biol. 9:1346–1350, 1989.
66. Arceci, R.J., Croop, J.M., Horwitz, S.B., and Housman, D. The gene encoding multidrug resistance is induced and expressed at high levels during pregnancy in the secretory epithelium of the uterus. Proc. Natl. Acad. Sci. USA 85:4350–4354, 1988.
67. Gottesman, M.M. Multidrug resistance during chemical carcinogenesis: a mechanism revealed? J. Natl. Cancer Inst. 80:1352–1353, 1989.
68. Kamimoto, Y., Gatmaitan, Z., Hsu, J., and Arias, I.M. The function of Gp170, the multidrug resistance gene product, in rat liver canalicular membrane vesicles. J. Biol. Chem. 264:11693–11698, 1989.
69. Yang, C.-P.H., DePinho, S.G., Greenberger, L.M., Arceci, R.J., and Horwitz, S.B. Progesterone interacts with P-glycoprotein in multidrug-resistant cells and in the endometrium of gravid uterus. J. Biol Chem. 264:782–788, 1989.
70. Benard, J., Da Silva, J., Teyssier, J.-R., and Riou, G. Over-expression of mdr1 gene with no DNA amplification in a multiple-drug-resistant human ovarian carcinoma cell line. Int. J. Cancer 43:471–477, 1989.
71. Chin, K.-V., Tanaka, S., Darlington, G., Pastan, I., and Gottesman, M.M. Heat shock and arsenite increase expression of the multidrug resistance (MDR1) gene in human renal carcinoma cells. J. Biol. Chem. 265:221–226, 1989.
72. Bates, S.E., Mickley, L.A., Chen, Y.-N., Richert, N., Rudick, J., Biedler, J.L., and Fojo, A.T. Expression of a drug resistance gene in human neuroblastoma cell lines: modulation by retinoic acid-induced differentiation. Mol Cell. Biol. 9:4337–4344, 1989.
73. Thorgiersson, S.S., Huber, B.E., Sorrell, S., Fojo, A., Pastan, I., and Gottesman, M.M. Expression of the multidrug resistance gene in hepatocarcinogenesis and regenerating rat liver. Science 236:1120–1122, 1987.
74. Burt, and Thorgierrson, S.S. Coinduction of MDR1 multidrug-resistance and cytochrome P-450 genes in rat liver by xenobiotics. J. Natl. Cancer. Inst. ●●:●●–●●, 1988.
75. Marino, P.A., Gottesman, M.M., and Pastan, I. Cell Growth Differen., in press, 1990.
76. Ueda, K., Cardarelli, C., Gottesman, M.M., and Pastan I. The human multidrug resistance (mdr1) gene: cDNA cloning and transcription initiation. J. Biol Chem. 262:505–508, 1987.
77. Ueda, K., Pastan, I., and Gottesman, M.M. Isolation and sequence of the promoter region of the human multidrug resistance (P-glycoprotein) gene. J. Biol. Chem. 262:17432–17436, 1987.
78. Rothenberg, M., Mickely, L.A., Cole, D.E., Balis, R.M., Tsuruo, T., Poplack, D.G., and Fojo, A.T. Expression of the mdr1/P-170 gene in patients with acute lymphoblastic leukemia. Blood 74:1388–1395, 1989.
79. Currier, S.J., Ueda, K., Willingham, M.C., Pastan, I., and Gottesman, M.M. Deletion and insertion mutants of the multidrug transporter. J. Biol. Chem. 264:14376–14381, 1989.
80. Azzaria, M., Schurr, E., and Gros, P. Discrete mutations introduced in the predicted nucleotide-binding sites of the mdr1 gene abolish its ability to confer multidrug resistance. Mol. Cell. Biol. 9:5289–5297, 1989.
81. Bruggemann, E.P., Germann, U.A., Gottesman, M.M., and Pastan, I. Two different regions of phosphoglycoprotein are photoaffinity-labeled by azidopine. J. Biol. Chem. 264:15483–15488, 1989.
82. Yoshimura, A., Kuwazuru, Y., Sumizawa, T., Ichikawa, M., Ikeda, S.-I., Uda, T., and Akiyama, S.-I. Cytoplasmic orientation and two-domain structure of the multidrug transporter, P-glycoprotein, demonstrated with sequence-specific antibodies. J. Biol. Chem. 264:16282–16291, 1989.
83. Choi, K., Chen, C., Krigler, M., and Roninson, I.B. An altered pattern of cross-resistance in multidrug resistant human cells results from spontaneous mutations in the mdr1 (P-glycoprotein) gene. Cell 53:519–529, 1988.

84. Moscow, J.A. and Cowan, K.H. Multidrug resistance. J. Natl. Cancer Inst. 80:14–20, 1988.
85. Greenberger, L.M., Williams, S.S., and Horwitz, S.B. Biosynthesis of heterogeneous forms of multidrug resistance-associated glycoproteins. J. Biol. Chem. 262:13685–13689, 1987.

4. Resistance to inhibitors of DNA topoisomerases

Daniel M. Sullivan and Warren E. Ross

Introduction

DNA topoisomerase II (EC 5.99.1.3) is a ubiquitous Mg^{2+}- and ATP-dependent enzyme that exists as a homodimer in eukaryotes (subunit molecular mass 131–180 kDa) and is encoded on human chromosome #17. This enzyme changes the linking number of DNA in steps of two and allows the interconversion of topological isomers of DNA by introducing a transient enzyme-bridged double-strand DNA break. Further details regarding the interaction of type II topoisomerases with DNA can be found in several recent reviews [1–6]. This enzyme has been purified to homogeneity from human Hela cells [7], *Saccharomyces cerevisiae* [8], *Drosophila melanogaster* [9], calf thymus [10–12], *Trypanosoma cruzi* [13], mouse leukemia P388 cells [14], *Crithidia fasciculata* [15], and Chinese hamster ovary cells [16]; and the gene has been cloned and sequenced from *Saccharomyces cerevisiae* [17], *Schizosaccharomyces pombe* [18], *Drosophila melanogaster* [19], HeLa cells [20], and human Burkitt lymphoma cells [21].

The reaction mechanism of topoisomerase II has been shown to involve five steps [9, 22–26]: 1) recognition and binding of the enzyme to its DNA substrate; 2) double-stranded cleavage of DNA, which appears to occur as two sequential single-strand breaks, resulting in covalent phosphotyrosyl bonds between the 5' end of each strand and a topoisomerase II monomer; 3) passage of a second DNA duplex through the break site (dependent on ATP binding of DNA); 4) religation of the cleaved DNA; and, 5) enzyme turnover, which depends on ATP hydrolysis. Topoisomerase II in vitro is able to knot/unknot double-strand circular DNA, relax closed circular DNA, and catenate/decatenate double-strand DNA circles. These changes in the topological state of DNA result in differences in electrophoretic mobility of the DNA products through agarose gels, thus allowing the quantitation of topoisomerase II catalytic activity by P4 DNA unknotting, relaxation of supercoiled plasmid DNA, and decatenation of kinetoplast DNA (kDNA). Topoisomerase II has been shown to be involved in several in vivo functions as well, including DNA replication [27–29], segregation of chromosomes during mitosis [30–32] and meiosis I [33], maintenance of the

Robert F. Ozols (ed.), MOLECULAR AND CLINICAL ADVANCES IN ANTICANCER DRUG RESISTANCE. Copyright © 1991.
Kluwer Academic Publishers, Boston. All right reserved. ISBN 0-7923-1212-0

structure and function of the nuclear matrix and scaffold [34–38], and assembly of transcriptionally active chromatin [39].

In addition to being involved in the various intracellular processes described above, topoisomerase II is the target of several of the intercalator and nonintercalator antitumor drugs. Drug-induced protein-associated DNA breaks were first observed in L1210 cells treated with doxorubicin and ellipticine [40–41], and that the protein involved might be DNA topoisomerase II was suggested in 1981 [42–43]. The subsequent work of several investigators [44–54] has demonstrated that anthracyclines (doxorubicin and daunomycin), anthracenediones (mitoxantrone), acridines (m-AMSA), actinomycin D, ellipticine derivatives, and the epipodophyllotoxins (VP-16 and VM-26) all inhibit DNA topoisomerase II. These drugs apparently block the religation of DNA [52–54] by topoisomerase II, and result in a substantial increase in apparent DNA damage, which can be measured as single-strand breaks (SSBs), double-strand breaks (DSBs), or DNA-protein corss-links (DPCs) by filter elution techniques. There is a good correlation between production of DNA DSBs and drug-induced cytotoxicity for the intercalators and nonintercalators listed above. The covalent DNA-topoisomerase II complex, which is increased in amount in the presence of drug, can also be quantified by prelabeling the DNA (with either [^{3}H]-thymidine or [^{32}P]-dATP) in vivo or in vitro, and then precipitating the complex with potassium chloride and SDS (K/SDS assay). It should be noted that the production of strand breaks in itself may not necessarily be directly responsible for cytotoxicity; rather a subsequent event, perhaps interference with replication fork progression [53], may be critical for lethality.

Several cells have either an intrinsic resistance to topoisomerase II inhibitors or have acquired resistance to these drugs during short-term exposure. The basis for the majority of this resistance depends on either quantitative or qualitative alterations in the target enzyme, topoisomerase II. Drug resistance to topoisomerase II inhibitors will be discussed under three broad headings. The first will focus on the mechanisms of resistance acquired by various cell lines selected in the presence of certain antineoplastic agents. This will be followed by a discussion of the cell cycle- and proliferation-dependent resistance to topoisomerase II inhibitors. Finally, the intrinsic resistance of human tumors to these same drugs will be explored.

Drug-resistant cell lines

A recent survey of the literature reveals that there are approximately 35 cell lines whose pleiotropic drug resistance is primarily dependent on an alteration in DNA topoisomerase II or its interaction with DNA and drug. These cell lines were generally isolated as resistant colonies during growth in the continuous presence of a single selecting agent [rarely cells were mutagenized with ethyl methanesulfonate (EMS) or N-methyl-N'-nitro-

N-nitrosoguanidine (MNNG) prior to selection]. These colonies are usually subcloned to ensure a homogeneous population, and can often be grown in culture in the absence of selecting without loss of resistance for several months. Evaluations of cell lines resistant to topoisomerase II inhibitors have included: 1) cytotoxicity assays (colony-forming or MTT) to determine the magnitude and patterns of resistance and cross-resistance to topoisomerase II-active drugs and other classes of antineoplastic agents; 2) drug transport studies with radiolabelled or fluorescent antitumor drugs to determine drug uptake, equilibrium concentration, or efflux; 3) depending on the results from 1 and 2, evaluation of the expression of the *mdr1* gene or its potein product (P-glycoprotein); 4) quantifying drug-induced DNA damage (SSBs, DSBs, DPCs) in cells and/or isolated nuclei by elution or sedimentation techniques; 5) finally, quantifying the amount of immuno-reactive topoisomerase II in cells and/or nuclear extracts and assaying these extracts for both topoisomerase II catalytic activity (P4 unknotting, decatenation of kDNA, etc.) and drug-induced enzyme-mediated DNA cleavage.

The mechanisms of resistance of the drug-resistant cell lines referred to above have been defined by various combinations of these assays; infrequently, the resistance mechanism has been precisely determined by more detailed and elaborate studies. These studies have centered around the biochemical characterization of homogeneous preparations of topoisomerase II or defining the resistance lesion at a genetic level. Mechanisms of resistance to topoisomerase II inhibitors delineated by the above investigations include: qualitative changes in DNA topoisomerase II, quantitative changes in this enzyme target, perturbantions in cellular transport of inhibitors (often in conjunction with alterations in tpoisomerase II), attenuated drug-induced DNA damage without a transport defect, changes in the processing of DNA strand breaks, and finally, suggestions that extrinsic factors may modulate topoisomerase II activity. These mechanisms have been listed from least equivocal to more speculative and will be discussed in that order. More than one of these mechanisms are often present in the same resistant cell line. It is uncommon for a drug-resistant cell line to have only one mechanism of resistance, even within the topoisomerase paradigm. Adr^{R}MCF-7 cells [55–58], for example, overexpress P-glycoprotein, have a decreased uptake of VP-16 with an unaltered efflux, demonstrate a twofold decrease (in nuclear extracts) of VP-16-induced DNA cleavage mediated by topoisomerase II, show a 140-fold cellular resistance to etoposide-induced SSBs, and have a 45-fold increase in an anionic GSH-S-transferase, which protects these cells from free radicals.

Qualitative alterations in the drug target

Equivalent immunoreactive topoisomerase II with altered activity. The cell lines that are multidrug resistant because they contain a "normal" amount of an abnormal topoisomerase II enzyme include the Chinese hamster ovary (CHO) Vpm R-5 cell line, HL-60/AMSA cells, and (likely) the CEM/VM-1 and CEM/VM-1-5 cell lines. The Vpm^R-5 cell line was isolated from EMS-mutagenized wild-type (WT) CHO cells in a single-step selection to VM-26 [59]. These cells are 20-fold resistant to VP-16 and 2.4-, 2.3-, 1.8-, 3- and 5-fold resistant to daunomycin, doxorubicin, ellimpticine, m-AMSA, and mitoxantrone, respectively [59,60]. The drug uptake of [^{3}H]-VP-16, [^{14}C]-m-AMSA, and [^{14}C]-daunomycin by the Vpm^R-5 cells is the same as WT cells [60,61], and immunoblotting with a polyclonal anti-topoisomerase II antibody demonstrates equivalent enzyme content relative to WT cells [16]. Resistance to VP-16-, m-AMSA-, mitoxantrone-, and doxorubicin-induced DNA damage (measured as SSBs by alkaline elution) correlates well with the cytotoxicity assays above [60, 61]. Crude 0.35 M NaCl nuclear extracts from these cells were found to have the same topoisosmerase II catalytic activity (decatenation of kDNA) as WT extracts, and these were inhibited by VP-16 equally. However, the nuclear extracts from the resistant cells had markedly diminished drug-stimulated DNA cleavage when measured as either conversion of supercoiled pBR322 DNA to linear form III, or as precipitation of covalent complexes formed between topoisomerase II and [^{32}P]-3'-end-labeled DNA using the K/SDS assay [22]. These results suggested that Vpm^R-5 cells contain an altered topoisomerase II molecule. Purification of the resistant and WT enzymes to homogeneity has allowed us to confirm this hypothesis [16].

Purified resistant and WT enzymes are similar in that they have the same native and monomeric molecular masses, have the same enzyme specific activity (decatenation of kDNA, which is inhibited equally by VP-16), bind and dissociate from DNA in a like manner, and share the same DNA cleavage sites. The purified Vpm^R-5 enzyme is unlike WT topoisomerase II in that it is heat labile and appears to show a dramatic reduction in drug-stimulated DNA cleavage (assayed as covalent DNA-topoisomerase II complexes by gel cleavage and the K/SDS assay). Our model suggests that the reduced cleavage is only "apparent"; that the resistant enzyme actually ligates cleaved DNA normally and is insensitive to the drug inhibition of religation normally seen. These results with the purified enzyme suggest that Vpm^R-5 cells are resistant because they contain drug-insensitive topoisomerase II. Proof that these cells contain a *mutant* enzyme awaits cloning and sequencing the topoisomerae II genes for the resistant and WT enzymes.

The drug-resistant HL-60/AMSA cell line was generated by pulsing cells with increasing doses of m-AMSA over several months [62]. These cells can be cultured in the absence of selecting agent and are 10- to 100-fold resistant to mAMSA [62–66]. HL-60/AMSA cells are minimally resistant to doxorubicin (1.6-fold) and VP-16 (2-fold), and demonstrate WT sensitivity to vinblastine and ellipticine. Uptake and efflux of [^{14}C]-m-AMSA is similar in WT and resistant cells, and immunoblotting has not detected overexpression of P-glycoprotein in HL-60/AMSA cells. DNA SSBs induced by m-AMSA were markedly reduced in whole cells and nuclei of HL-60/AMSA cells [63], whereas the DNA damage induced by VP-16 was similar to that seen in parental cells [66]. Topoisomerase II catalytic activity (decatenation of kDNA) in 0.35 M NaCl nuclear extracts was similar in sensitive and resistant extracts, as was the inhibition of this activity by VP-16. However, the catalytic activity of the HL-60/AMSA nuclear extract was somewhat resistant to inhibition by m-AMSA. These findings regarding catalytic activity suggest that the two drugs, VP-16 and m-AMSA, interact differently with the HL-60/AMSA enzyme. DNA cleavage studies with these same nuclear extracts paralleled the cytotoxicity data, i.e., HL-60/AMSA extracts were very resistant to m-AMSA-induced DNA cleavage (measured by K/SDS precipitation of covalent DNA-enzyme complexes), and demonstrated VP-16-induced cleavage that was similar to WT cleavage. These initial studies suggested that HL-60/AMSA cells contain an altered or mutated topoisomerase II enzyme similar to the Vpm^R-5 cells. Further molecular studies and experiments with near-purified enzyme have confirmed this [66]. Purified topoisomerase II from drug-resistant cells demonstrates the same catalytic activity as purified parental enzyme. Drug-stimulated DNA cleavage by purified topoisomerase II confirmed the HL-60/AMSA resistance to m-AMSA seen in nuclear extracts. The molecular mass of purified WT and resistant topoisomerase II enzymes were found to be the same (149 kDa) by Western blotting with a polyclonal anti-topoisomerase II antibody; likewise, the amount of immunoreactive topoisomerase II in nuclear extracts and whole cells was shown to be similar in resistant and sensitive cell lines (detected predominately as a doublet on SDS-PAGE gels at 156 and 149 kDa). Southern blots of HpaII- and XmnI-restricted total cellular DNA from HL-60/AMSA and WT cells with a topoisomerase II cDNA probe (ZII69) are very suggestive of a mutation in the resistant topoisomerase II gene. These two restriction enzymes gave different patterns on Southern blots. The data with HpaII may simply reflect a change in methylation rather than a base change, however, the XmnI data are consistent with either an allele-specific restriction fragment length polymorphism or a mutation. Thus, the drug resistance of HL-60/AMSA cells appears to be secondary to a mutation in the resistant topoisiomerase II gene, which results in an enzyme that is resistant to m-AMSA-induced DNA cleavage. This lack of drug-stimulated covalent DNA-enzyme complex formation (which may reflect, as proposed for Vpm^R-5 cells, normal religation in the presence of m-AMSA) appears to confer resistance to these cells. As with the Vpm^{R-5} cell line, it will be necessary to clone and sequence the resistant topoisomerase II gene to definitively demonstrate a mutation.

Support for the hypothesis that a mutation in the topoisomerase II gene can result in resistance to topoisomerase II inhibitors exists in E. coli DNA gyrase mutants [67]. Four E. coli KL-16 spontaneous gyrA mutants have been isolated and characterized. These mutants are resistant to the gyrase (topoisomerase II) inhibitors, nalidixic acid and ciprofloxacin, with levels of resistance over 100-fold. Single base changes in the *gyrA* gene have been identified (one per mutant) and found to result in the following single amino acid changes in the 97 kDa GyrA polypeptide: Ser to Leu, Ser to Trp, Gln to His, and Ala to Ser at amino acid positions 83, 83, 106, and 67, respectively. Interestingly, these mutations are all fairly close to Tyr 122, the site where DNA covalently binds gyrase in a transient phosphotyrosine bond.

The CEM/VM-1 line was selected from parental CCRF-CEM cells by growth in the intermittent presence of sublethal concentrations of VM-26 [68]. Further selection of drug-resistant CEM/VM-1 cells with intermittent VM-26 resulted in the isolation of CEM/VM-1-5 cells [69]. CEM/VM-1 cells are 50-fold resistant to VM-26 by cytotoxicity assays, while CEM/VM-1-5 cells demonstrate 141-fold resistance to VM-26 [68–71]. These cell lines have similar magnitudes of cross-resistance to m-AMSA, doxorubicin, and VP-16. In addition, CEM/VM-1 cells are cross-resistant to actinomycin D (3-fold), daunomycin (6.6-fold), and mitoxantrone (16-fold), whereas CEM/VM-1-5 cells are 11-fold resistant to actinomycin D and 7-fold resistant to vincristine. Alterations in drug transport (including overexpression of the *mdr1* gene) do not appear to contribute significantly to the drug resistance of these cell lines. Neither can the drug resistance be explained by a simple decrease in topoisomerase II, as immunoblots of crude nuclear extracts of both resistant cell lines and WT cells demonstrate the same amount of immunoreactive enzyme [69,71]. However, the topoisomerase II present in 0.35 M and 1.0 M NaCl nuclear extracts from CEM/VM-1 and CEM/VM-1-5 cells appears to have both altered catalytic and cleavage activity. Relative to parental CCRF-CEM cells, the P4 unknotting activity of CEM/VM-1 nuclear extract was decreased twofold, while that of CEM/VM-1-5 extracts were decreased fourfold; this unknotting activity from the resistant cell lines was also less sensitive to inhibition by VM-26. Catenation of pBR322 DNA by nuclear extracts from WT and CEM/VM-1 cells was similar, while this activity was decreased four- to sixfold in CEM/VM-1-5 extracts. VM-26-stimulated DNA cleavage activity (measured as formation of covalent DNA-enzyme complexes) of nuclear extracts was likewise altered in the two resistant extracts. It was reduced 1.5-fold and 4-fold in the extracts from CEM/VM-1 and CEM/VM-1-5 cells, respectively. In summary, these two resistant cell lines have normal amounts of what is apparently an altered topoisomerase II enzyme. The more resistant the cell line (CEM/VM-1-5), the greater the alteration in activity. The drug resistance described here is different than that seen in Vpm[R]-5 and HL-60/AMSA cells in that both topoisomerase II cleavage and *catalytic* activity are apparently altered in the resistant CEM cell lines. The possibility that a factor(s) extrinsic to the topoisomerase II molecule modulates enzyme activity in crude nuclear extracts needs to be excluded by repeating the enzyme assays with homogeneous preparations of topoisomerase II from the resistant cell lines.

These same investigators have also presented preliminary evidence that the drug resistance of these cell lines may depend in part on either an alteration in ATP binding by topoisomerase II [72,73] or an altered intracellular distribution of topoisomerase II [74]; see below for further discussion regarding these two possibilities. Finally, hybrid cell lines produced by fusing drug-resistant CEM/VM-1 cells with a drug-sensitive CEM cell line demonstrate that VM-26 resistance is expressed recessively [71]. Cytotoxicity assays with VM-26 demonstrated WT sensitivity of the hybrids, while nuclear extracts from WT and hybrid cells had both equivalent VM-26-induced DNA cleavage activity and equal amounts of immunoreactive topoisomerase II. The normal topoisomerase II activity of the hybrid may be due to the restoration of an unaltered enzyme or the addition/deletion of a modulating factor.

Isoforms of DNA topoisomerase II. P388 tumors resistant to m-AMSA (P388/amsacrine) have been cloned in soft agar and the individual clones further characterized [75]. The A20 clone is 19-fold resistant to m-AMSA and cross-resistant to VM-26 (10-fold), doxorubicin (10-fold), actinomycin D (8-fold), and vinblastine (10-fold); it remains sensitive to cisplatinum and camptothecin. A20 cells have the same uptake of [^{14}C]-m-AMSA as cloned WT P388 cells (WT20), but only 50% [^{3}H]-vinblastine uptake compared to WT20 cells. VM-26- and m-AMSA-induced DNA damage (measured as SSBs by alkaline elution) was found to be attenuated in both whole cells and nuclei of the A20 line. Finally, 0.35 M NaCl nuclear extracts from WT20 cells demonstrate 2.3-fold more topoisomerase II activity (P4 DNA unknotting) than A20 extracts. A polyclonal anti-topoisomerase II antibody reacted with two proteins (164 and 173 kDa) from A20 and WT20 cells during Western blot analysis. When total immunoreactive enzyme was determined, three times more topoisomerase II was measured in the WT20 cells. The topoisomerase II activity from P388/A20 and WT20 cells has now been purified to homogeneity and further characterized [14,21,76]. This activity apppears to exist as two isoforms, with molecular mass 170 and 180 kDa, that are well separated by either cation- [14] or anion-exchange [76] column chromatography. When purified to >90% homogeneity, these two forms of topoisomerases II have been found to have similar catalytic activity (P4 DNA unknotting), the same ATP requirements for relaxation of supercoiled pBR322 DNA (which is inhibited equally by both novobiocin and the ATPase inhibitor orthovanadate), as well as qualitatively similar m-AMSA-stimulated covalent binding of DNA. These two isozymes are functionally distinct by the following criteria: the p170 enzyme relaxes supercoiled DNA in a distributive manner while p180 is processive, they have different KCl concentration optima for unknotting P4 DNA, the p180 catalytic activity is twice as heat labile as p170 and is threefold more resistant to VM-26 inhibition of this activity, and finally, the p180 form is 3- to 25-fold more resistant to VM-26-induced DNA cleavage. The K/SDS DNA cleavage assay has shown that the two enzymes have common and different cleavage sites, where p170 appears to prefer AT-rich areas and p180 GC-rich areas. These investigators have also provided the following evidence that these two isozymes are in fact distinct molecules. First, proteolysis of the two enzymes by *Staphylococcus* V8 protease produced significantly different cleavage patterns and, second, polyclonal anti-p170 and anti-p180 antibodies do not cross-react with the isozymes by western blotting. In addition, the anti-p170 antibody inhibits the catalytic activity of p170 topoisomerase II but not that of p180. The possible relevance of topoismoerase II isozymes to drug resistance is suggested by the observation that drug-resistant P388/A20 cells contain very little p170 topoisomerase II (relative to WT20) but similar amounts of p180. Variations in isozyme ratios may also be important in proliferation-dependent resistance (see below).

Further genetic characterization of the isozymes of topoisomerase II has been accomplished by studying the p170 and p180 forms in a hypersensitive Burkitt lymphoma cell line (Raji-HN$_2$). This cell line was isolated after intermittent exposure to mechlorethamine and is sevenfold resistant to this agent [77]. However, these cells are 4- to 11-fold hypersensitive to m-AMSA, VP-16, VM-26, and novobiocin. They are also 2.5-fold hypersensitive to the topoisomerase I inhibitor, camptothecin. Raji-HN$_2$ cells have a threefold increase in topoisomerase II catalytic activity (P4 unknotting), most likely due to increased transcription of p180 topoisomerase II [77–79]. Immunoblotting demonstrates the same p170 content as parental cells, but dramatically increased p180 isozyme, in the hypsensitive cells. Thus, the increased sensitivity of Raji-HM$_2$ cells to topoisomerase II-active drugs appears to result from an augmentation of the drug target. A Raji-HN$_2$ library has been screened with a cDNA probe encoding *Drosophila* topoisomerase II and two classes of cDNAs have been described [21]. The SP1 cDNA (class I) is identical to the 3031-bp *Eco*R1-*Eco*R1 fragment of the HeLa topoisomerase II sequence. SP11 cDNA (class II) is different from the HeLa map, with 75% overall identity with SP1. The SP1 and SP11 peptide sequences have 92% similarity, and the SP11 protein spans the first 59% (895 amino acids) of HeLa protein. The unique patterns observed when restricted genomic DNA from Raji-HN$_2$ cells was probed with the SP1 and SP11 cDNAs suggests that the two classes of cDNAs are from different genomic sequences and that there is a different gene for each topoisomerase II enzyme. Specific oligonucleotide probes for SP1 (probe I) and SP11 (probe II) were made (where sequences of the two cDNAs differed greatly); both detected a 6.5-kb mRNA. However, only unlabelled probe I could compete for hybridization to RNA with ^{32}P-labelled proble I, suggesting the presence of two different comigrating RNAs. Finally, polyclonal antibodies were generated to synthetic dodecapeptides, representing corresponding but dissimilar protein stretches of SP1 and SP11. Antibodies to class (SP1) dodecapeptides recognized only the 170 kDa topoisomerase II on western blot, and the antibodies to class II (SP11) recognized p180 and a 145 kDa protein. These elaborate genetic and immunologic studies provide good

64

evidence that there are separate genes encoding two distinct forms of DNA topoisomerase II. An altered ratio of expression of these isozymes may result in drug resistance or hypersensitivity. The frequency with which the p170 and p180 isozymes occur is unknown. They have been found (in various ratios) in P388 cells, U937 human monoblast cells, Raji cells, human colon carcinoma COLO 201 cells, and in mouse fibroblast 3T3 cells.

Altered interaction of ATP with DNA topoisomerase II. The strand passage activity of DNA topoisomerase II is dependent upon binding of ATP, whereas enzyme turnover depends on ATP hydrolysis [6]. Studies with VM-26-resistant CEM/VM-1 and CEM/VM-1-5 cells have shown that strand passage (unknotting of P4 DNA) is half-maximal at $67\,\mu M$ and $300\,\mu M$ ATP, respectively, whereas the parental cell line (CEM) requires $38\,\mu M$ ATP [72,73]. These investigators have also shown that unknotting activity from all three cell lines is sensitive to inhibition by novobiocin, a competitive inhibitor of ATP binding. VM-26- and m-AMSA-induced covalent DNA-enzyme complex formation was also found to be reduced in nuclear extracts from both resistant cell lines. In the presence of 100 μM -AMSA, 1 mM ATP stimulated covalent complex formation ~2.5-fold in the sensitive and CEM/VM-1 cell lines (compared to assays in the presence of m-AMSA but no ATP). The addition of ATP to assays with CEM/VM-1-5 did not stimulate complex formation in the presence of m-AMSA. While not conclusive, these observations suggest that alterations in ATP binding by topoisomerase II may have a role in drug resistance to topoisomerase II inhibitors.

Quantitative changes in the drug target

Decreased content of DNA topoisomerase II with or without aberrant enzyme activity. The drug resistant cell lines VpmR-5, HL-60/AMSA, and CEM/VM-1 and -1-5 (discussed above) have "normal" amounts of cellular immunoreactive topoisomerase II and are resistant to topoisomerase II inhibitors becuase of an altered or mutated enzyme molecule. P388 A20 cells appear to be resistant because of a quantitative change in the ratio of functionally distinct topoisomerase II isozymes. The cell lines to be discussed in this section appear to be resistant to topoisomerase II inhibitors, primarily because of a decrease in immunoreactive enzyme. The contribution of altered enzyme activity is either minor or not well defined.

Four drug-resistant human nasopharyngeal carcinoma KB cell lines were isolated in the presence of progressively increasing doses of VP-16 [80,81]. KB/1c, KB/7d, KB/20a, and KB/40a cells are 29-, 145-, 187-, and 287-fold resistant to VP-16 respectively. A parallel increase in resistance from least resistant (KB/1c) to most resistant (KB/40a) was also seen for m-AMSA (2- to 10-fold), doxorubicin (8 to 34-fold), and mitoxantrone (2- to 6-fold). All four cell lines demonstrate both parental sensitivity to 10-hydroxycamptothecin and roughly equivalent (13- to 16-fold) resistance to vincristine. Immunoblots of these cells with monoclonal antibody C219 did not demonstrate overexpression of P-glycoprotein, however, $10\,\mu M$ verapamil significantly reversed the drug resistance to vincristine (by 92–98%) and partially reversed VP-16 resistance (by 54–78%). Equilibrium intracellular concentrations of $[^3H]$-VP-16 were reduced 50–75% in all four resistant cell lines relative to WT accumulation, whereas the efflux of this same drug was similar in parental and resistant cells. Topoisomerase I activity (relaxation of pBR322 DNA in the absence of ATP) was found to be increased approximately 150% in all four drug-resistant cell lines, and western blots for topoisomerase I with a monoclonal antibody demonstrated 133–178% of the 97kDa protein (relative to WT cells). Topoisomerase II activity (unknotting P4 DNA) was uniformally decreased by 50%, while immunoreactive enzyme was decreased to 22–60% of the parental enzyme level. In summary, these four drug-resistant cell lines have a significant decrease in DNA topoisomerase II activity and content, which undoubtedly contributes to their resistance to topoisomerase II inhibitors. There is no evidence that the topoisomerase II in these cells has altered activity; in fact, VP-16 inhibition of equal unknotting activity from these cell lines was equivalent and was similar to WT inhibition. A drug-transport defect also contributes to the resistance of these cells to both topoisomerase II inhibitors and vincristine. The reciprocal increase in DNA topoisomerase I has been observed in other resistant cell lines (see below).

A cell line of P388 leukemia resistant to doxorubicin was developed by treating $B6D2F_1$ mice bearing ascitic tumor with doxorubicin over several transplant generatiions [82]. Two drug-resistant clones, P388/ADR/3 and P388/ADR/7, have been isolated and their mechanisms of resistance well described [83–87]. P388/ADR/3 and P388/ADR/7 are 5- and 10-fold resistant to doxorubicin, respectively, and exhibit cross-resistance to daunomycin (11- and 16-fold), mitoxantrone (13- and 11-fold), VP-16 (4- and 6-fold), and actinomycin D (18-fold each). The P388/ADR/7 line is also 15-fold resistant to vincristine. Both resistant cell lines demonstrate a decreased uptake of $[^{14}C]$-doxorubicin and overexpress P-glycoprotein (~2-fold in both cell lines by Northern and western blots). Interestingly, the efflux of $[^{14}C]$-doxorubicin from these cells is similar to WT efflux. Perhaps a low level (twofold) of P-glycoprotein overexpression is not sufficient to increase drug efflux. Immunoblotting with a polyclonal rabbit anti-recombinant topoisomerase II antibody has shown a substantial decrease in topoisomerase II in both of these resistant cell lines [86]. Accompanying this is a three- to fivefold decrease in topoisomerase II catalytic activity (decatenation of kDNA), was well as a marked decrease in drug-induced DNA cleavage (measured as either covalent DNA-enzyme complexes by the K/SDS method or as SSBs and DSBs by alkaline or neutral elution). Recent evidence suggests that a decreased copy number of the normal topoisomerase II allele accounts for the diminution of protein product [87]. These investigators identified two mRNA transcripts by probing total RNA from sensitive and resistant cells with the 1.8-kb (λhTOP2-Z2) and 5.6-kb (pBS-hTOP2) human topoisomerase II cDNAs. The 6.6-kb message was present in all three cell lines but reduced 7- to 8-fold in both P388/ADR/3 and P388/ADR/7 cells, whereas the 5.5-kb message was found only in the two resistant cell lines. Southern blot analyses of restriction fragments from genomic DNA treated with BamH1, Stul, and Pvull with both cDNAs demonstrate a fragment from the native allele (which is decreased in copy number in the resistant cells), and fragments unique to the resistant cells. These studies suggest that a decrease in the 6.6-kb message from the normal topoisomerase II allele in the drug-resistant cells is responsible for the quantitative change in enzyme. The 5.5-kb message is likely from a mutant allele and is either not translated, the protein product is rapidly degraded, or the antibodies used for immunoblotting simply do not recognize the protein product. The drug resistance of P388/ADR/3 and P388/ADR/7 cells is multifactorial; over-expression of P-glycoprotein and underexpression of DNA topoisomerase II are certainly involve. A qualitative change in the topoisomerase II present has not been excluded, and the role of anionic glutathione transferase, which is increased 1.5- to 2-fold in activity and content in the resistant cells, is unknown. Finally, the contribution of altered DNA repair is discussed below.

A genetic mechanism that controls the amount of topoisomerase II produced in m-AMSA-resistant P388 cells has been described [88]. Nuclear extracts from these cells demonstrate a twofold decrease in topoisomerase II catalytic activity and immunoreactivity, as well as a 1.6-fold increase in topoisomerase I activity. Northern blots with both a human Hela cDNA (λhTOPI-D2) probe for topoisomerase I and a human Raji-HN$_2$ cDNA (SP1) probe for topoisomerase II have demonstrated mRNAs of 4 kb and 6 kb, respectively. The 4 kb transcript was increased 130% relative to WT cells, and the 6 kb message decreased by 50%; these changes correlate fairly well with the alterations in activity/content seen in topoisomerase I and II above. Southern blot analyses, with the SP1 cDNA, of Bgl1- and BamHI-restricted DNA, have shown a 50% reduction in the resistant cells of a fragment present in the sensitive cells, as well as the presence of new fragments from the resistant cells. Southern blot analyses have also shown that the topoisomerase II gene is hypermethylated. In short, it appears that the reduction in topoisomerase II protein is due to inactivation of one topoisomerase II allele by gene rearrangement and/or hypermethylation. This quantitative change in "normal" topoisomerase II certainly contributes to the resistance of these cells. The reciprocal increase in topoisomerase I activity may in part compensate in vivo for the topoisomerase II required for normal cellular functioning.

A multiple drug-resistant Chinese hamster lung cell line, DC3F/9-OHE, was isolated in the presence of stepwise increments of 9-hydroxyellipticine [89–97]. These cells are approximately 100-fold resistant to the selecting agent, and cross-resistant to actinomycin D, m-AMSA, daunomycin, doxorubicin, VP-16, and vincristine. Drug uptake by these resistant cells of [^{14}C]-2-methyl-9-hydroxyelliptcine and [^{14}C]-mAMSA is equivalent to that of the WT cells, while uptake of [^{3}H]-actinomycin D and [^{14}C]-doxorubicin is reduced approximately twofold. Drug-induced DNA damage (DPCs, SSBs, and DSBs) is reduced in DC3F/9-OHE cells and nuclei in response to VP-16, m-AMSA, and 2-methyl-9-hydroxyellipticine. Nuclear extracts from the resistant cells have shown a two to threefold decrease in topoisomerase II by western blot analysis, with a 3.5-fold decrease in decatenation activity. Topoisomerase I catalytic activity is equivalent in sensitive and resistant cells. This drug-resistant cell line is also reported to contain an unusual drug-independent DNA-protein linking activity that copurifies with topoisomerase I. The diminution of drug target in this cell line is a mechanism of resistance. The contribution of either an altered topoisomerase II enzyme or a modulating factor to resistance awaits the further characterization of homogeneous preparations of these proteins.

From the discussion presented above, it is apparent that a decrease in nuclear topoisomerase II plays a major role in multiple drug resistance not attributable to P-glycoprotein. Recent studies have demonstrated that an increase in nuclear topoisomerase II can result in a hypersensitive phenotype [98–99]. CHO cells were mutagenized with EMS, and a hyper-sensitive cell line (ADR-1) was isolated by the "toothpick" replica plate method in the presence of a low concentration of doxorubicin. ADR-1 cells are 3.6-fold hypersensitive to doxorubicin and cross-hypersensitive to m-AMSA, daunomycin, mitoxantrone, VP-16, and ellipticine (3.2- to 4.4-fold). These cells have the same sensitivity to cisplatinum and vincristine as WT cells. Uptake of [^{3}H]-daunomycin is unaltered in ADR-1 cells. Western blot analysis of nuclear extracts has demonstrated a threefold increase in topoisomerase II in ADR-1 cells. Assays for topoisomerase II catalytic activity and drug-induced DNA cleavage activity have shown concomitant increases. Studies with hybrids of ADR-1 and CHO-K1 cells demonstrate that the hypersensitivity of ADR-1 cells is due to an over-production of topoisomerase II. The CHO-K1/ADR-1 hybrid has the paren-tal sensitivity to both m-AMSA and doxorubicin, as well as the WT content of immunoreactive topoisomerase II. These studies with a hypersensitive cell line complement those above and underscore the importance of nuclear topoisomerase II in determining the sensitivity of a cell to several anti-neoplastic agents.

Intracellular distribution of DNA topoisomerase II. The cell lines discussed in the previous section all have as a major contribution to their multiple drug resistance a significant reduction in DNA topoisomerase II, the target of several antineoplastic agents. Recent evidence suggests that an altered intracellular partioning of topoisomerase II may also be important in resist-ance, without a decrease in toal enzyme amount. Studies have shown that nuclear matrix preparations from CCRF-CEM cells contain fourfold more newly synthesized DNA compared to the high salt-soluble nonmatrix DNA [100]. Treatment of these cells with topoisomerase II inhibitors (VP-16, VM-26, and m-AMSA) was found to reduced the specific activity of nascent DNA on the nuclear matrix by 60%. Therefore, the inhibition of matrix DNA topoisomerase II by these antitumor drugs appears to interfere with the replication of DNA. In another study, CEM/VM-1 cells (discussed above) were found to be resistant to several topoisomerase II inhibitors while containing WT amounts of immunoreactive enzyme. Pretreatment of these cells with either VM-26 or m-AMSA did not affect the specific activity of nascent DNA isolated from the nuclear matrices of these cells (compared with CEM parental matrices that had a 50–75% reduction in newly replicated DNA). Topoisomerase II activity in nuclear matrices of the resistant cells (decatenation of kDNA and P4 unknotting) was diminished sevenfold, and decreased enzyme was also seen by western blot analysis [74]. If nuclear matrix DNA topoisomerase II is a major target of these inhibitors, it is likely that CEM/VM-1 cells are resistant because of their altered intra-cellular distribution of topoisomerase II. The primary drug target has been substantially reduced.

Alterations in cellular transport of topoisomerase II inhibitors

Overexpression of P-glycoprotein associated with alterations in DNA topoisomerase II. The cell lines to be discussed in this section are resist-ant to several classes of topoisomerase II inhibitors, contain increased amounts of the classic P-glycoprotein drug efflux pump, and have aberrant topoisomerase II activity. LIa5µM cells were selected from parental mouse leukemia L1210 cells in the presence of increasing concentration of VM-26 (101). They are 1300-fold resistant to VM-26 and are cross-resistant to actinomycin D (596-fold), m-AMSA (41-fold), doxorubicin (183-fold), VP-16 (214-fold), and vincristine (1500-fold). Western blot analysis has demonstrated overexpression of P-glycoprotein [101,102] and transport studies with VM-26 have shown a fourfold decrease in both drug uptake and steady-state levels, as well as an increased efflux of VM-26. Nuclear extracts from sensitive and resistant cells have similar topoisomerase II activity (P4 unknotting), and this is inhibited equally by VM-26. At equitoxic doses of VM-26 (which gives much higher drug levels in LIa5µM cells), there remains a marked resistance to VM-26-induced DNA damage in the resist-ant cells; contrasted with equitoxic doses of doxorubicin, which result in near-equal DNA strand breaks. Equitoxic drug doses were used, rather than equivalent intracellular drug levels, because 60% of the resistant cells contain lipid vesicles (as opposed to 3% of the parental cells). The drug resistance of LIa5µM cells likely depends on a cleavage-resistant topoisomerase II enzyme, in addition to the overexpression of P-glycoprotein. The above studies with VM-26 also suggest that this drug may be cytotoxic, independent of its action on topoiosmerase II, i.e., the fact that *equitoxic* doses of VM-26 did not result in equivalent DNA damage suggests that VM-26 is lethal to LIa5μM cells, in spite of diminished DNA scission.

P388/ADR/3 and P388/ADR/7 cells (discussed in detail above) are cross-resistant to all classes of topoisomerase II inhibitors, overexpress P-glycoprotein, demonstrate decreased uptake of doxorubicin, and have decreased topoisomerase II immunoreactivity and catalytic activity. Similar to LIa5μM cells, there remains a four- to ninefold decrease in doxorubicin-induced DNA DSBs after intracellular drug concentrations are equalized (not here that concentration and not cytotoxicity was the basis for drug levels). This would suggest that these cells also contain a drug-resistant topoisomerase II enzyme.

Multiple drug-resistant cell lines L1210/DOX0.05 (or R1) and L1210/DOX0.25 (or R2) were isolated from L1210 cells exposed to increasing concentrations of doxorubicin [103,104]. R1 cells are 10-fold resistant to both doxorubicin and VP-16, and 2-fold resistant to m-AMSA; while R2 cells are 40-fold resistant to both doxorubicin and VP-16, and 7-fold resistant to m-AMSA. R1 and R2 cells overexpress P-glycoprotein 4-fold, respectively, by immunoblotting. Uptake and retention of doxorubicin by R1 cells is similar to WT cells, while R2 cells show a 50% reduction in uptake and retention. Topoisomerase II activity (decatenation) of nuclear extracts was shown to be reduced twofold and fourfold in R1 and R2 extracts, respectively. VP-16-induced DNA cleavage was significantly reduced in these resistant cell lines, out of proportion to the attenuated topoisomerase II catalytic activity. These studies, as well as those with LIa5μM and P388/ADR cells, suggest that resistance to topoisomerase II inhibitors in these cell lines correlates better with resistance to drug-induced DNA cleavage than drug transport differences. A qualitative change in topoisomerase II may be more critical than overexpression of P-glycoprotein.

Non-P-glycoprotein alterations in drug transport. Several drug-resistant cell lines have been described that are cross-resistant to various topoisomerase II inhibitors, do not overexpress P-glycoprotein, yet have a perturbation in drug transport and (when looked for) an alteration in topoisomerase II activity. The drug-resistant human small-cell lung carcinoma cell line, GLC₄/ADR, was isolation in the presence of doxorubicin and is 44- to 123-fold resistant to this agent [105–107]. These cells are also cross-resistant to VP-16, VM-26, mitoxantrone, m-AMSA, vincristine, and vindesine. Overexpression of the *mdr1* gene was not found by Western, Northern, or Southern blot analyses. However, these cells have a 45% reduction in the steady-state concentration of adriamycin. Whether the threefold decrease in topoisomerase II catalytic activity and the decrease in drug-induced DNA cleavage are the result of a quantitative or qualitative alteration in topoisomerase II is unknown.

The drug-resistant human nasopharyngeal carcinoma cell lines discussed in detail above (KB/1c, 7d, 20a, and 40a) are P-glycoprotein negative by immunoblotting yet have a verapamil-responsive perturbation in VP-16 uptake. These cell lines also have a quantitative change in topoisomerase II that contributes to their resistance. HT1080/DR4 human fibrosarcoma cells [108] are 222-fold resistant to their selecting agent, doxorubicin, and are cross-resistant to VP-16 (837-fold), actinomycin D (17-fold), vincristine (25-fold), and cytosine arabinoside (18-fold). Again, these cells are P-glycoprotein negative yet have a twofold decrease in equilibrium concentrations of doxorubicin and an increased efflux of this drug. Treatment with verapamil increases intracellular doxorubicin by 12.6% and augments cytotoxicity by 340%. It is likely these cells have an alteration in topoisomerase II activity, but this is yet to be determined. The mitoxantrone-resistant human colon carcinoma cell line, WiDr/R, is 21-fold resistant to mitoxantrone, 8-fold resistant to doxorubicin, and 2-fold resistant to vinblastine [109,110]. Western, Southern, and Northern blots failed to detect overexpression of the classic MDR genotype. The initial uptake of [^{3}H]-mitoxantrone by the resistant cells is equivalent to that of parental cells, while the equilibrium level of this drug is reduced 20% in WiDr/R cells; efflux of mitoxantrone is increased. Verapamil did not affect drug transport or cytotoxicity in the resistant cells. An alteration in nuclear topoisomerase II may contribute to the resistance of this cell line. The significance of the homogeneously staining region on the short arm of chromosome 7 in WiDr/R cells is also unknown.

Two distinct HL-60 resistant cell lines were isolated in the presence of increasing concentrations of doxorubicin. HI-60/Adr [111–113] and HL-60/AR [114–117] cells are 80- and 111-fold resistant to the selecting agent, respectively, as well as 75- and 50-fold resistant to daunomycin, 15- and 6-fold resistant to actinomycin D, and 25- and 8-fold resistant to vincristine. Western blot analyses did not detect overexpression of P-glycoprotein in either cell line, although HL-60/Adr cells have a decreased uptake of [^{3}H]-vincristine, and HL-60/AR cells have a diminished uptake and increased efflux of [^{14}C]-daunomycin. Alterations in topoisomerase II levels/activity have not been explored in either cell line. The HI-60/Adr cells appear to have a change in phosphorylation state of a non-MDR glycoprotein (see below), and the HL-60/AR cells demonstrate an alteration in the subcellular distribution of daunomycin (see below). These findings may also contribute to the drug resistance of these multiple drug-resistant cell lines.

Multiple cell lines have a resistance phenotype suggestive of an alteration in topoisomerase II, are P-glycoprotein negative, yet demonstrate significant significant alterations in drug transport. Further characterization of these cell lines will determine the contribution of a quantitative or qualitative change in topoisomerase II to drug resistance.

Altered subcellular distribution of DNA topoisomerase II inhibitor. A cell can be resistant to a topoisomerase II inhibitor if the drug does not reach the target. This type of resistance could theoretically occur in the presence of normal topoisomerase II content/activity. The HL-60/AR cell line (discussed above) and parental HL-60 cells have been examined for the intracellular distribution of daunomycin by fluorescence microscopy [115, 117]. Sensitive HL-60 cells initially localize daunomycin in the golgi region; later the majority of drug is found in the nucleus. Drug resistant cells translocate daunomycin from the golgi region to lysosomes and mitochondria; little is found in the nucleus. The drug resistance of HL-60/AR cells may be a consequence of the drug not reaching the target enzyme, as almost all topoisomerase II resides in the nucleus. B16VDXR-resistant mouse melanoma cells are 200-fold resistant to the selecting agent, doxorubicin, and are cross-resistant to daunomycin and vincristine [118,119]. They demonstrate decreased uptake and increased efflux of doxorubicin. At the same intracellular concentration of doxorubicin as WT cells, B16VDXR cells display decreased drug-induced DNA SSBs. Fluorescence microscopy has demonstrated that the nuclear/cytoplasmic ratio of doxorubicin is much reduced in the resistant cells. It is likely that a qualitatively different topoisomerase II enzyme and/or diminished nuclear drug uptake may contribute to the resistance of these cells.

Incompletely characterized cell lines that express the topoisomerase II inhibitor phenotype with unaltered drug transport

There are cell lines described in the literature that are resistant to several classes of topoisomerase II inhibitors and do not have a perturbation in drug transport. They are included in this section because, although they may have an alteration in topoisomerase II activity or control, their mechanism(s) of resistance are as yet poorly defined.

Drug-resistant C25X cells were isolated from doxorubicin-treated CCRF-CEM cells [120] and are 24-fold resistant to this agent. They have approximately the same level of resistance (15- to 20-fold) to VP-16, mitoxantrone, daunomycin, and m-AMSA. They are sensitive to vincristine. Western bolt analysis failed to detect overexpression of P-glycoprotein, and uptake of [^{3}H]-daunomycin and [^{3}H]-VP-16 by C25X cells was the same as WT cells. DNA strand breaks induced by the above agents were quantified by a fluorometric assay and were found to be diminished in the resistant cells. The rate of repair of these strand breaks was found to be similar in sensitive and resistant cells. Another drug-resistant cell line (C80X), isolated at the same time as C25X, is 83-fold resistant to doxorubicin (with a proportional increase in resistance to other topoisomerase II inhibitors) and is 100-fold resistant to vincristine. Immunoblots show a dramatic increase in P-glycoprotein. Uptake of daunomycin and VP-16 were found to be greatly reduced. The higher levels of resistance to topoisomerase II-active drugs seen in C80X cells are accompanied by an increase in the MDR efflux pump, with accompanying resistance to vincristine.

The HL-60/MX2 cell line was generated by treating HL-60 cells with increasing concentrations of mitoxantrone [121]. These cells are 35-fold resistant to mitoxantrone and are cross-resistant to m-AMSA (32-fold), VM-26 (24-fold), VP-16 (15-fold), daunomycin (4-fold) doxorubicin (4-fold), and actinomycin D (2-fold). In addition, they are approximately three-fold hypersensitive to blemonycin. Overexpression of P-glycoprotein was not found in these cells, and there was no difference in [^{14}C]-mitoxantrone uptake or efflux when compared to WT cells. Cytogenetic analysis failed to find double-minute chromosomes or homogeneously staining regions, suggesting gene amplification is not involved in the resistance of this cell line. Although it is likely that a quantitative or qualitative alteration in DNA topoisomerase II contributes to the resistance of HL-60/MX2 cells, this has not yet been determined.

BHK 21/13 cells were mutagenized with MNNG, and resistant mutants were selected in the presence of novobiocin [122,123]. One drug-resistant cell line (Nov^{r}A2) is 4.3-fold resistant to novobiocin and 3.4-, 3.5-, 7.5- and 13-fold cross-resistant to vinblastine, m-AMSA, doxorubicin, and VP-16, respectively. It has the same uptake of [^{3}H]-VP-16 as parental cells, and topoisomerase II catalytic activity (P4 unknotting) from cytoplasmic and nuclear extracts is equivalent from sensitive and resistant cells. Partially purified topoisomerase II from parental and resistant cells, likewise, have equivalent catalytic activity (decatenation), which is inhibited to the same extent by VP-16. VP-16-induced DNA cleavage mediated by partially purified topoisomerase II was no different in WT versus Nov^{r}A2 cells. However, VP-16-stimulated DNA strand breaks in whole cells and nuclei, quantified by sedimentation analyses, were dramatically reduced in number in Nov^{r}A2 cells compared to parental BHK cells. In summary, assays of topoisomerase II (either partially purified or in nuclear extracts) suggest that there is no difference in catalytic activity or cleavage activity in sensitive versus resistant cells. Drug-induced DNA damage in the intact cell, however, is markedly reduced in the resistant cells. This implicates an alteration in intracellular drug partitioning or the presence of a topoisomerase II modulating factor as being pivotal in the mechanism of drug resistance of these cells. The mechanism(s) of resistance of the three cell lines discussed in this section are not well defined, but probably involve an alteration in topoisomerase II activity (or the control thereof), and are apparently not the result of drug-transport perturbations.

Processing topoisomerase II-mediated DNA damage induced by drugs

Several investigators have shown that the number of DNA DSBs (as opposed to DNA SSBs) induced by topoisomerase II inhibitors correlates better with drug-induced cytotoxicity. It is reasonable to assume that an increased or decreased DNA repair capacity (i.e., religation by topoisomerase II) could affect the sensitivity of a cell to topoisomerase II inhibitors. The multiple drug-resistant P388/ADR/3 and P338/ADR/7 cell lines (discuessed above) demonstrate decreased DNA DSB formation in response to topoisomerase II inhibitors. In addition, the sensitive and resistant cell lines process doxorubicin-induced DSBs differently [84]. The onset of repair DSBs (which is actually religation of cleaved DNA by topoisomerase II) after drug removal occurs at 1 hr for both resistant cell lines and at 4 hr in the WT cells. The rate of repair is similar in all three cell lines, but at 24 hr the sensitive cells still contain more DSBs than either resistant cell line. P388/ADR/3 and P388/ADR/7 cells demonstrate decreased drug-induced DNA damage, which is likely due to a quantitative or qualitative alteration in topoisomerase II, but may also be drug resistant because they repair (religate) the potentially lethal DNA damage sooner.

The drug-resistant human small-cell lung cancer line, GLC$_4$/ADR, has been found to have a two- to fourfold decrease in doxorubicin-stimulated DNA DSBs (see discussion above). The stability of these DSBs has also been investigated [105]. One hour after a treatment with doxorubicin, the GLC$_4$/ADR cells have repaired 80% of the DSBs, while at 2 hr post-treatment the parental cells have more than 100% DSBs remaining. The repair of DNA damage after x-ray treatment was also examined in these cell lines. At 20 minutes post-irradiation, the sensitive cells have repaired 30% of the DSBs, while the resistant cells have repaired 70% of the DNA damage. GLC$_4$/ADR cells, similar to the resistant P388/ADR lines above, probably have an alteration in topoisomerase II that contributes to the resistant phenotype. The [apparent] increased repair of drug-induced DSBs by GLC$_4$/ADR cells may be due to the fact that they have an increased rate of efflux of doxorubicin from the cell (a decresed steady state of this drug has already been shown). This would result in less inhibition of DNA religation, or faster "repair." An augmented DNA DSB repair capacity by the resistant cells after x-ray treatment may represent a non-topoisomerase II mechanism of resealing DNA breaks.

That a more efficient DNA repair process can confer resistance to topoisomerase II inhibitors has been suggested [84,105]. However, in each case it is likely that faster religation of strand breaks caused by topoisomerase II inhibitors is a result of a greater rate of drug efflux by enhanced cellular transport mechanism(s). Interestingly, recent studies have indicated that the converse may be true, i.e., a defective DNA repair capacity can increase the drug sensitivity of cells. The CHO-K1 mutant strain, xrs-1, has been shown to be hypersensitive to ionizing radiation but not to UV or alkylating agents. This is likely due to the defective DNA DSB rejoining mechanism present in this cell line [124–127]. The xrs-1 cell line is 25-, 7.1-, and 4.3-fold hypersensitive to VP-16, m-AMSA, and ellipticine, respectivly. It is also 9.5-fold hypersensitive to γ-rays and has the same sensitivity as WT cells to novobiocin. The sensitive and resistant cells have equivalent topoisomerase II activity in nuclear extracts (unknotting P4 DNA), as well as the same VP-16- and m-AMSA-induced enzyme-DNA complex formation. Preliminary experiments have apparently shown that drug-induced DNA DSB formation is equal in the sensitive and hypersensitive cell lines. Thus, hypersensitive xrs-1 cells appear to have normal topoisomerase II activity, which results in the same amount of drug-stimulated DNA damage initially; a slower repair of these DSBs results in hypersensitivity of this cell line to topoisomerase II inhibitors. This slower repair may involve alterations in drug efflux or changes in the topoisomerase II molecule itself, which result in slower religation of cleaved DNA. Studies that actually examine the onset and rate of repair after drug treatment need to be done. Strain LY-S from mouse lymphoma L5178Y cells is 1.8-fold hypersensitive to x-radiation relative to LY-R, again due to a deficiency in DNA DSB repair [128]. This cell line is also 3.2-, 2.1-, and 1.4-fold hypersensitive to m-AMSA, ellipticine, and VP-16, respectively, and approximately 2.5-fold resistant to both novobiocin and camptothecin. VP-16- and m-AMSA-induced DNA DSBs are increased in the LY-S cell line, and repair of these DSBs at 1 hr is slightly reduced in LY-S when induced by VP-16. Repair of m-AMSA-induced DSBs is equivalent in LY-S and LY-R. It is most likely that this cell line has an increased nuclear content of topoisomerase II, which accounts for its hypersensitivity to topoisomerase II inhibitors.

Modulators of DNA topoisomerase II activity

Phosphorylation and poly(ADP ribosylation) of DNA topoisomerase II have been shown to increase and decrease, respectively, the activity of this enzyme. The evidence for this will be discussed, as will the theoretical roles of these modification in drug resistance. In addition, a few drug-resistant cell lines appear to overproduce or modify proteins that may be involved in the control of topoisomerase II activity. In vitro experiments have shown that *Drosophila melanogaster* topoisomerase II has a cAMP-independent protein kinase activity tightly associated with in that is able to phosphorylate topoisomerase II, histones, and casein on serine or threonine [129]. This topoisomerase II is also a substrate for phosphorylation by casein kinase II, which results in a threefold increase in catalytic activity [130]. Finally, homogeneous *Drosophila* topoisomerase II is a substrate for in vitro phosphorylation by rat brain protein kinase C with a $K_{M(topo\ II)}$ of approximately 100 nM [131]. These studies demonstrated one phosphorylation site/subunit topoisomerase II, which occured only on serine. Phosphorylation by protein kinase C stimulated topoisomerase II catalytic activity, when measured as unknotting of P4 DNA and relaxation of supercoiled pBR322 DNA. Finally, cAMP-dependent protein kinase did not phosphorylate *D. Melanogaster* topoisomerase II, whereas serine phosphorylation by calmodulin-dependent protein kinase type II did occur at high concentrations of this kinase. Phosphorylation of topoisomerase II from the sponge *Geodia cydonium* by protein kinase C also augments its activity by 2.5-fold [132].

The in vivo phosphorylation of topoisomerase II has been studied in detail [133,134]. *Drosophila* Kc cells were labeled in vivo with [^{3}u22P]-orthophosphate, and immunoprecipitates of topoisomerase II from nuclear extracts of these cells were analyzed. These studies showed that topoisomerase II is indeed phosphorylated in vivo in *Drosophila* embryonic cells, and that serine is the only amino acid residue that is phosphorylated. Phosphorylation studies with purified topoisomerase II from *Drosophila* Kc cells and either homogenates of Kc cells of purified protein kinases have conclusively identified casein kinase II as the kinase involved in this modification. Phosphorylation in these cells occurs as one phosphate group/homodimer. MSB-1 (chicken lymphoblastoid) cells have also been labelled in log phase in vivo by [^{32}P]-orthophosphate [134]. Topoisomerase II was immunoprecipitated from the various phases of the cell cycle (which had been separated by centrifugal elutriation) in MSB-1 cells, and after electrophoresis on an SDS-PAGE gel the enzyme was transferred to nitrocellulose. Autoradiography of this nitrocellulose identified ^{32}P-labeled topoisomerase II, and subsequent immunoblotting of this same nitrocellulose developed with ^{125}I-protein A allowed quantitation of total topoisomerase II. These studies demonstrated that topoisomerase II is phosphorylated in vivo and that the phosphorylated species is 170 kDa. In the log phase cells, phosphoryation steadily increases during G_1 and S to reach a maximum in G_2 and mitosis that is 3.5-fold greater than G_1. In summary, phosphorylation of DNA topoisomerase II does occur in vivo (we have also observed the phosphorylation of 170 kDa topoisomerase II in vivo in WT and drug-resistant Chinese hamster ovary cells; unpublished observation). This phosphorylation appears to stimulate topoisomerase II activity approximate threefold. Although not yet reported, it is easy to envision an alteration in phosphorylation that could result in resistance to topoisomerase II inhibitiors. For example, a mutant kinase that hypophosphorylates topoisomerase II such that its activity is not augmented in G_2/M might appear to be a topoisomerase II that is resistant to drug, and indeed result in decrease DNA damage.

Inhibition of calf thymus topoisomerase II activity by poly(ADP ribosyla-tion) has been observed in vitro [135]. P4 unknotting, relaxation of super-coiled PM2 DNA, catenation of DNA, and cleavable complex formation by topoisomerase II were all inhibited when the assay included NAD and poly(ADP ribose) synthetase. The only suggestion that poly(ADP ribosylation) might have a role in drug resistance comes from P388/R cells [136,137]. These cells are 170-fold resistant to doxorubicin and have a decreased uptake of this drug. Doxorubicin-induced DNA SSBs are reduced four- to fivefold in P388/R cells, and although 15 µM verapamil augments doxorubicin retention by twofold, it does not increase DNA SSBs. The baseline synthesis of poly(ADP ribose) in P388/R cells is twofold greater than in WT cells and does not change in either cell line in response to doxorubicin treatment. These studies suggest that the activity of poly(ADP ribose) synthetase is increased in the resistant cells. This could possibly alter the activity of topoisomerase II in these cells such that they appear resistant to drug-stimulated DNA cleavage. Obviously more definitive studies are needed here.

Evidence for protein factors that may be involved in the drug resistance to topoisomerase II inhibitors is scant and comes from three sources. When nuclei from K21 murine mastocytoma cells are treated with $10 \mu M$ m-AMSA, a threefold increase in topoisomerase II-DNA complex formation is detected by the K/SDS method [138]. The addition of $20-30 \mu g$ (protein) of cytoplasmic extracts from these same cells resulted in a 10-fold stimulation of complex formation (similar to intact cells). This enhancing activtity is apparently not topoisomerase I or II, is lost in extracts from cells pretreated with cycloheximide, is heat labile, and has a molecular mass $>50 kDa$. It is likely a protein (kinase?) whose loss could hypothetically result in diminished DNA cleavage in response to m-AMSA. P-glycoprotein negative drug-resistant HL-60/Adr cells contain a membrane glycoprotein of molecular mass 150 kDa [111–113]. This protein is present in equal amount in sensitive and resistant cells, but is only phosphorylated in vivo in the HL-60/Adr line. This protein may contribute to the resistance phenotype of these cells. Finally, the role of a 22 kDa protein, found only in the membrane-cytosol factions of VM-26-resistant LIa5 μM cells, in the resistance to topoisomerase II inhibitors has not yet been explored [101,102]. Factors that are extrinsic to topoisomerase II and modulate its activity, which may include phosphorylation or poly(ADP ribosylation), are beginning to be defined. Alterations in this control of topoisomerase II activity will undoubtedly contribute to the drug resistance to inhibitors of this enzyme.

Proliferation-dependent resistance to topoisomerase II inhibitors

Several investigators have shown that the nuclear content of DNA topoisomerase II may vary as a function of 1) proliferative stage (exponential versus quiescent growth), 2) developmental stage (embryonic versus adult), 3) phase of the cell cycle (G_1, S, G_2/M content of DNA), 4) degree of transformation (normal versus malignant phenotype), and 5) difference in topoisomerase II isozymes (p170 and p180), combined with the other factors. In general, topoisomerase II content is increased in rapidly dividing cells. Those cells with diminished enzyme content, for whatever reason, are functionally resistant to the DNA-damaging and cytotoxic effects of topoisomerase II inhibitors.

Early studies demonstrated a 10-fold increase in topoisomerase II activity (catenation and decatenation) in regenerating rat livers 40 hr after partial hepatectomy [139]. EGF-stimulated human fibroblasts and Swiss/3T3 mouse fibroblasts [140], as well as concanavation A-stimulated guinea-pig lymphocytes [141], were found to have dramatic increases in topoisomerase II activity following stimulation. In contrast, C3H 10T1/2 mouse embryo fibroblasts were shown to have the same topoisomerase II activity in log and plateau growth, as well as in all phases of the cell cycle [142]. Topoisomerase I activity in these same cells increased fourfold in log phase cells, and maximum activity (in synchronized cell populations) occurred at mid-S phase.

The proliferation-dependent cytotoxic and DNA-damaging effects of VP-16 and m-AMSA in CHO cells, HeLa cells, human lymphoblastic CCRF cells, and mouse leukemia L1210 cells were investigated by Sullivan et al. [143,144]. We have found that relative to log phase cells, plateau CHO and CCRF cells are resistant to the cytotoxic effects of these drugs, demonstrate decreased drug-induced DNA SSBs, have decreased topoisomerase II catalytic and cleavage activity, and have substantial decreases in immunoreactive enzyme by western blot analysis. These quiescent cells have primarily a G_0-G_1 content of DNA. Quiescent HeLa and L1210 cells, however, have the same topoisomerase II content as their log phase counterparts, similar drug-induced DNA SSBs, and near-equal log and plateau cell-cycle distribution by flow cytometry (with a high S fraction). However, quiescent L1210 cells remain fairly resistant to VP-16-induced cytotoxicity. These studies demonstrate that topoisomerase II is not proliferation dependent in all cell lines, and that equivalent DNA cleavage does not necessary result in the same degree of cytotoxicity. A decrease in topoisomerase II activity, which results in decreased sensitivity to topoisomerase II inhibitors, as well as diminished drug-induced DNA damage, has also been found in quiescent human fibrobasts and human glioblastoma cells [145], in plateau-phase Chinese hamster fibroblasts [146], and in quiescent Chinese hamster ovary AA8 cells [147]. Human skin fibroblasts (NIH 3T3 and 3T6 cells) that are either quiescent because of serum deprivation or confluent because they are density arrested have a substantial decrease in topoisomerase II by immunoblotting, without a change in immunoreactive topoisomerase I [148]. Transformed cell lines, including HeLa, L1210, and cos-1 cells, in plateau phase because of serum deprivation or increased cell densities, were found to have no fluctuations in immunoreactive topoisomerase I or II (similar to above). Dunning rat prostatic adenocarcinoma R3327-G has both an increased growth rate and an increased rate of DNA synthesis compared to normal rat prostate [149]. Accompanying this rapid proliferation is an increase in topoisomerase II levels (fivefold) and an increase in P4 unknotting by R3327-G topoisomerase II. In summary, rapidly proliferating cells (exponential growth) in culture or in tumor models have augmented levels of topoisomerase II and are generally more susceptible to the cytotoxic action of drugs because of this increase in target enzyme. Quiescent cells, with a lower S fraction, are relatively resistant to topoisomerase II inhibitors.

The developmental regulation of topoisomerase II has also been examined. Early proliferating chicken erythroblasts have approximately 1.5×10^5 copies of topoisomerase II/cell [150]. As these erythrocytes age, they have a decrease in topoisomerase II content by immunobloting (to 2% by day 10). A mature chicken erythrocyte has at most 300 copies of topoisomerase II/cell. The regulation of topoisomerase II has also been followed during the development of *Drosophila melanogaster* embryos into adults [151]. Western and Northern blot analyses for topoisomerase II correlate fairly well and show an increase in topoisomerase II during early and mid-embryogenesis and during pupation, and essentially none in the adult. The increases in enzyme are coincident with an increase in mitotic activity. Northern blot analysis of log and plateau *Drosophila* Kc cells demonstrated 10–20 topoisomerase II mRNA transcripts/cell in exponential growth and only 1 transcript/cell in the quiescent stage [151].

Etoposide-induced cytotoxicity and DNA damage varies as a function of cell-cycle phase in BALB/c 3T3 cells released from serum-deprived quiescent growth into fresh media [152]. These cells achieve maximum immunoreactive topoisomerase II levels 20–24 hr after release, and this is accompanied by peak drug-stimulated DNA SSBs during this same G_2/M period. VP-16-induced DNA damage can be prevented if cells are pretreated with cycloheximide. Maximum cytotoxicity, however, occurs at 18 hr postrelease, during S phase. Maximum cytotoxicity and peak DNA cleavage induced by VP-16 thus appear to be separate events. These same observations have also been made in synchronized HeLa cells [153], where maximum m-AMSA-induced DNA SSBs wre found to occur in M and early G_1 phases, whereas peak cytotoxicity was in the S phase. Topoisomerase II activity, as seen before, did not vary across the cell cycle in HeLa cells. Chicken lymphoblastoid MSB-1 cells also have augmented topoisomerase II levels before mitosis, with a peak in immunoreactive enzyme occurring in the $G_/M$ phase [154]. Topoisomerase II levels were found to decrease substantially after mitosis, during G_1, to levels that were lower than could be accounted for by distribution to two daughter cells. To account for this, the half-life of topoisomerase II was determined. The $t_{1/2}$ of topoisomerase II in chicken hepatoma cells is 12 hr, and during the M to G_1 transition is 1.8 hr. In primary chicken embryo fibroblasts, the $t_{1/2}$ of topoisomerase II is 3.3 hr, and 1.3 hr during the M to G_1 transition. These results suggest that topoisomerase II is lost during G_1 secondary to degradation, and that the increased $t_{1/2}$ of topoisomerase II in transformed cells (12 versus 3.3 hours) may explain why the enzyme is not decreased during the cell cycle. At odds with the above studies is one that found decreased DPCs in plateau L1210 nuclei treated with m-AMSA or VP-16 [155]. These investigators also found the increase in topoisomerase II activity, drug-induced cytotoxicity, and drug-induced DNA damage all to be maximal during S phase in NIH 3T3 fibroblasts released from quiescence [155]. In agreement with others, these investigators found diminished m-AMSA and VP-16-induced DNA damage in quiescent whole cells and nuclei of NIH 3T3 cells.

Maximum topoisomerase II activity and drug-stimulated DNA damage appear to occur shortly before or during mitosis; during the M to G_1 transition this enzyme is rapidly degraded. Peak cytotoxicity, however, has been observed to occur during S phase, and cells are relatively resistant during other phases of the cell cycle.

Isozymes of topoisomerase II (p170 and p180) have also been found to vary as a function of the proliferative state of the cell [76,156]. In P388 cells the content of p170 topoisomerase II is the same in log and plateau stages, while p180 has been found to increase as cells reach quiescent growth. Human monoblast U937 cells show a dramatic decrease in p170 and an increase in p180 in plateau stage. More detailed studies with normal and *ras*-transformed NIH 3T3 cells show an increase in both topoisomerase II activity and VM-26-induced SSBs in log phase transformed cells [156]. Northern and western blot analyses of log and plateau normal and transformed 3T3 cells for total topoisomerase II, p170, and p180 have demonstrated: 1) increased levels of total topoisomerase II in whole cells and 0.425 M NaCl nuclear extracts from log and quiescent *ras*-transformed cells relative to normal cells at the same proliferative stage; 2) a decrease in total topoisomerase II in plateau growth in both cell lines, which is mostly due to a decrease in the p170 form (decreased 40% in transformed and 70% in normal cells); and 3) an increase in p180 as a percent of total topoisomerase II in quiescent growth due to the decrease in p170. As log phase *ras*-transformed cells have more p170 isozyme, nuclear extracts from these cells were more susceptible to inhibition of topoisomerase II activity by VM-26 and merbarone, drugs that preferentially inhibit p170, than were extracts from normal cells. This preferential inhibition of p170 was reflected in the cytotoxicity data with these same drugs. Novobiocin inhibition of topoisomerase II activity and its cytotoxic effect on normal and transformed cells was equivalent; it demonstrated no isozyme preference. Thus, topoisomerase II isozymes may fluctuate in response to proliferation and, because of a differential inhibition of these isozymes by topoisomerase II inhibitors, may alter the sensitivity/resistance of a cell to these agents.

Resistance of human tissues to topoisomerase II inhibitors

Several human tissues, both malignant and benign, have been assayed for topoisomerase II activity or response to inhibitors of this enzyme. Four human lung carcinoma cell lines, including two small-cell lung cancers (SW900 and SW1271), an adenocarcinoma (A549), and a large-cell cancer (H157), have been studied for sensitivity to VP-16 [157]. These four human tumors show a gradation in response to both the cytotoxic effects of the epipodophyllotoxins and their DNA-damaging effects. SW1271 cells are the most sensitive by cytotoxicity assays and also have the greatest number of VP-16-stimulated SSBs and DSBs. SW900 are the most resistant and nuclei from these cells have the least number of VP-16-induced SSBs. The differences in resistance of these cells to topoisomerase II inhibitors likely result from differences in nuclear topoisomerase II activity, either quantitative or qualitative.

80

Freshly isolated human leukemic myeloblasts demonstrate a variable response to the cytotoxic effects of m-AMSA [158]. IC_{50}s for m-AMSA range from 0.25 to 5.0 μM and are comparable to that seen with peripheral blood lymphocytes (1 μM). Over this same concentration range of m-AMSA, DNA strand breaks are formed in both myeloblasts and peripheral blood lymphocytes (PBL). These investigators observed a tendency for those patients most sensitive to m-AMSA in vitro to be more likely to achieve a remission. Other investigators have found no topoisomerase II activity (relaxation of supercoiled DNA or catenation of DNA) in PBL [159]. We have also examined cell lines, freshly isolated patient leukemic cells, and PBL for topoisomerase II activity [160]. CCRF-CEM, HL-60, and RPMI 7666 cells have easily measured DNA strand breaks in response to treatment with VP-16, while the leukemic patients (6 CLL, 3 ALL, 3 AML, 1 CML, 1 hairy cell leukemia) had relatively few VP-16 induced strand breaks. The uptake of [³H]-VP-16 by both patient cells and established cell lines was variable but covered the same range. Topoisomerase II was easily detected in CCRF cells by immunoblotting with a polyclonal mouse anti-HeLa topoisomerase II antibody, but was undetectable in patient leukemic cells and PBL. Interestingly, normal human PBL stimulated with phytohemagglutinin and IL-2 demonstrate increased VP-16-induced DNA strand breaks and a topoisomerase II content that was detectable by immunoblotting. PBL from chickens also have undetectable topoisomerase II until they are stimulated with phytohemagglutinin and concanavalin A. Five to 30% of cells have topoisomerase II 72 hr after stimulation, and all of these cells are in S phase [150].

Several other hematologic malignancies have been examined for topoisomerase II activity and response to inhibitors of this enzyme [161, 162]. Forty-seven patients with untreated B-cell CLL and 17 normal PBL were studied. None of the 28 patients examined with CLL, nor 7 PBL, had detectable topoisomerase II levels by immunoblotting. These same patients demonstrated no doxorubicin-induced DNA damage at concentrations of doxorubicin that were 0.17–86.2 μM. Increased doses of m-AMSA and VP-16 did result in DNA cleavage in these same cells. Uptake of doxorubicin, m-AMSA, and VP-16 by CLL cells and PBL was in the same range as L1210 cells, whereas flow cytometry revealed a normal cell cycle distribution of L1210 cells but only a G_0/G_1 DNA content in CLL cells and PBL. Other patient cells, including prolymphocytic leukemia, Burkitt's lymphoma, diffuse histiocytic lymphoma, nodular mixed lymphoma, and nodular poorly differentiated lymphoma, had measurable topoisomerase II activity and immunoreactivity by Western blot analysis. In summary, human hematologic malignancies demonstrate a wide range in topoisomerase II activity and content, and because of this, a wide range of sensitivities to topoisomerase II inhibitors. CLL should probably not be treated with topoisomerase II inhibitors. As topoisomerase I was easily detected by both western blot analysis and assays of catalytic activity in all of the above cells (including

CLL cells), it is likely that a topoisomerase I inhibitor (camptothecin) would be more efficacious in treating these malignancies.

In addition to the quantitative alterations in topoisomerase II seen in the human tumors above, recent evidence suggests that human tissues may contain a drug-resistant topoisomerase II. A very sensitive topoisomerase II assay, which measures catenation of relaxed ^{3}H-labelled M13 RF DNA by filter binding, has been used to determine enzyme catalytic activity in normal and malignant human tissues [163]. Relatively high topoisomerase II activity was found in normal spleen and thymus gland, as well as in breast cancer, leiomyosarcoma, and aggressive lymphomas. The malignant tissues had an S fraction of 14–39% and the normal tissues had S fractions of 1–5%. Topoisomerase I activity was approximately the same in all benign and malignant tissues examined. An unexpected finding was that aggressive lymphoma, tonsil, placenta, and thymus nuclear extracts contain a topoisomerase II activity that is resistant to inhibition by VM-26. Significant decatenation activity was present in thymus nuclear extracts in the presence of 609 μM VM-26. Perhaps a VM-26-resistant topoisomerase II isozyme is present in these tissues.

Summary

The evidence presented above suggests that very few cell lines have only one mechanism of resistance when selected in the presence of DNA topoisomerase II inhibitors. Combinations of mechanisms are common and may involve perturbations that have nothing to do with topoisomerase II (e.g., overexpression of P-glycoprotein or increased GSH-S-transferase activity). Those mechanisms that involve topoisomerase II directly or indirectly include 1) alterations in the enzyme molecule itself that result in a change in catalytic or cleavage activity or, perhaps, a change in the ATPase activity of topoisomerase II; 2) the existence of isozymes that respond differently to antineoplastic agents and are present in different ratios in sensitive and resistant cells; 3) a quantitative change in nuclear topoisomerase II such that less drug target is available (secondary to gene inactivation or changes in the distribution of enzyme); 4) alterations in either topoisomerase II inhibitor transport (P-glycoprotein or otherwise) or intracellular distribution, such that less drug reaches the target enzyme; 5) altered processing of drug-induced topoisomerase II-mediated DNA strand breaks; and 6) the presence of activators and inhibitors of enzyme activity (the control of phosphorylation most likely involved in drug resistance). Studies have demonstrated the importance of proliferative stage and cell-cycle phase in determining the resistance to topoisomerase II inhibitors. Both proliferation-dependent resistance and the intrinsic resistance of the few fresh tumor cells examined are primarily the result of a decrease in cellular content of topoisomerase II.

Overcoming resistance in vivo to topoisomerase II inhibitors is dependent upon, first, accurately defining (both quantitatively and qualitatively) the mechanisms that exist in human malignancies. A single determination of topoisomerase II activity is unlikely to be helpful. Meaningful information will be obtained when tumors in vivo are followed over time (before treatment and at relapse) for topoisomerase II activity, ratios of isozymes, and mutations. The availability of molecular probes that recognize mutations in the topoisomerase II gene will facilitate the latter. Treatment options for overcoming resistance to topoisomerase II inhibitors will likely include new and more specific enzyme inhibitors, techniques to augment the amount (or activity) of target enzyme in vivo, and perhaps, concurrent treatment will both topoisomerase I and II inhibitors.

Resistance to inhibitors of DNA topoisomerase I

Introduction

The enzyme topoisomerase I catalyzes the isomerization of topologically restrained DNA by breaking and rejoining a single strand of DNA. Its mechanism of action has been well characterized and is reviewed elsewhere [164]. Briefly, the enzyme becomes covalently bound to the 3′ terminus of the break site. It is independent of ATP and functions in DNA replication and transcription. It likely provides the principal swivelling mechanism required for advancement of the replication fork during DNA synthesis [29,164]. Topoisomerase I deletion mutants are viable in yeast [165]. Apparently, the functions of the enzyme can be subserved by DNA topoisomerase II, although there is no evidence to support the converse. In contrast to DNA topoisomerase II, intracellular content of topoisomerase I does not vary with the state of cellular proliferation. Quiescent cells appear to contain the same amount of enzyme as proliferating ones. Increased topoisomerase I content has been observed in ex vivo samples and xenografts of human colon carcinoma when compared to normal colonic epithelium [166].

Early work on activity and mechanism

The plant alkaloid camptothecin was studied as a potential anticancer agent approximately 15 years before it was recognized that its mechanism of action was the inhibition of DNA topoisomerase I [167]. It is derived from the heartwood of the *Camptotheca acuminata* tree, which is native to northern China. Camptothecin demonstrated significant activity in L1210 leukemia and rat walker 256 carcinoma [168]. A Phase I trial in nine patients with large bowel cancer reported objective responses in eight patients [169]. Subsequent studies failed to confirm this early promise and toxicities of the compound, including myelosuppression, diarrhea, stomatitis, and hemorrhagic cystitis were not considered predictable [170–172]. Whether the toxicities were related to the principle mechanism of action of the drug or to problems in formulation has not been resolved.

Early studies on camptothecin's mechanism of action revealed that it inhibits RNA and DNA synthesis reversibly [173,174] and that its cytotoxicity is highly S-phase specific [175,176]. Not surprisingly, therefore, the drug is lethal only to those cells that are actively cycling. The molecular basis for camptothecin's antitumor activity was enigmatic, however. The best hints were the studies that demonstrated that although the drug does not directly inhibit DNA or RNA polymerases [177], it does induce significant DNA strand breakage in treated cells [178]. An excellent structure-activity relationship exists between camptothecin and its analogs with respect to inhibition of nucleic acid synthesis, DNA strand breakage, and in vivo tumor activity [178].

Identification of the intracellular target

The renaissance of camptothecin began in 1985 with the report that this drug, in a fashion similar to that of topoisomerase II inhibitors, induces site-specific cleavage of DNA in the presence of purified mammalian topoisomerase I [179]. As would be predicted by the mechanism of the enzyme, and in contrast to that of topoisomerase II, the enzyme is found linked to the 3' end of the broken DNA strands. In addition to inducing a form of cleavable complex via topoisomerase I, camptothecin also was found to inhibit the catalytic activity of the enzyme. No evidence of inhibition of catalytic activity or induction of cleavable complexes by mammalian topoisomerase II by camptothecin was observed. Studies of DNA damage in cells exposed to camptothecin following this initial report have confirmed that the DNA strand breakage is stoichiometrically a protein-DNA crosslink [180,181]. Immunoblot analysis confirmed that the protein is most likely DNA topoisomerase I [182]. Somewhat unexpectedly, it has been shown that the protein associated DNA breaks can form and reverse within minutes at 4°C [181]. Recent structure-activity relationship studies using camptothecin analogs have confirmed the original observations above and demonstrated that inhibition of topoisomerase I correlates well with the ability to induce strand breaks in vivo and to inflict cytotoxicity [183,184]. The mechanism by which camptothecin inhibits topoisomerase I appears to involve inhibition of the rejoining step of the enzyme [185].

Some of the basis for camptothecin's renaissance is attributable to the suspicion that many of the original problems encountered by the drug in clinical trials related to its poor water solubility. A host of new more soluble derivatives have been reported in recent years, and some of these exhibit striking antitumor activity in animal models. CPT-11, (7-ethyl-10-[4-(1-piperidino)-1-piperidino]carbonyloxycamptothecin) is a water-soluble camptothecin analog synthesized by Japanese investigators [186]. The compound exhibits excellent antitumor activity in a broad spectrum of experimental tumor models by intraperitoneal, intravenous, or oral administration. Cures of several solid tumors were observed. The drug also inhibited spontaneous and experimental metastasis in mice [187]. Of particular interest, CPT-11 was shown to be effective against P388 leukemia cells that exhibit the multidrug-resistant (MDR) phenotype [188]. A recent report demonstrated that 20-(RS)-9-amino-camptothecin has excellent activity against xenografts of colon cancer and immunodeficient mice [166]. Indeed in this model, the drug was found to induce prolonged disease-free remissions, an unusual degree of activity for any drug in this system. Drug toxicity was mild and allowed for repeated treatment. Finally, another water-soluble camptothecin derivative, currently designated SK&F 104,864, shares the property of being active against a wide variety of animal solid tumor models [189]. Its activity is also undiminished by the MDR phenotype.

Several groups have developed yeast mutants that have contributed handsomely to understanding the action of camptothecin and to the screening process for new more active derivatives. *Saccharomyces cerevisiae* mutants, selected for permeability to camptothecin, exhibited growth inhibition in the presence of drug [190]. Capitalizing on a previous observation that topoisomerase I was not essential for growth or survival of yeast [165], these investigators constructed a mutant in which the TOP 1 gene responsible for encoding DNA topoisomerase I was deleted. As a consequence to this deletion, they yeast cells became highly resistant to the cytotoxicity of camptothecin. Similar studies reported at the same time [191] observed that an *S. cervisiae* DNA repair mutant, RAD52, is hypersensitive to the cytotoxicity of camptothecin. When they prepared topoisomerase I deletion mutants from these yeasts, resistance to camptothecin was observed. In addition, a mutant bearing a temperature-sensitive topoisomerase I exhibited corresponding temperature sensitivity to the lethal effect of camptothecin. Interestingly, another strain, this one overproducing topoisomerase I, exhibited hypersensitivity to camptothecin. Camptothecin sensitivity has been reconstituted in a yeast TOP1 deletion mutant by expressing human DNA topoisomerase I in the yeast via a plasmid-borne human complementary DNA clone [192]. In this case, the human gene was under the control of a galactose-inducible, glucose-repressible promoter. Camptothecin cytotoxicity, as one might predict, was observed in the presence of galactose, but not glucose.

The observation that camptothecin could cause cell death by inhibition of an enzyme that was apparently not essential for cell growth created a seeming paradox. Hints of the resolution of this paradox were apparent in the results of yeast studies that indicated that the cleavable complex formed by topoisomerase I and DNA in the presence of camptothecin may be recognized as DNA damage by the cell. As noted, cytotoxicity of camptothecin in yeast is exaggerated in strains that contain a RAD52 DNA repair mutant

[190,191]. Furthermore, exposure of sensitive yeast to camptothecin induces the expression of a DNA damage inducible gene DIN3 and high levels of homologous DNA recombination [192]. Recent studies have provided important additional evidence bearing on the mechanism of camptothecin cytotoxicity [193]. As predicted from the phase specificity of the drug, they observed that cotreatment of leukemia cells with aphidicolin, an inhibitor of DNA polymerase, completely abolished camptothecin cytotoxicity. This group then employed a cell-free SV40 DNA replication system to further elucidate the relationship between the effects of camptothecin and DNA replication. They found that camptothecin inhibited replication only in the presence of topoisomerase I. Further, in the enviroment of excess topoisomerase I, not only was replication inhibited, but there was also accumulation of linearized replication products containing covalently bound DNA topoisomerase I. They hypothesized that the camptothecin-induced cleavable complexes collided with moving replication forks, causing fork arrest and/or breakage. Camptothecin-induced DNA breakage at the replication fork of SV40 has also been observed by electron microscopy [194]. Summarizing the available evidence regarding the molecular mechanisms of camptothecin's antitumor effect, it is likely that the drug induces cleavable complexes in the vicinity of moving DNA replication forks during the DNA synthetic phase of the cell cycle. Anomalous interaction, perhaps even a physical encounter, between the replication fork and the cleavable complex disrupts the replication machinery in such a way that the normally reversible cleavable complex induced by camptothecin is rendered irreversible, and thereupon recognized by the cell as a form of DNA damage. Events following this recognition remain unclear.

Camptothecin-resistant cell lines

Only a few studies of cell lines resistant to camptothecin or its analogs have been reported. A human T-cell derived acute lymphoblastic leukemia line, RPMI 8402, resistant to CPT-11 has been isolated [195]. Details of cell line isolation were not provided, and the degree of resistance to CPT-11 could not be quantified using the data provided. The basis for resistance of this cell line has been reported in detail. Intracellular content of immunoreactive topoisomerase I in resistant cells was less than half of that in WT cells. Enzyme catalytic activity was similarly reduced, indicating that specific activities of the two enzymes were similar. When topoisomerase I from WT and CPT-resistant cells were purified to homogeneity, they were found to have identical molecular weights. Striking differences in the two enzymes, however, were noted in their response to camptothecin and water-soluble analogs. Topoisomerase I from the drug-resistant cell line did not exhibit inhibition of catalytic function nor induction of cleavable complex formation in the presence of camptothecin or its analogs, whereas the WT enzyme was highly sensitive to both, as expected. The degree of resistance at the enzymatic level was greater than 125-fold, but again could not be precisely quantitated. Although the specific activity of the resistant enzyme, with respect of catalytic function, was similar to WT enzyme, potentially important differences were observed in DNA cleavage [196]. The resistant enzyme demonstrated a greater capacity for DNA cleavage in the absence of drug than did WT, suggesting that the cleavable complex formed by this enzyme was more stable. This was further supported by the observation that enzyme-DNA complexes formed by the resistant enzyme were less salt-reversible than were those formed by the WT.

A Chinese hamster ovaery (CHO) cell line has been isolated and characterized [197] that exhibits 250- to 350-fold resistance to camptothecin. It was isolated in a single step by cloning in the presence of drug. The cells exhibit no cross-resistance towards colchicine, vinblastine, taxol, or puromycin, but are slightly hypersensitive to topoisomerase II inhibitors. Somatic cell hybrids formed by sensitive and resistance cell lines were found to be sensitive to camptothecin. The dominance of sensitivity in this model is comparable to that observed with some cell lines resistant to topoisomerase II inhibitors [59] and is consistant with a mechanism of action in which a sensitive enzyme is required to inflict DNA damage in the presence of drug. The basis of resistance of this cell line was examined at the biochemical and molecular level. Camptothecin-induced DNA breakage was undectable in the resistant cell line, but readily observed in WT cells. Enzyme activity, as well as immunoreactive protein content of topoisomerase I, was reduced approximately 50% in the resistant cells as compared to WT cells when nuclear extracts were examined. Enzyme purified to homogeneity from the two cell lines exhibited qualitative differences, despite having similar molecular weights. Elution of the enzyme from resistant cells on a phenyl sepharose column occurred at a higher ammonium sulfate concentration, suggesting that it may be less hydrophobic than WT enzyme. In addition, both inhibition of catalytic activity and induction of cleavable complex formation by camptothecin was at least 10-fold greater in WT enzymes than that from resistant cells.

The CHO cell line just described [197] exhibits some similarities to the RPMI 8402 cell line previously described [195]. In both cases there was a quantitative reduction in intracellular enzyme content as well as a qualitative alteration in the enzyme. A recent report [88] suggests a mechanism by which at least the quantitative differences might have occurred. Camptothecin-resistant P-388 leukemia cells were derived in mice by repeated exposure to sublethal doses of drug administered by the intraperitoneal route. Compared with WT P-388 cells, the camptothecin-resistant cells demonstrated approximately one-third the topoisomerase I activity and a similar reduction in immunoreactive protein. The basis for these reductions was revealed at the genetic level. Topoisomerase I mRNA in the resistant cell line was reduced compared to that of the WT cells to an extent comparable to that of immunoreactive protein. Examination of the topoisomerase I gene using restriction digests and a human topoisomerase I cDNA probe revealed rearrangement in one allele. In addition, the remaining allele was found to be hypermethylated in the resistant cell line when compared to the alleles of the WT cells. This data suggest that the reduction in transcription was a function of both rearrangement of a single allele and reduced transcription in the remaining allele secondary to hypermethylation.

Summary

Studies examining the mechanisms of resistance to camptothecin and its water-soluble analogs have been reported only recently. None of these studies have involved resistance derived in vivo in humans. Some of the mechanisms already describe could be predicted from the mechanism of action of the drug and from prior studies in yeast. It is interesting that, to date, the only mechanisms of resistance relate directly to the target of the drug, DNA topoisomerase I, and that the drugs are active in cell lines exhibiting the multidrug-resistant phenotype. Should camptothecin analogs prove as active in human clinical trials as animal tests predict, it will be interesting to see if additional mechanisms of resistance emerge from studies in treated patients. On the other hand, if clinical activity is similar to that demonstrated by camptothecin 15 years ago, the issue will be of academic interest only.

References

1. Liu, L.F. DNA topoisomerase-enzymes that catalyse the breaking and rejoining of DNA. CRC Crit. Rev. Biochem. 15:1–24, 1983.
2. Wang, J.C. DNA topoisomerases. Annu. Rev. Biochem. 54:665–697, 1985.
3. Vosberg, H.-P. DNA topoisomerases: enzymes that control DNA conformation. Curr. Topics Microbiol. Immunol. 114:19–102, 1985.
4. Maxwell, A. and Gellert, M. Mechanistic aspects of DNA topoisomerases. Adv. Prot. Chem. 38:69–107, 1986.
5. Wang, J.C. Recent studies of DNA topoisomerases. Biochim. Biophys. Acta. 909:1–9, 1987.
6. Osheroff, N. Biochemical basis for the interactions of type I and type II topoisomerases with DNA. Pharmacol. Ther. 41:223–241, 1989.
7. Miller, K.G., Liu, L.F., and Englund, P.T. A homogeneous type II DNA topoisomerase from HeLa cell nuclei. J. Biol. Chem. 256:9334–9339, 1981.
8. Goto, J. and Wang, J.C. Yeast DNA topoisomerase II. An ATP-dependent type II topoisomerase that catalyzes the catenation, decatenation, unknotting, and relaxation of double-strand DNA rings. J. Biol. Chem. 257:5866–5872, 1982.
9. Shelton, E.R. Osheroff, N., and Brutlag, D.L. DNA topoisomerase II from *Drosophila melanogaster*. Purification and physical characterization. J. Biol. Chem. 258:9530–9535, 1983.

10. Halligan, B.D., Edwards, K.A., and Liu, L.F. Purification and characterization of a type II DNA topoisomerase from bovine calf thymus. J. Biol. Chem. 260:2475–2482, 1985.

11. Schomburg, W. and Grosse, F. Purification and characterization of DNA topoisomerase II from calf thymus associated with polypeptides of 175 and 150 kDa. Eur. J. Biochem. 160:451–457, 1986.

12. Strausfeld, U. and Richter, A. Simultaneous purification of DNA topoisomerase I and II from eukaryotic cells. Prep. Biochem. 19:37–48, 1989.

13. Douc-Rasy, S., Kayser, A., Riou, J., and Riou, G. ATP-independent type II topoisomerase from typanosomes. Proc. Natl. Acad. Sci. USA. 83:7152–7156, 1986.

14. Drake, F.H., Zimmerman, J.P., McCabe, F.L., Bartus, H.F., Per, S.R., Sullivan, D.M., Ross, W.E., Mattern, M.R., Johnson, R.K., Crooke, S.T., and Mirabelli, C.K. Purification of topoisomerase II from amsacrine-resistant P388 leukemia cells. Evidence for two forms of the enzyme. J. Biol. Chem. 262:16739–16747, 1987.

15. Melendy, T. and Ray, D.S. Novobiocin affinity purification of a mitochondrial type II topoisomerase from the trypanosomatid Crithidia fasciculata. J. Biol. Chem. 264: 1870–1876, 1989.

16. Sullivan, D.M., Rowe, T.C., Latham, M.D., and Ross, W.E. Purification and characterization of an altered topoisomerase II from a drug-resistant Chinese hamster ovary cell line. Biochemistry, 28:5680–5687, 1989.

17. Giaever, G., Lynn, R., Goto, T., and Wang, J.C. The complete nucleotide sequence of the structural gene TOP2 of yeast DNA topoisomerase II. J. Biol. Chem. 261: 12448–12454, 1986.

18. Uemura, T., Morikawa, K., and Yanagida, M. The nucleotide sequence of the fission yeast DNA topoisomerase II gene: structural and functional relationships to other DNA topoisomerases. EMBO J. 5:2355–2361, 1986.

19. Wyckoff, E., Natalie, D., Nolan, J.M., Lee, M., and Hsieh, T. Structure of the Drosophila DNA topoisomerase II gene. Nucleotide sequence and homology among topoisomerases II. J. Mol. Biol. 205:1–13, 1989.

20. Tsai-Pflugfelder, M., Liu, L.F., Liu, A.A., Tewey, K.M., Whang-Peng, J., Knutsen, T., Huebner, K., Croce, C.M., and Wang, J.C. Cloning and sequencing of cDNA encoding human DNA topoisomerase II and localization of the gene to chromosome region 17q21–22. Proc. Natl. Acad. Sci. USA 85:7177–7181, 1988.

21. Chung, T.D., Drake, F.H., Tan, K.B., R., P.S., Crooke, S.T., and Mirabelli, C.K. Characterization and immunological identification of cDNA clones encoding two human DNA topoisomerase II isozymes. Proc. Natl. Acad. Sci. USA 86:9431–9435, 1989.

22. Liu, L.F., Rowe, T.C., Yang, L., Tewey, K.M., and Chen, G.L. Cleavage of DNA by mammalian DNA topoisomerase II. J. Biol. Chem. 258:15365–15370, 1983.

23. Osheroff, N. Eukaryotic topoisomerase II. Characterization of enzyme turnover. J. Biol. Chem. 261:9944–9950, 1986.

24. Osheroff, N. Role of the divalent cation in topoisomerase II mediated reactions. Biochemistry 26:6402–6406, 1987.

25. Zechiedrich, E.L., Christiansen, K., Andersen, A.H., Westergaard, O., and Osheroff, N. Double-stranded DNA cleavage/religation reaction of eukaryotic topoisomerase II: evidence for a nicked DNA intermediate. Biochemistry 28:6229–6236, 1989.

26. Andersen, A.H., Christiansen, K., Zechiedrich, E.L., Jensen, P.S., Osheroff, N., and Westergaard, O. Strand specificity of the topoisomerase II mediated double-stranded DNA cleavage reaction. Biochemistry 28:6237–6244, 1989.

27. Sundin, O. and Varshavsky, A. Arrest of segregation leads to accumulation of highly intertwined catenated dimers: dissection of the final stages of SV40 DNA replication. Cell 25:659–669, 1981.

28. Nelson, W.G., Liu, L.F., and Coffey, D.S. Newly replicated DNA is associated with DNA topoisomerase II in cultured rat prostatic adenocarcinoma cells. Nature 322: 187–189, 1986.

29. Brill, S.J., DiNardo, S.K., V.-M., and Sternglanz, R. Need for DNA topoisomerase activity as a swivel for DNA replication for transcription of ribosomal RNA. Nature 326:414–416, 1987.

30. DiNardo, S., Voelkel, K., and Sternglanz, R. DNA topoisomerase II mutant of *Saccharomyces cerevisiae*: topoisomerase II is required for segregation of daughter molecules at the termination of DNA replication. Proc. Natl. Acad. Sci. USA 81: 2616–2620, 1984.

31. Holm, C., Goto, T., Wang, J.C., and Botstein, D. DNA topoisomerase II is required at the time of mitosis in yeast. Cell. 41:553–563, 1985.

32. Uemura, T., Ohkura, H., Adachi, Y., Morino K., Shiozaki, K., and Yanagida, M. DNA topoisomerase II is required for condensation and separation of mitotic chromosomes in *S.pombe*. Cell 50:917–925, 1987.

33. Rose, D., Thomas, W., and Holm, C. Segregation of recombined chromosomes in meiosis I requires DNA topoisomerase II. Cell 60:1009–1017, 1990.

34. Berrios, M., Osheroff, N., and Fisher, P.A. *In situ* localization of DNA topoisomerase II, a major polypeptide component of the *Drosophila* nuclear matrix fraction. Proc. Natl. Acad. Sci. USA 82:4142–4146, 1985.

35. Earnshaw, W.C., Halligan, B., Cooke, C.A., Heck, M.M., and Liu, L.F. Topoisomerase II is a structural component of mitotic chromosome scaffolds. J. Cell Biol. 100:1706–1715, 1985.

36. Schroder, H.C., Trolltsch, D., Friese, U., Bachmann, M., and Muller, W.E. Mature mRNA is selectively released from the nuclear matrix by an ATP/dATP-dependent mechanism sensitive to topoisomerase inhibitors. J. Biol. Chem. 262:8917–8925, 1987.

37. Tsutsui, K., Tsutsui, K., and Muller, M.T. The nuclear scaffold exhibits DNA-binding sites selective for supercoiled DNA. J. Biol. Chem. 263:7235–7241, 1988.

38. Adachi, Y., Kas, E., and Laemmli, U.K. Preferential, cooperative binding of DNA topoisomerase II to scaffold-associated regions. EMBO J. 8:3997–4006, 1989.

39. To, R.Q. and Kmiec, E.R. Assembly of transcriptionally active chromatin *in vitro*: a possible role for topoisomerase II. Cell Growth Different. 1:39–45, 1990.

40. Ross, W.E., Glaubiger, D.L., and Kohn, K.W. Protein-associated DNA breaks in cells treated with adriamycin or ellipticine. Biochim. Biophys. Acta 519:23–30, 1978.

41. Ross, W.E., Glaubiger, D., and Kohn, K.W. Qualitative and quantitative aspects of intercalator-induced DNA strand breaks. Biochim. Biophys. Acta 562:41–50, 1979.

42. Ross, W.E. and Bradley, M.O. DNA double-strand breaks in mammalian cells after exposure to intercalating agents. Biochim. Biophys. Acta 654:129–134, 1981.

43. Zwelling, L.A., Michaels, S., Erickson, L.C., Ungerleider, R.S., Nichols, M., and Kohn, K.W. Protein-associated deoxyribonucleis acid strand breaks in L1210 cells treated with the deoxyribonucleic acid intercalating agents 4'-(9-acridinylamino) methanesulfon-m-anisidide and adriamycin. Biochemistry 20:6553–6563, 1981.

44. Wozniak, A.J. and Ross, W.E. DNA damage as a basis for 4'-demethylepipodophyllotoxin-9-(4,6-O-ethylidene-beta-D-glucopyranoside) (etoposide) cytotoxicity. Cancer Res. 43:120–124, 1983.

45. Ross, W., Rowe, T., Glisson, B., Yalowich, J., and Liu, L. Role of topoisomerase II in mediating epipodophyllotoxin-induced DNA cleavage. Cancer Res. 44:5857–5860, 1984.

46. Pommier, Y., Mattern, M.R., Schwartz, R.E., Zwelling, L.A., and Kohn, K.W. Changes in deoxyribonucleic acid linking number due to treatment of mammalian cells with the intercalating agent 4'-(9-acridinylamino) methanesulfon-m-anisidide. Biochemistry 23: 2927–2932, 1984.

47. Tewey, K.M., Chen, G.L., Nelson, E.M., and Liu, L.F. Intercalative antitumor drugs interfere with the breakage-reunion reaction of mammalian DNA topoisomerase II. J. Biol. Chem. 259:9182–9187, 1984.

48. Chen, G.L., Yang, L., Rowe, T.C., Halligan, B.D., Tewey, K.M., and Liu, L.F. Nonintercalative antitumor drugs interfere with the breakage-reunion reaction of mammalian DNA topoisomerase II. J. Biol. Chem. 259:13560–13566, 1984.

90

49. Tewey, K.M., Rowe, T.C., Yang, L., Halligan, B.D., and Liu, L.F. Adriamycin-induced DNA damage mediated by mammalian DNA topoisomerase II. Science 226:466–468, 1984.

50. Nelson, E.M., Tewey, K.M., and Liu, L.F. Mechanism of antitumor drug action: poisoning of mammalian DNA topoisomerase II on DNA by 4'-(9-acridinylamino) methanesulfon-m-anisidide. Proc. Natl. Acad. Sci. USA 81:1361–1365, 1984.

51. Pommier, Y., Minford, J.K., Schwartz, R.E., Zwelling, L.A., and Kohn, K.W. Effects of the DNA intercalators 4'-(9-acridinylamino) methanesulfon-m-anisidide and 2-methyl-9-hydroxyellipticinium on topoisomerase II mediated DNA strand cleavage and strand passage. Biochemistry 24:6410–6416, 1985.

52. Osheroff, N. Effect of antineoplastic agents on the DNA cleavage/religation reaction of eukaryotic topoisomerase II: inhibition of DNA religation by etoposide. Biochemistry 28:6157–6160, 1989.

53. Holm, C., Covey, J.M., Kerrigan, D., and Pommier, Y. Differential requirement of DNA replication for the cytotoxicity of DNA topoisomerase I and II inhibitors in Chinese hamster DC3F cells. Cancer Res. 49:6365–6368, 1989.

54. Robinson, M.J. and Osheroff, N Stabilization of the topoisomerase II-DNA cleavage complex by antineoplastic drugs: inhibition of enzyme-mediated DNA religation by 4'-(9-acridinylamino) methanesulfon-m-anisidide. Biochemistry 29:2511–2515, 1990.

55. Batist, G., Tulpule, A., Sinha, B.K., Katki, A.G., Myers, C.E., and Cowan, K.H. Overexpression of a novel anionic glutathione transferase in multidrug-resistant human breast cancer cells. J. Biol. Chem. 261:15544–15549, 1986.

56. Sinha, B.K., Haim, N., Dusre, L., Kerrigan, D., and Pommier, Y. DNA strand breaks produced by etoposide (VP-16, 213) in sensitive and resistant human breast tumor cells: implications for the mechanism of action. Cancer Res. 48:5096–5100, 1988.

57. Politi, P.M. and Sinha, B.K. Role of differential drug, efflux, and binding of etoposide in sensitive and resistant human tumor cell lines: implications for the mechanisms of drug resistance. Mol. Pharmacol. 35:271–278, 1989.

58. Mimnaugh, E.G., Dusre, L., Atwell, J., and Myers, C. Differential oxygen radical susceptibility of adriamycin-sensitive and -resistant MCF-7 human breast tumor cells. Cancer Res. 49:8–15, 1989.

59. Gupta, R.S. Genetic, biochemical, and cross-resistance studies with mutants of Chinese hamster ovary cells resistant to the anticancer drugs, VM-26 and VP16-213. Cancer Res. 43:1568–1574, 1983.

60. Glisson, B., Gupta, R., Hodges, P., and Ross, W. Cross-resistance to intercalating agents in an epipodophyllotoxin-resistant Chinese hamster ovary cell line: evidence for a common intracellular target. Cancer Res. 46:1939–1942, 1986.

61. Glisson, B.R., Gupta, S.S., S.-K., and Ross, W. Characterization of acquired epipodophyllotoxin resistance in a Chinese hamster ovary cell line: loss of drug-stimulated DNA cleavage activity. Cancer Res. 46:1934–1938, 1986.

62. Beran, M. and Andersson, B.S. Development and characterization of a human myelogenous leukemia cell line resistant to 4'-(9' acridinylamino)-3-methanesulfon-m-anisidide. Cancer Res. 47:1897–1904, 1987.

63. Bakic, M., Beran, M., Andersson, B.S., Silberman, L., Estey, E., and Zwelling, L.A. The production of topoisomerase II-mediated DNA cleavage in human leukemia cells predicts their susceptibility to 4'-(9-acridinylamino) methanesulfon-m-anisidide (m-AMSA). Biochem. Biophys. Res. Commun. 134:638–645, 1986.

64. Bakic, M., Chan, D., Andersson, B.S., Beran, M., Silberman, L., Estey, E., Ricketts, L., and Zwelling, L.A. Effect of 1-B-D-arabinofuranosylcytosine (ara-C) on nuclear topoisomerase II activity and on the DNA cleavage and cytotoxicity produced by 4'-(9-acridinylamino)-methanesulfon-m-aniside (m-AMSA) and etoposide in m-AMSA-sensitive and -resistant human leukemia cells. Biochem. Pharmacol. 36:4067–4078, 1987.

65. Estey, E.H., Silberman, L., Beran, M., Andersson, B.S., and Zwelling, L.A. The interaction between nuclear topoisomerase II activity from human leukemia cells,

exogenous DNA, and 4'-(9-acridinylamino) methanesulfon-*m*-anisidide (m-AMSA) or 4-(4,6-O-ethylidene-B-D-glucopyranoside) (VP-16) indicates the sensitivity of the cells to the drugs. Biochem. Biophys. Res. Commun. 144:787–793, 1987.

66. Zwelling, L.A., Hinds, M., Chan, D., Mayes, J., Sie, K.L., Parker, E., Silberman, L., Radcliffe, A., Beran, M., and Blick, M. Characterization of an amsacrine-resistant line of human leukemia cells. J. Biol. Chem. 264:16411–16420, 1989.

67. Yoshida, H.T., Kojima, T., Yamagishi, J, and Nakamura, S. Quinolone-resistant mutations of the *gyrA* gene of *Escherichia coli*. Mol. Gen. Genet. 211:1–7, 1988.

68. Danks, M.K., Yalowich, J.C., and Beck, W.T. Atypical multiple drug resistance in a human leukemic cell line selected for resistance to teniposide (VM-26). Cancer Res. 47:1297–1301, 1987.

69. Danks, M.K., Schmidt, C.A., Cirtain M.C., Suttle, D.P., and Beck, W.T. Altered catalytic activity of and DNA cleavage by DNA topoisomerase II from human leukemic cells selected from resistance to VM-26. Biochemistry 27:8861–8869, 1988.

70. Beck, W.T., Cirtain, M.C., Danks, M.K., Felsted Safa, A.R., Wolverton, J.S., Suttle, D.P., and Trent, J.M. Pharmacological, molecular, and cytogenetic analysis of "atypical" multidrug-resistant human leukemic cells. Cancer Res. 47:5455–5460, 1987.

71. Wolverton, J.S., Danks, M.K., Schmidt, C.A., and Beck, W.T. Genetic characterization of the multidrug-resistant phenotype of VM-26-resistant human leukemic cells. Cancer Res. 49:2422–2426, 1989.

72. Danks, M.K., Schmidt, C.A., Deneka, D.A., and Beck, W.T. Altered interaction of ATP with DNA topoisomerase II from VM-26-resistant CEM cells. Proc. Am. Assoc. Cancer Res. 30:524, 1989.

73. Danks, M.K., Schmidt, C.A., Deneka, D.A., and Beck, W.T. Increased ATP requirement for activity of and complex formation by DNA topoisomerase II from human leukemic CCRF-CEM cells selected for resistance to teniposide. Cancer Commun. 1: 101–109, 1989.

74. Fernandes, D.J., Danks, M.K., and Beck, W.T. Decreased nuclear matrix DNA topoisomerase II (topo II) in VM-26 resistant human leukemia cells. Proc. Am. Assoc. Cancer Res. 30:502, 1989.

75. Per, S.R., Mattern, M.R., Mirabelli, C.K. Drake, F.H., Johnson, R.K., and Crooke, S.T. Characterization of a subline of P388 leukemia resistant to amsacrine: evidence of altered topoisomerase II function. Mol. Pharmacol. 32:17–25, 1987.

76. Drake, F.H., Hofmann, G.A., Bartus, H.F., Mattern, M.R., Crooke, S.T., and Mirabelli, C.K. Biochemical and pharmacological properties of p170 and p180 forms of topoisomerase II. Biochemistry 28:8154–8160, 1989.

77. Tan, K.B., Mattern, M.R., Boyce, R.A., and Schein, P.S. Elevated DNA topoisomerase II activity in nitrogen mustard-resistant human cells. Proc. Natl. Acad. Sci. USA 84: 7668–7671, 1987.

78. Tan, K.B., Mattern M.R., Boyce, R.A., and Schein, P.S. Unique sensitivity of nitrogen mustard-resistant human Burkitt lymphoma cells to novobiocin. Biochem. Pharmacol. 37:4411–4413, 1988.

79. Tan, K.B., Per, S.R., Boyce, R.A., Mirabelli, C.K., and Crooke, S.T. Altered expression and transcription of the topoisomerase II gene in nitrogen mustard-resistant human cells. Biochem. Pharmacol. 37:4413–4416, 1988.

80. Ferguson, P.J., Fisher, M.H., Stephenson, J., Li, D., Zhou, B., and Cheng, Y. Combined modalities of resistance in etoposide-resistant human KB cell lines. Cancer Res. 48:5956–5964, 1988.

81. Liu, S.Y., Hwang, B.D., Haruna, M., Imakura, Y., Lee, K.H., and Cheng, Y.C. Podophyllotoxin analogs: effects on DNA topoisomerase II, tubulin polymerization, human tumor KB cells, and their VP-16 resistant variants. Mol. Pharmacol. 36:78–82, 1989.

82. Johnson, R.K., Ovejera, A.A., and Goldin, A. Activity of anthracyclines against an adriamycin (NSC-123127)-resistant subline of P388 leukemia with special emphasis on

cinerubin A (NSC-18334). Cancer Treat. Rep. 60:99–102, 1976.

83. Goldenberg, G.J., Wang, H., and Blair, G.W. Resistance to adriamycin: relationship of cytotoxicity to drug uptake and DNA single- and double-strand breakage in cloned cell lines of adriamycin-sensitive and -resistant P388 leukemia. Cancer Res. 46:2978–2983, 1986.

84. Deffie, A.M., Alam, T., Seneviratne, C., Beenken, S.W., Batra, J.K., Shea, T.C., Henner, W.D., and Goldenberg, G.J. Multifactorial resistance to adriamycin: relationship of DNA repair, glutathione transferase activity, drug efflux, and P-glycoprotein in cloned cell lines of adriamycin-sensitive and resistant P388 leukemia. Cancer Res. 48:3595–3602, 1988.

85. Seneviratne, C. and Goldenberg, G.J. Further characterization of drug-sensitivity and cross-resistance profiles of cloned cell lines of adriamycin-sensitive and -resistant P388 leukemia. Cancer Commun. 1:21–27, 1989.

86. Deffie, A.M., Batra, J.K., and Goldenberg. G.J. Direct correlation between DNA topoisomerase II activity and cytotoxicity in adriamycin-sensitive and -resistant P388 leukemia cell lines. Cancer Res. 49:58–62, 1989.

87. Deffie, A.M., Bosman, D.J., and Goldenberg, G.J. Evidence for a mutant allele of the gene for DNA topoisomerase II in adriamycin-resistant P388 murine leukemia cells. Cancer Res. 49:6879–6882, 1989.

88. Tan, K.B., Mattern, M.R., Eng, W., McCabe, F.L., and Johnson, R.K. Nonproductive rearrangement of DNA topoisomerase I and II genes: correlation with resistance to topoisomerase inhibitors. J. Natl. Cancer Inst. 81:1732–1735, 1989.

89. Salles, B., Charcosset, J.Y., and Jacquemin-Sablon, A. Isolation and properties of Chinese hamster lung cells resistant to ellipticine derivatives. Cancer Treat. Rep. 66: 327–338, 1982.

90. Charcosset, J.Y., Bendirdjian, J.P., Lantieri M.F., and Jacquemin-Sablon, A. Effects of 9-OH-ellipticine on cell survival, macromolecular syntheses, and cell cycle progression in sensitive and resistant Chinese hamster lung cells. Cancer Res. 45:4229–4236, 1985.

91. Pommier, Y., Schwartz, R.E., Zwelling, L.A., Kerrigan, D., Mattern, M.R., Charcosset, J.Y., Jacquemin-Sablon, A., and Kohn, K.W. Reduced formation of protein-associated DNA strand breaks in Chinese hamster cells resistance to topoisomerase II inhibitors. Cancer Res. 46:611–616, 1986.

92. Pommier, Y., Kerrigan, D., Schwartz, R.E., Swack, J.A., and McCurdy, A. Altered DNA topoisomerase II activity in Chinese hamster cells resistant to topoisomerase II inhibitors. Cancer Res. 46:3075–3081, 1986.

93. Pommier, Y., Kerrigan, D., and Kohn, K.W. Topoisomerase alterations associated with drug resistance in a line of Chinese hamster cells. NCI Monogr. 4:83–7, 1987.

94. Pommier, Y., Kerrigan, D., Covey, J.M., Kao-Shan, C.S., and Whang-Peng, J. Sister chromatid exchanges, chromosomal aberrations and cytotoxicity produced by antitumor topoisomerase II inhibitors in sensitive (DC3F) and resistant (DC3F/9-OHE) Chinese hamster cells. Cancer Res. 48:512–516, 1988.

95. Charcosset, J.Y., Saucier, J.M., and Jacquemin-Sablon, A. Reduced DNA topoisomerase II activity and drug-stimulated DNA cleavage in 9-hydroxyellipticine resistant cells. Biochem. Pharmacol. 37:2145–2149, 1988.

96. Delaporte, C., Charcosset, J.Y., and Jacquemin-Sablon, A. Effects of verapamil on the cellular accumulations and toxicity of several antitumor drugs in 9-hydroxy-ellipticine-resistant cells. Biochem. Pharmacol. 37:613–619, 1988.

97. Markovits, J., Linassier, C., Fosse, P., Couprie, J., Pierre, J., Jacquemin-Sablon, A., Saucier, J.M., Le Pecq, J.B., and Larsen, A.K. Inhibitory effects of the tyrosine kinase inhibitor genistein on mammalian DNA topoisomerase II. Cancer Res. 49:5111–5117, 1989.

98. Robson, C.N., Hoban, P.R., Harris, A.L., and Hickson, I.D. Cross-sensitivity to topoisomerase II inhibitors in cytotoxic drug-hypersensitive Chinese hamster ovary cell lines. Cancer Res. 47:1560–1565, 1987.

99. Davies, S.M., Robson, C.N., Davies, S.L., and Hickson, I.D. Nuclear topoisomerase II levels correlate with the sensitivity of mammalian cells to intercalating agents and epipodophyllotoxins. J. Biol. Chem. 263:17724–17729, 1988.

100. Fernandes, D.J., Smith-Nanni, C., Paff, M.T., and Neff, T.A. Effects of antileukemia agents on nuclear matrix-bound DNA replication in CCRF-CEM leukemia cells. Cancer Res. 48:1850–1855, 1988.

101. Roberts, D., Lee, T., Parganas, E., Wiggins, L., Yalowich, J., and Ashmun, R. Expressions of resistance and cross-resistance in teniposide-resistant L1210 cells. Cancer Chemother. Pharmacol. 19:123–130, 1987.

102. Roberts, D., Foglesong, D., Parganas, E., and Wiggins, L. Reduced formation of lesions in the DNA of a multidrug-resistant L1210 subline selected for teniposide resistance. Cancer Chemother. Pharmacol, 23:161–168, 1989.

103. Ganapathi, R., Grabowski, D., Ford, J., Heiss, C., Kerrigan, D., and Pommier, Y. Progressive resistance to doxorubicin in mouse leukemia L1210 cells with multidrug resistance phenotype: reductions in drug-induced topoisomerase II-mediated DNA cleavage. Cancer Commun. 1:217–224, 1989.

104. Ganapathi, R. and Grabowski, D. Differential effect of the calmodulin inhibitor trifluoperazine in modulating cellular accumulation, retention and cytotoxicity of doxorubicin in progressively doxorubicin-resistant L1210 mouse leukemia cells. Biochem. Pharmacol. 37:185–193, 1988.

105. ZijIstra, J.G., de Vries, E.G., and Mulder, N.H. Multifactorial drug resistance in an adriamycin-resistant human small cell lung carçinoma cell line. Cancer Res. 47:1780–1784, 1987.

106. ZijIstra, J.G., de Vries, E.G.E., Muskiet, F.A.J., Martini, I.A., Timmer-Bosscha, H., and Mulder, N.H. Influence of docosahexaenoic acid in vitro on intracellular adriamycin concentration in Iymphocytes and human adriamycin-sensitive and -resistant small-cell lung cancer cell lines, and on cytotoxicity in the tumor cell lines. Int. J. Cancer. 40: 850–856, 1987.

107. de Jong, S., ZijIstra, J.G., de Vries, E.G.E., and Mulder, N.H. Reduced DNA topoisomerase II activity and drug-induced DNA cleavage activity in an adriamycin-resistant human small cell lung carcinoma cell line. Cancer Res. 50:304–309, 1990.

108. Slovak, M.L., Hoeltge, G.A., Dalton W.S., and Trent, J.M. Pharmacological and biological evidence for differing mechanisms of doxorubicin resistance in two human tumor cell lines. Cancer Res. 48:2793–2797, 1988.

109. Wallace, R.E., Lindh, D., and Durr, F.E. Studies on the development of resistance to mitoxantrone in human colon carcinoma cells in vitro. Proc. Am. Assoc. Cancer Res. 23:767, 1982.

110. Dalton, W.S., Cress, A.E., Alberts, D.S., and Trent, J.M. Cytogenetic and phenotypic analysis of a human colon carcinoma cell line resistant to mitoxantrone. Cancer Res. 48:1882–1888, 1988.

111. Marsh, W., Sicheri, D., and Center, M.S. Isolation and characterization of adriamycin-resistant HL-60 cells which are not defective in the initial intracellular accumulation of drug. Cancer Res. 46:4053–4057, 1986.

112. Marsh, W. and Center, M.S. Adriamycin resistance in HL60 cells and accompanying modification of a surface membrane protein contained in drug-sensitive cells. Cancer Res. 47:5080–5086, 1987.

113. McGrath, T. and Center, M.S. Mechanisms of multidrug resistance in HL60 cells: evidence that a surface membrane protein distinct from P-glycoprotein contributes to reduced cellular accumulation of drug. Cancer Res. 48:3959–3963, 1988.

114. Lutzky, J., Astor, M.B., Taub, R.N., Baker, M.A., Bhalla, K., Gervasoni, J., J. E., Rosado, M., Stewart, V., Krishna, S, and Hindenburg, A.A. Role of glutathione and dependent enzymes in anthracycline-resistant HL60/AR cells. Cancer Res. 49:4120–4125, 1989.

115. Hindenburg, A.A., Gervasoni, J., J.E., Krishna, S., Stewart, V.J., Rosado, M., Lutzky,

J., Bhalla, K., Baker, M.A., and Taub, R.N. Intracellular distribution and pharmacokinetics of daunorubicin in anthracycline-sensitive and-resistant HL-60 Cells. Cancer Res. 49:4607–4614, 1989.

116. Bhalla, K., Hindenburg, A., Taub, R.N., and Grant, S. Isolation and characterization of an anthracycline-resistant human leukemic cell line. Cancer Res. 45:3657–3662, 1985.

117. Remnick, R.A., Gervasoni, J., J. E., Hindenburg, A.A., Lutzky, Krishna, S., Rosado, M., and Taub, R.N. The subcellular distribution of daunorubicin in drug resistant cell lines that do and do not overexpress the P-glycoprotein. Proc. Am. Assoc. Cancer Res. 30:511, 1989.

118. Supino, R., Prosperi, E., Formelli, F., Mariani, M., and Parmiani, G. Characterization of a doxorubicin-resistant murine melanoma line: studies on cross-resistance and its circumvention. Br. J. Cancer 54:33–42, 1986.

119. Supino, R., Mariani, M., Capranico, G., Colombo, A., and Parmiani, G. Doxorubicin cellular pharmacokinetics and DNA breakage in a multi-drug resistant B16 melanoma cell line. Br. J. Cancer 57:142–146, 1988.

120. McGrath, T., Marquardt, D., and Center, M.S. Multiple mechanisms of adriamycin resistance in the human leukemia cell line CCRF-CEM. Biochem. Pharmacol. 38: 497–501, 1989.

121. Harker, W.G., Slade, D.L., Dalton W.S., Meltzer, P.S., and Trent, J.M. Multidrug resistance in mitoxantrone-selected HL-60 leukemia cells in the absence of P-glycoprotein overexpression. Cancer Res. 49:4542–4549, 1989.

122. Ishida, R., Nishizawa, M., Fukami, K., Maekawa, K., Takahashi, T., and Nishimoto, T. Isolation and characterization of novobiocin-resistant BHK cells. Somat. Cell Mol. Genet. 13:11–20, 1987.

123. Ishida, R., Nishizawa, M., Nishimoto, T., and Takahashi, T. Cross-resistance of novobiocin-resistant BHK cell line to topoisomerase II inhibitors. Somat. Cell Mol. Genet. 14:489–497, 1988.

124. Jeggo, P.A. and Kemp, L.M. X-ray-sensitive mutants of Chinese hamster ovary cell line. Isolation and cross-sensitivity to other DNA-damaging agents. Mutat. Res. 112:313–327, 1983.

125. Kemp, L.M., Sedgwick, S.G., and Jeggo, P.A. X-ray sensitive mutants of Chinese hamster ovary cells defective in double-strand break rejoining. Mutat. Res. 132:189–196, 1984.

126. Weibezahn, K.F., Lohrer, H., and Herrlich, P. Double-strand break repair and G2 block in Chinese hamster ovary cells and their radiosensitive mutants. Mutat. Res. 145:177–183, 1985.

127. Jeggo, P.A., Caldecott, K., Pidsley, S., and Banks, G.R. Sensitvity of Chinese hamster ovary mutants defective in DNA double strand break repair to topoisomerase II inhibitors. Cancer Res. 49:7057–7063, 1989.

128. Evans, H.H., Ricanati, M., Horng, M.F., and Mencl, J. Relationship between topoisomerase II and radiosensitivity in mouse L5178Y lymphoma strains. Mutat. Res. 217:53–63, 1989.

129. Sander, M., Nolan J.M., and Hsieh, T.S. A protein kinase activity tightly associated with Drosophila type II DNA topoisomerase. Proc. Natl. Acad. Sci. USA 81:6938–6942, 1984.

130. Ackerman, P., Glover, C.V., and Osheroff, N. Phosphorylation of DNA topoisomerase II by casein kinase II: modulation of eukaryotic topoisomerase II activity in vitro. Proc. Natl. Acad. Sci. USA 82:3164–3168, 1985.

131. Sahyoun, N., Wolf, M., Besterman, J., Hsieh, T.S., Sander, M., LeVine, I., H., Chang, K.J., and Cuatrecasas, P. Protein kinase C phosphorylates topoisomerase II: topoisomerase activation and its possible role in phorbol ester-induced differentiation of HL-60 cells. Proc. Natl. Acad. Sci. USA 83:1603–1607, 1986.

132. Rottmann, M., Schroder, H.C., Gramzow, M., Renneisen, K., Kurelec, B., Dorn, A., Friese, U., and Muller, W.E.G. Specific phosphorylation of proteins in pore complex-laminae from the sponge Geodia cydonium by the homologous aggregation factor and

phorbol ester. Role of protein kinase C in the phosphorylation of DNA topoisomerase II. EMBO J. 6:3939–3944, 1987.

133. Ackerman, P., Glover, C.V.C., and Osheroff, N. Phosphorylation of DNA topoisomerase II *in vivo* and in total homogenates of *Drosophila* Kc cells. J. Biol. Chem. 263: 12653–12660, 1988.

134. Heck, M.M.S., Hittelman, W.N., and Earnshaw, W.C. *In vivo* phophorylation of the 170-kDa form of eukaryotic DNA topoisomerase II. J. Biol. Chem. 264:15161–15164, 1989.

135. Darby, M.K., Schmitt, B., Jongstra-Bilen, J., and Vosberg, H.P. Inhibition of calf thymus type II DNA topoisomerase by poly(ADP-ribosylation). EMBO J. 4:2129–2134, 1985.

136. Maniar, N., Krishan, A., Israel, M., and Samy, T.S.A. Anthracycline-induced DNA breaks and resealing in doxorubicin-resistant murine leukemic P388 cells. Biochem. Pharmacol. 37:1772, 1988.

137. Krishan, A., Sauerteig, A., and Wellham, L.L. Flow cytometric studies on modulation of cellular adriamycin retention by phenothiazines. Cancer Res. 45:1046–1051, 1985.

138. Darkin, S.J. and Ralph, R.K. A protein factor that enhances amsacrine-mediated formation of topoisomerase II-DNA complexes in murine mastocytoma cell nuclei. Biochim. Biophys. Acta. 1007:295–300, 1989.

139. Duguet, M., Lavenot, C., Harper, F., Mirambeau, G., and DeRecondo, A.M. DNA topoisomerases from rat liver: physiological variations. Nucleic Acid Res. 11:1059–1075, 1983.

140. Miskimins, R., Miskimins W.K., Bernstein, H., and Shimizu, N. Epidermal growth factor-induced topoisomerase(s). Exp. Cell Res. 146:53–62, 1983.

141. Taudou, G., Mirambeau, G., Lavenot, C., A., D. G., Vermeersch, J., and Duguet, M. DNA topoisomerase activities in concanavalin A-stimulated lymphocytes. FEBS. 176: 431–435, 1984.

142. Tricoli, J.V., Sahai, B.M., McCormick, P.J., Jarlinski, S.J., Bertram, J.S., and Kowalski, D. DNA topoisomerase I and II activities during cell proliferation and the cell cycle in cultured mouse embryo fibroblast (C3H 10T1/2) cells. Exp. Cell Res. 158:1–14, 1985.

143. Sullivan, D.M., Glisson, B.S., Hodges, P.K., Smallwood-Kentro, S., and Ross, W.E. Proliferation dependence of topoisomerase II mediated drug action. Biochemistry 25: 2248–2256, 1986.

144. Sullivan, D.M., Latham, M.D., and Ross, W.E. Proliferation-dependent topoisomerase II content as a determinant of anti-neoplastic drug action in human, mouse, and Chinese hamster ovary cells. Cancer Res. 47:3973–3979, 1987.

145. Zwelling, L.A., Estey, E., Silberman, L., Doyle, S., and Hittelman, W. Effect of cell proliferation and chromatin conformation on intercalator-induced, protein-associated DNA cleavage in human brain tumor cells and human fibroblasts. Cancer Res. 47: 251–257, 1987.

146. Robbie, M.A., Baguley, B.C., Denny, W.A., Gavin, J.B., and Wilson, W.R. Mechanism of resistance of noncycling mammalian cells to 4'-(9-acridinylamino) methanesulfon-*m*-anisidide: comparison of uptake, metabolism, and DNA breakage in log- and plateau-phase Chinese hamster fibroblast cell cultures. Cancer Res. 48:310–319, 1988.

147. Schneider, E., Darkin, S.J., Robbie, M.A., Wilson, W.R., and Ralph, R.K. Mechanism of resistance of non-cycling mammalian cells to 4'-[9-acridinylamino] methanesulphon-*m*-anisidide: role of DNA topoisomerase II in log- and plateau-phase CHO cells. Biochim. Biophys. Acta 949:264–272, 1988.

148. Hsiang, Y.H., Wu, H.Y., and Liu, L.F. Proliferation-dependent regulation of DNA topoisomerase II in cultured human cells. Cancer Res. 48:3230–3235, 1988.

149. Nelson, W.G., Cho, K.R., Hsiang, Y.H., Liu, L.F., and Coffey, D.S. Growth-related elevations of DNA topoisomerase II levels found in Dunning R3327 rat prostatic adenocarcinomas. Cancer Res. 47:3246–3250, 1987.

150. Heck, M.M. and Earnshaw, W.C. Topoisomerase II: a specific marker for cell proliferation. J. Cell Biol. 103:2569–2581, 1986.

151. Fairman, R. and Brutlag, D.L. Expression of the *Drosophila* type II topoisomerase is

96

developmentally regulated. Biochemistry 27:560–565, 1988.

152. Chow, K.C. and Ross, W.E. Topoisomerase-specific drug sensitivity in relation to cell cycle progression. Mol. Cell. Biol. 7:3119–3123, 1987.

153. Estey, E., Adlakha, R.C., Hittelman, W.N., and Zwelling, L.A. Cell cycle stage dependent variations in drug-induced topoisomerase II mediated DNA cleavage and cytotoxicity. Biochemistry 26:4338–4344, 1987.

154. Heck, M.M.S., Hittelman, W.N., and Earnshaw, W.C. Differential expression of DNA topoisomerases I and II during the eukaryotic cell cycle. Proc. Natl. Acad. Sci. USA 85:1086–1090, 1988.

155. Markovits, J., Pommier, Y., Kerrigan, D., Coery, J.M., Tilchen, E.J., and Kohn, K.W. Topoisomerase II-mediated DNA breaks and cytotoxicity in relation to cell proliferation and the cell cycle in NIH 3T3 fibroblasts and L1210 leukemia cells. Cancer Res. 47: 2050–2055, 1987.

156. Woessner, R.D., Chung, T.D.Y., Hofmann, G.A., Mattern, M.R., Mirabelli, C.K., Drake, F.H., and Johnson, R.K. Differences between normal and ras-transformed NIH-3T3 cells in expression of the 170kD and 180kD forms of topoisomerase II. Cancer Res. 50:2901–2908, 1990.

157. Long, B.H., Musial, S.T., and Brattain, M.G. DNA breakage in human lung carcinoma cells and nuclei that are naturally sensitive or resistant to etoposide and teniposide. Cancer Res. 46:3809–3816, 1986.

158. Brox, L.W., Belch, A., Ng, A., and Pollock, E. Loss of viability and induction of DNA damage in human leukemic myeloblasts and lymphocytes by m1-AMSA. Cancer Chemother. Pharmacol. 17:127–132, 1986.

159. Priel, E., Aboud, M., Feigelman, H., and Segal, S. Topoisomerase II activity in human leukemic and lymphoblastoid cells. Biochem. Biophys. Res. Comm. 130:325–332, 1985.

160. Edwards, C.M., Glisson, B.S., King, C.K., Smallwood-Kentro, S., and Ross, W.E. Etoposide-induced DNA cleavage in human leukemia cells. Cancer Chemother. Pharmacol. 20:162–168, 1987.

161. Potmesil, M., Hsiang, Y.H., Liu, L.F., Wu, H.Y., Traganos, F., Bank, B., and Silber, R. DNA topoisomerase II as a potential factor in drug resistance of human malignancies. NCI Monogr. 4:105–109, 1987.

162. Potmesil, M., Hsiang, Y.H., Liu, L.F., Bank, B., Grossberg, H., Kirschenbaum, S., Forlenzar, T.J., Penziner, A., Kanganis, D., Knowles, D., Traganos, F., and Silber, R. Resistance of human leukemic and normal lymphocytes to drug-induced DNA cleavage and low levels of DNA topoisomerase II [published erratum appears in Cancer Res. 48:4716, 1988]. Cancer Res. 48:3537–3543, 1988.

163. Holden, J.A., Rolfson, D.H., and Wittwer, C.T. Human DNA topoisomerase II: evaluation of enzyme activity in normal and neoplastic tissues, Biochemistry 29:2127–2134, 1990.

164. Liu, L.F. DNA topoisomerase poisons as antitumor drugs. Ann Rev. Biochem. 58: 351–375, 1989.

165. Trash, C., Voelkel, K., DiNardo, S., and Sternglanz, R. Identification of Saccharomyces cerevisiae mutants deficient in DNA topoisomerase I activity. J. Biol. Chem. 259: 1375–1377, 1984.

166. Giovanella, B.C., Stehlin, J.S., Wall, M.E., Wani, M.C., Nicholas, A.W., Liu, L.F., Siber, R., and Potmesil, M. DNA topoisomerase I — targeted chemotherapy of human colon cancer in xenografts. Science 246:1046–1048, 1989.

167. Wall, M.E., Wani, M.C., and Cook, C.E. Plant antitumor agents. I. The isolation and structure of camptothecin, a novel alkaloidal leukemia and tumor inhibitor from Camptotheca acuminata. J. Am. Chem. Soc. 83:3888–3890, 1966.

168. Gallo, R.C., Whang, P.J., and Adamson, R.H. Studies on the antitumor activity, mechanism of action, and cell cycle effects of camptothecin. J. Natl Cancer Inst. 46:789–795, 1971.

169. Gottlieb, J.A., Guarino, A.M., and Call, J.B. Preliminary pharmacological and clinical

evaluation of camptothecin sodium (NSC-100880). Cancer Chemotherap. Rep. 54: 461–470, 1970.

170. Gottlieb, J.A. and Luce, J.K. Treatment of malignant melanoma with camptothecin (NSC-100880). Cancer Chemother. Rep. 56:103–105, 1972.

171. Muggia, F.M., Creaven, P.J., Hansen, H.H., Cohen, M.H., and Selawry, O.S. Phase I clinical trial of weekly and daily treatment with camptothecin (NSC-100880): correlation with preclinical studies. Cancer Chemotherap. Rep. 56:515–521, 1972.

172. Moertel, C.G., Schutt, A.J., Reitemeier, R.J., and Hahn, R.G. Phase II study of camptothecin (NSC-100880) in the treatment of advanced gastrointestinal cancer. Cancer Chemother. Rep. 56:95–101, 1972.

173. Bosmann, H.B. Camptothecin inhibits macromolecular synthesis in mammalian cells but not in isolated mitochondria or E.coli. Biochem. Biophys. Res. Comm. 41:1412–1420, 1970.

174. Kessel, D., Bosmann, H.B., and Lohr, K. Camptothecin effects on DNA synthesis in murine leukemia cells. Biochim. Biophys. Acta 269:210–216, 1972.

175. Drewinko, B., Freireich, E.J., and Gottlieb, J.A. Lethal activity of camptothecin sodium on human lymphoma cells. Cancer Res. 34:747–750, 1974.

176. Li, L.H., Fraser, T.J., Olin, E.J., and Bhuyan, B.K., Action of camptothecin on mammalian cells in culture. Cancer Res. 32:2643–2650, 1972.

177. Horwitz, S.B., Chang, C.K., and Grollman, A.P. Studies on camptothecin: I. Effects on nucleic acid and protein synthesis. Molec. Pharmacol. 7:632–644, 1971.

178. Horwitz, M.S. and Horwitz, S.B. Intracellular degradation of HeLa and adenovirus type 2 DNA induced by camptothecin. Biochem. Biophys. Res. Comm. 45:723–727, 1971.

179. Hsiang, Y.H., Hertzberg, R., Hecht, S., and Liu, L.F. Camptothecin induces protein-linked DNA breaks via mammalian DNA topoisomerase I. J. Biol. Chem. 260: 14873–14878, 1985.

180. Mattern, M.R., Mong, S.M., Bartus, H.F., and Mirabelli, C.K. Relationship between the intracellular effects of camptothecin and the inhibition of DNA topoisomerase I in cultured L1210 cells. Cancer Res. 47:1793–1798, 1987.

181. Covey, J.M., Jaxel. C., Kohn, K.W., and Pommier, Y. Protein-linked DNA strand breaks induced in mammalian cells by camptothecin, an inhibitor of topoisomerase I. Cancer Res. 49:5016–5022, 1989.

182. Hsiang, Y.H. and Liu, L.F. Identification of mammalian topoisomerase I as an intra-cellular target of the anticancer drug camptothecin. Cancer. Res. 48:1722–1726, 1988.

183. Hsiang, Y.H., Liu, L.F., Wall, M.E., Wani, M.C., Nicholas, A.W., Manikumar, G., Kirschenbaum, S., Silber, R., and Potmesil, M. DNA topoisomerase l-mediated DNA cleavage and cytotoxicity of camptothecin analogues. Cancer Res. 49:4385–4389, 1989.

184. Jaxel, C., Kohn, K.W., Wani, M.C., Wall, M.E., and Pommier, Y. Structure-activity study of the actions of camptothecin derivatives on mammalian topoisomerase I: evidence for a specific receptor site and a relation to antitumor activity. Cancer Res. 49:1465–1469, 1989.

185. Porter, S.E. and Champoux, J.J. The basis for camptothecin enhancement of DNA breakage by eukaryotic topoisomerase I. Nucleic Acids Res. 17:8521–8532, 1989.

186. Kunimoto, T., Nitta, K., Tanaka, T., Uehara, N., Baba, H., Takeuchi, M., Yokokura, T., Sawada, S., Miyasaka, T., and Mutai, M. Antitumor activity of a 7-ethyl-10-[4-(1-piperidino)-1-piperidino]carbonyloxycamptothecin, a novel water-soluble derivative of camptothecin, against murine tumors. Cancer Res. 47:5944–5947, 1987.

187. Matsuzaki, T., Yokokura, T., Mutai, M., and Tsuruo, T. Inhibition of spontaneous and experimental metastasis by a new derivative of camptothecin, CPT-11, in mice. Cancer Chemother. Pharmacol. 21:308–312, 1988.

188. Tsuruo, T., Matsuzaki, T., Matsushita, M., Saito, H., and Yokokura, T. Antitumor effect of CPT-11, a new derivative of camptothecin, against pleiotropic drug-resistant tumors in vitro and in vivo. Cancer Chemother. Pharmacol. 21:71–74, 1988.

98

189. Johnson, R.K., McCabe, F.L., Faucette, L.F., Hertzberg, R.P., Kingsbury, W.D., Boehm, J.C., Caranfa, M.J., and Holden, K.G. SK&F 104864, a water soluble analog of camptothecin with broad spectrum activity in preclinical tumor models. Proc. Am. Assoc. Cancer. Res. 30:623, 1989.

190. Nitiss, J. and Wang, J.C. DNA topoisomerase-targeting antitumor drugs can be studies in yeast. Proc. Natl. Acad. Sci. USA 85:7501–7505, 1988.

191. Eng, W.K., Faucette, L., Johnson, R.K., and Sternglanz, R. Evidence that DNA topoisomerase I is necessary for the cytotoxic effects of camptothecin. Mol. Pharmacol. 34:755–760, 1988.

192. Bjornsti, M.A., Benedetti, P., Viglianti, G.A., and Wang, J.C. Expression of human DNA topoisomerase I in yeast cells lacking yeast DNA topoisomerase I: restoration of sensitivity of the cells to the antitumor drug camptothecin. Cancer Res. 49:6318–6323, 1989.

193. Hsiang, Y.H., Lihou, M.G., and Liu, L.F. Arrest of replication forks by drug-stabilized topoisomerase I-DNA cleavable complexes as a mechanism of cell killing by camptothecin. Cancer Res. 49:5077–5082, 1989.

194. Avemann, K., Knippers, R., Koller, T., and Sogo, J.M. Camptothecin, a specific inhibitor of type I DNA topoisomerase, induces DNA breakage at replication forks. Mol. Cell Biol. 8:3026–3034, 1988.

195. Andoh, T., Ishi, K., Suzuki, Y., Ikegami, Y., Kusunoki, Y., Takemoto, Y., and Okada, K. Characterization of a mammalian mutant with a camptothecin-resistant DNA topoisomerase I. Proc. Natl. Acad. Sci. USA 84:5565–5569, 1987.

196. Kjeldsen, E., Bonven, B., Andoh, T., Ishii, K., Okada, K., Bolund, L., and Westergaard, O. Characterization of a camptothecin-resistant human DNA topoisomerase I. J. Biol. Chem. 263:3912–3916, 1988.

197. Gupta, R.S., Gupta, R., Eng, B., Lock, R.B., Ross, W.E., Hertzberg, R.P., Caranfa, M.J., and Johnson, R.K. Camptothecin-resistant mutants of Chinese hamster ovary cells containing a resistant form of topoisomerase I. Cancer Res. 48:6404–6410, 1988.

5. Expression of the *MDR1* gene in human cancers

Lori J. Goldstein, Michael M. Gottesman, and Ira Pastan

Multidrug resistance in human malignancies

Although chemotherapy can result in the cure of many malignancies, such as testicular cancer, Hodgkin's disease, and childhood leukemias, we are continually faced with the obstacle of tumors that respond poorly to chemotherapy, such as non-small-cell lung cancer and gastrointestinal malignancies. In addition, there are many cancers, such as breast cancer and non-Hodgkins lymphoma, that initially may respond to chemotherapy and then relapse either during or after therapy.

To overcome this perplexing problem of intrinsic and acquired drug resistance, chemotherapeutic regimens have been optimized both on the basis of the Goldie-Coldman hypothesis [1] and dose intensity [2]. However, in many situations we are still confronted with the problem that some tumors remain refractory to this strategy and that subpopulations of cells may be resistant to intense combination chemotherapy.

Extensive investigation by many laboratories has led to an increasing understanding of at least one mechanism by which tumor cells may become simultaneously resistant to many different drugs, that is, multidrug resistance (MDR). This phenomenon was first described when malignant cell lines that were selected for single chemotherapeutic agent resistance were found to be resistant to other structurally unrelated natural products [3–7]. Cell lines that display the MDR phenotype are usually resistant to the *Vinca* alkaloids, anthracyclines, epipodophyllotoxins, taxol, and actinomycin D. Resistance to these products was found to be secondary to increased drug efflux, causing decreased intracellular drug accumulation [4,8]. These malignant cell lines demonstrating the MDR phenotype usually contained an amplified gene, *MDR1* which encodes a 4.5 kb mRNA [9–14]. The protein product of this gene is a 170 kd membrane glycoprotein, called P-glycoprotein, which functions as an energy-dependent drug efflux pump [15–18].

Cloning of the cDNA for the human *MDR1* gene [19] has allowed the identification of *MDR1* RNA in both normal and malignant human tissues. Using a region of this cDNA as a probe, *MDR1* expression has been dem-

Robert F. Ozols (ed.), *MOLECULAR AND CLINICAL ADVANCES IN ANTICANCER DRUG RESISTANCE.* Copyright © 1991.
Kluwer Academic Publishers, Boston. All rights reserved. ISBN 0-7923-1212-0

onstrated in the normal human kidney, adrenal gland, liver, and colon [20]. By immunohistochemical studies, the *MDR1* gene product, P-glycoprotein, has been localized on the apical surface of epithelial cells in liver, kidney, colon, jejunum, and pancreatic ductule cells, which is consistent with the possible normal function of P-glycoprotein as a transporter [21]. More recently, P-glycoprotein has also been detected on specialized endothelial cells in the brain and testis, and in human placenta [22–24].

While expression of the *MDR1* gene cannot theoretically account for the broad range of drug resistance seen in human tumors refractory to agents outside the MDR phenotype, it is thus far the best understood mechanism of multidrug resistance. We present here evidence that indicates that *MDR1* gene expression has clinical significance in a large number of malignancies, and we suggest that methods of reversing this mechanism of multidrug resistance may successfully be incorporated into clinical trials.

Evidence suggesting that expression of the *MDR1* gene in human cancers results in drug resistance

To determine whether **MDR1** gene expression in human malignancies is significant, it is important to establish that expression of the *MDR1* gene results in drug resistance. First, it has been demonstrated that when full-length cDNAs for human or mouse *MDR1* genes are transfected [25,26], or infected into human cells [27,28], these cells become multidrug resistant. Second, in renal adenocarcinoma, there is a correlation between *MDR1* RNA levels and resistance of tumor explants to vinblastine [29]. A third piece of evidence is that in permanent unselected renal adenocarcinoma cell lines that express *MDR1* RNA, the resistance is reversed by verapamil and quinidine [30]. More recently a transgenic mouse model has been generated using a plasmid carrying a human *MDR1* cDNA under the control of chicken β-actin promoter that expressed the transgene primarily in the bone marrow and spleen. By immunofluorescence localization studies, P-glycoprotein was demonstrated on the bone marrow cells. Most importantly, in vivo experiments showed that the transgenic mice were resistant to daunomycin-induced leukopenia [31]. This transgenic system can potentially be used as a model for evaluating new reversing agents and to determine whether dose intensification improves response rates and survival. Another study demonstrated that positive staining for P-glycoprotein in multiple myeloma, lymphoma, and breast cancer predicts intrinsic cellular resistance to doxorubicin in vitro [32]. These results imply that *MDR1* gene expression in human tumors may indeed account for at least one kind of drug resistance.

It is possible that, under unusual circumstances, such as the induction by retinoic acid of *MDR1* expression in colon cancer cells in vitro, expression of *MDR1* RNA and P-glycoprotein may not result in the full phenotype of multidrug resistance [33]. Such results suggest the possibility that, under some circumstances, such as after in vitro induction, a post-translational modification of P-glycoprotein may be needed for its functional activation. In contrast, induction of the *MDR1* gene in renal adenocarcinoma cell lines in vitro by heat-shock, sodium-arsenite, or cadmium-chloride treatment results in increased P-glycoprotein levels that confer transient resistance to vinblastine [34].

The ultimate test of the hypothesis that expression of the *MDR1* gene contributes to multidrug resistance in human cancer will be the demonstration that agents that inhibit the multidrug transporter act clinically to sensitize cancers to therapy with natural product drugs. Once preclinical animal models are completed, then rational clinical trials using methods of reducing *MDR1* expression or inhibiting function will be needed to determine if tumor cytotoxicity can be enhanced.

Molecular diagnosis of multidrug resistance

There are several methodologies available to determine gene expression. At the RNA level, expression can be measured using Northern blot analysis, RNA slot blot analysis, RNase protection assays, primer extension assays, in situ hybridization, and the polymerization chain reaction (PCR) following reverse transcription of RNA. The protein product of a gene can be detected with western blot analysis and immunohistochemistry. While each of these methods carries its own advantages, disadvantages, specificities, and sensitivities, we established our database for *MDR1* expression using RNA slot blot analysis. This technique in our hands was reproducible, reliable, and semiquantitaive [35].

For convenience and to assure that the RNA was of good quality, all of the solid tumor samples were frozen in liquid nitrogen or dry ice and stored at −70°C. Samples of hematologic malignancies were prepared on Ficoll-hypaque gradients and stored at −70°C in 10% DMSO. RNA was isolated by homogenization in guanidinium isothiocyanate, followed by either a cesium-chloride gradient [36] or acid-phenol [37] extraction. Agarose gel electrophoresis was performed for all RNA samples to assure that the RNA was of good quality. Using a slot blot apparatus, total RNA in serial dilutions was transferred to nitrocellulose filters. The blots were hybridized with the *MDR1* cDNA probe, 5A [19]. Duplicate blots were hybridized with an actin probe to calibrate for RNA loading. Using on each blot RNA from a drug-sensitive cell line, KB-3-1, and a three to six fold resistant cell line, KB-8-5, which has a 30- to 40-fold increase in *MDR1* mRNA [20], we were able to quantify the level of *MDR1* expression. We assigned a value of 30 units to the amount of MDR1 RNA from this drug-resistant cell line, KB-8-5, and by comparison established relative values to the individual RNA samples by comparing the intensity of hybridization to the drug-resistant line. These results were confirmed by RNase protection assays to assure the specificity of the mRNA for *MDR1*. Using this method, over 600 tumors were analyzed and the results were divided into three categories for untreated tumors: 1) those malignancies that have high expression of *MDR1*; 2) tumors that occasionally express *MDR1*, and 3) tumors with low or undetectable levels of *MDR1* RNA. A fourth group consists of those tumors that have increased expression of *MDR1* after treatment with at least one of the agents affected by the MDR phenotype [38].

Intrinsic resistance of cancers not treated with chemotherapy

We began our analysis of *MDR1* gene expression with cancers from patients who had not yet received chemotherapy. These data have indicated the widespread expression of the *MDR1* gene, particularly in solid tumors derived from tissues that normally express this gene. In addition, *MDR1* expression was found in many other types of cancer as well.

Tumors with high MDR1 *expression*

Certain cancers were found to have consistently elevated levels of *MDR1* RNA, comparable to or higher than the multidrug-resistant cell line, KB-8-5. Untreated cancers that have these high levels of *MDR1* RNA in at least 50% of cases include colon cancer, renal cell carcinoma, hepatoma, adrenocortical carcinoma, pheochromocytoma, islet cell tumors of the pancreas, carcinoid tumors, and non-small-cell carcinoma with neuroendocrine properties (NSCLC-NE) (Table 1).

All of these tumors are relatively unresponsive to chemotherapy. In addition, many of these tumors are derived from tissues that normally express the *MDR1* gene, e.g., colon, liver, kidney, pancreas, and adrenal gland. This finding suggests that one of the reasons these tumors are refractory to chemotherapy with natural product cytotoxic agents is because their tissues of origin express the *MDR1* gene. These findings are explained by assuming that when a normal cell undergoes malignant transformation,

Table 1. Generally high *MDR1* RNA levels in untreated tumors

Tumor	Total	Positive ≥30 Units	Low Positive 2–29 Units	% Positive
Colon	41	10	25	85
Renal	53	36	6	80
Hepatoma	12	7	5	100
Adrenocortical carcinoma	9	6	1	77
Pheochromycytoma	20	11	4	75
Pancreatic carcinoma	4	2	0	50
NSCLC-NE (cell lines)	6	2	3	83
Carcinoid	9	2	5	77

the *MDR1* gene continues to be expressed. The level of *MDR1* RNA observed in these tissues is similar to the level of expression in the bone marrow of transgenic mice carrying the *MDR1* gene that are resistant to daunomycin-induced myelosuppression [31], which is significant because these tumor samples contain some cells that do not express *MDR1* RNA.

Within this group of tumors, renal cell carcinoma has been studied most extensively. First, immunohistochemical localization studies have shown that in the kidney, *MDR1* is expressed in the proximal tubules, which is the histological site of origin of most renal cell carcinomas [30]. In addition, in situ hybridization studies have detected *MDR1* RNA only in the proximal tubules of the kidney [40]. Second, since *MDR1* RNA is expressed in normal kidneys, kidney tumors and adjacent normal renal parenchyma were evaluated and compared for *MDR1* expression. Expression in normal tissues did not correlate with the expression of the tumor of an individual patient [30]. It has also been demonstrated that the most differentiated renal adenocarcinomas have the highest levels of *MDR1* [41]. This suggests that since *MDR1* RNA is detected in the proximal tubules, from which most renal adenocarcinomas arise, P-glycoprotein may normally function as a transporter in these differentiated cells.

Another tumor that has been extensively investigated is colon carcinoma. Since colon cancer is the second most common cause of cancer deaths in the United States, methods to improve therapy are extremely important [42]. Although recent regimens of 5-fluorouracil modified by agents such as leucovorin [43] and levamisole [44] have shown significant response rates, there is a large fraction of affected patients who will not enjoy a complete response and prolonged survival. In colon cancer the response to doxorubicin as a single agent is poor (approximately 9%) [45]. Since *MDR1* RNA is found in normal colon, colon cancer was also evaluated. As for renal-cell carcinoma, when colon tumors and adjacent normal colon tissue were compared for *MDR1* gene expression, no correlation in samples from an individual patient was established [20]. As noted in Table 1, most colon carcinoma samples had easily detectable levels. Based on these data, clinical trials at the NCI using quinidine or amiodarone as inhibitors of the multidrug transporter are currently underway in an effort to modulate the activity of anthracyclines and *Vinca* alkaloids in renal-cell carcinoma, colon cancer, adrenocortical carcinoma, and pheochromocytoma.

Intermediate expression of the MDR1 *gene*

Other untreated tumors have occasionally high or intermediate levels of *MDR1* RNA. This group includes adult acute lymphocytic leukemia (ALL), adult nonlymphocytic leukemia (ANLL), non-Hodgkin's lymphoma (NHL), neuroblastoma, astrocytoma, and chronic myelogenous leukemia (CML) in blast crisis (Table 2).

This is an intriguing group of malignancies. Many of these usually are

Table 2. Occasionally high expression of *MDR1* RNA in untreated tumors

Tumor	Total	Positive >30 Units	Low Positive 2–20 Units	% Positive
ALL (adult)	15	2	0	13
ANLL (adult)	25	4	0	16
Non-Hodgkins lymphoma	20	1	3	20
Neuroblastoma	34	1	16	58
CML — blast crisis	4	3	0	75
Astrocytoma	3	1	1	66

initially sensitive to chemotherapy. However, a significant percentage of all of these tumors will not respond to chemotherapy. The agents used in the treatment of many of these tumors are a combination of drugs affected by the multidrug-resistance phenotype and drugs that are not. Therefore, the percentage of the nonresponders should be consistent with the fraction of those expressing *MDR1*. For example, in adult ANLL, most patients are initially treated with cytosine-arabinoside, an agent not affected by the MDR phenotype, and daunomycin, a classic substrate for the P-glycoprotein pump. The complete response rate for each as a single agent is 25% and 40–50%, respectively, while in combination a response rate of 65% can be seen [46]. Therefore the 35% of ANLL patients whose leukemias fail to respond to chemotherapy may include the 20% of such leukemias that express the *MDR1* gene and may indeed be secondary to anthracycline resistance based on drug efflux. In adult ANLL, early date suggest that *MDR1* gene expression may be one of the best prognostic predictors for response to a daunomycin-based regimen [47,48]. Clearly other mechanisms of anthracycline resistance may be contributing to clinical resistance, such as an alteration in the killing pathway involving topoisomerase II and changes in the glutathione system. The anionic glutathione transferase gene was evaluated in ANLL and was found to be uniformly expressed at the same level, regardless of anthracycline sensitivity or clinical response [48].

Consistently elevated levels of *MDR1* RNA were also found in CML in blast crisis. One interesting aspect of this result is that there is little to no detectable expression of *MDR1* RNA in samples of CML in chronic phase, though most of these samples were not obtained sequentially from the same patient. This suggests that some event, such as oncogene activation, may be involved in both the activation of *MDR1* expression and in malignant transformation. A recent follow-up study of a small number of patients with CML in blast crisis demonstrated that the presence or absence of *MDR1* expression correlated with clinical resistance and response, respectively [49]. In another study of CML in chronic and blast phase, elevated *MDR1* RNA levels were seen in the cells of some patients in blast crisis, but when the immature myeloid cells present in the samples from chronic phase patients were isolated, some *MDR1* RNA was also found [48]. These results suggest that elevated expression of *MDR1* RNA in CML in blast crisis may reflect the enrichment of immature myeloid cells in this disease.

In a study in which untreated neuroblastoma samples were examined, 55% of the tumors expressed *MDR1*, RNA; however, the level of expression did not correlate with any of the other established prognostic criteria for this disease, such as age, stage, grade, and *N-myc* amplification [50]. Bourhis et al. found similar levels of *MDR1* expression in their study of neuroblastoma [51].

Low or undetectable MDR1 *gene expression*

While many untreated malignancies do express *MDR1* RNA, there are a host of others that have low or undetectable levels of this RNA. This group includes breast cancer, non-small-cell lung cancer (NSCLC), small-cell lung cancer (SCLC), bladder cancer, CML in chronic phase, esophageal carcinoma, head and neck cancer, melanoma, mesothelioma, ovarian cancer, prostate cancer, sarcoma, thymoma, thyroid cancer, and Wilm's tumor (Table 3). In another earlier study, by immunoblotting P-glycoprotein was detected in both pre- and post-treatment sarcoma samples [52]. Although

Table 3. Low expression of *MDR1* RNA in untreated tumors

Tumor	Total	Positive >30 Units	Low Positive 2–29 Units	% Positive
Breast	57	0	9	15
NSCLC				
Tissue	19	0	7	36
Cell lines	30	0	5	16
Bladder	10	0	1	10
CML — chronic phase	3	0	0	0
	14	0	0	0
Esophageal	2	0	0	0
Gastric	14	0	0	0
Head and neck	3	0	0	0
Melanoma				
Mesothelioma				
Cell lines	20	0	1	5
Ovarian	35	0	0	0
Prostate	4	0	0	0
Sarcoma	13	0	1	7
SCLC				
Tissue	1	0	0	0
Cell lines	20	0	0	0
Thymoma	1	0	0	0
Thyroid	4	0	0	0
Wilm's	20	0	0	0

Wilm's tumor is an example of a drug-sensitive malignancy with correspondingly low *MDR1* RNA levels, other members of this group, such as melanoma and head and neck cancer, are clearly clinically resistant to the cytotoxic agents that are substrates for P-glycoprotein and yet do not express *MDR1* RNA.

Since lung cancer is the leading cause of cancer death in the United States, we were interested in investigating the possible role of expression of the *MDR1* gene in these tumors. Primary lung tumors and cell lines derived

MDR1 Expression in Human Tumor Cell Lines

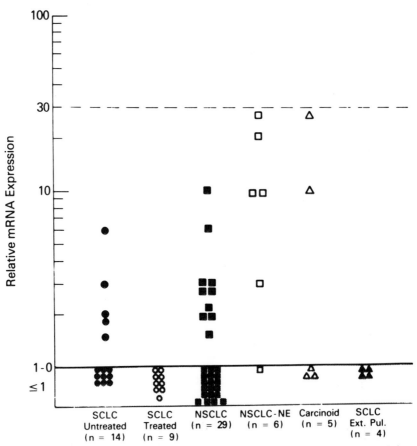

Figure 1. MDR1 levels in lung cancer cell lines displayed on a semilogarithmic scale. Subtypes of lung cancer are represented by symbols and identified below the horizontal axes: control drug-resistant KB-8-5 cell line expresses *MDR1* at a level of 30 units, which is represented by the dashed line. Cell lines with values of 2–29 units were considered to be intermediate expressors, whereas those with values of ≥30 units were high expressors. Ext. pul. = extrapulminary. (From J. Natl. Cancer Inst. 81:1144–1150, 1989, with permission.)

from primary lung tumors were evaluated for *MDR1* RNA levels [53]. Similar levels of *MDR1* RNA were measured in squamous cell carcinoma samples and the cell lines derived from these specimens, demonstrating that the establishment of a cell line did not select for altered gene expression, at least in the case of the *MDR1* gene. As shown in Figure 1, almost all of the SCLC and NSCLC samples expressed low levels of *MDR1* RNA, except NSCLC-NE. *MDR1* expression in lung cancer cell lines was also compared to the clinical response of the patients from whom they were derived in 21 previously untreated patients. Only four patients, all of whom had NSCLC-NE, had intermediate to high levels of *MDR1* expression, and the differences in *MDR1* RNA levels between responders and nonresponders were not significant. Since the response rates to combination chemotherapy for SCLC and NSCLC are 57–81% and 14–40%, respectively [54], with few durable responses, it is clear that mechanisms other than drug efflux secondary to *MDR1* must be responsible for the drug resistance seen in most lung cancer.

Breast cancer is the most common malignancy among women in the United States, and although there is a significant response to adriamycin-based regimens, resistance and subsequent relapse affect a significant number of individuals. As noted in Table 3, the expression of *MDR1* is generally low in breast cancer. A separate study of 248 breast cancer specimens, of which 219 were previously untreated, evaluated by Southern, Northern, and western blot analysis, showed no evidence of amplification, expression of *MDR1* RNA, or P-glycoprotein [55]. In contrast to these data, a preliminary study done in Glascow showed that 50% of untreated breast cancer samples expressed the *MDR1* gene [56]. Despite this study, overall it appears that in breast cancer the *MDR1* gene is not expressed at easily detectable levels, at least given the limitations of population methods for analyzing *MDR1* gene expression in highly heterogenous tumors like breast cancer (see below).

Clearly, there are many tumors in this category that are clinically resistant to most classes of chemotherapeutic drugs. This indicates that there must be mechanisms other than *MDR1* to explain why these malignancies resist chemotherapy.

Acquired resistance after chemotherapy

Malignancies that may initially be sensitive to chemotherapy have also been studied at relapse. Tumors that have high levels of *MDR1* RNA at relapse after exposure to at least one drug affected by the MDR phenotype include NHL, neuroblastoma, pheochromocytoma, breast cancer, CML in blast crisis, adult and childhood ALL, adult ANLL, and ovarian cancer (Table 4). Even though many of these tumors, such as ALL and NHL, may have a significant response to chemotherapy, upon relapse the response to chemotherapy is significantly diminished. Ma et al. have also reported

Table 4. MDR1 RNA in tumors relapsing after treatment

Tumor	Chemotherapy	Total	Positive >30 Units	Low Positive 2–29 Units	% Positive
Non-Hodgkins lymphoma	−	20	1	3	20
	+	6	1	2	50
Neuroblastoma	−	34	1	16	50
	+	16	5	11	100
CML					
Chronic phase	−	3	0	0	0
Blast crisis	−	4	3	0	75
Blast crisis	+	3	2	0	66
ALL (adult)	−	15	2	0	13
	+	1	1	0	100
ANLL (adult)	−	25	4	0	16
	+	9	5	2	80
Breast	−	57	0	9	15
	+	2	0	2	100
ALL (childhood)	−	9[a]	n	n	11
	+	20[a]	n	n	15
Pheochromocytoma	−	20	11	4	75
	+	1	1	0	100
Ovarian	−	35	0	0	0
	+	15	1	2	20

[a] Samples analyzed by Northern blot and RNase protection.
n = not evaluated.

immunohistochemically detectable P-glycoprotein in two patients with drug-resistant ANLL [57]. In contrast, Ito et al. studied 19 adult acute leukemia cases with Southern blot, Northern blot, and immunohistochemical analysis and found infrequent MDR1 expression, both at initial presentation and at relapse [58].

Another hematologic malignancy that expresses the MDR1 gene is multiple myeloma, a plasma cell dyscrasia that is characterized by a high initial response rate to chemotherapy, followed by clinical drug resistance and relapse. Dalton et al., using immunohistochemical techniques found that 2 of 4 refractory myeloma patients expressed the MDR1 gene [59].

In most cases samples pre- and post-treatment from the same patient were unavailable. However, there are a few illustrative cases where this information was obtained. Untreated pheochromocytoma may show over-expression of the MDR1 gene, which would be expected, since it is derived from the adrenal gland, which normally expresses MDR1 RNA. However, there are some pheochromocytomas that do not express MDR1 [20]. In one pheochromocytoma that initially responded to chemotherapy and had low levels of MDR1 RNA at diagnosis, MDR1 RNA levels at relapse were sixfold higher [60]. Another example of this increase postchemotherapy is a patient with NHL whose lymphoma had an MDR1 RNA level of 8 at diagnosis. After chemotherapy with PROmace-MOPP (cyclophosphamide, doxorubicin, etoposide, prednisone, mechlorethamine, vincristine, and procarbazine), the relapsed lymphoma that had the same histology had a level of 24 [38]. Expression of *MDR1* in refractory NHL has been corroborated by Moscow et al. [61].

Conclusions derived from many of the tumors studied in this group by us and others have been limited both by small sample numbers and the unavailability of pre- and post-treatment samples from the same patient. More extensive experience with both ovarian cancer and neuroblastoma indicates an association between resistance to chemotherapy and increased *MDR1* gene expression. Limited studies in ovarian cancer include western blot analysis of six untreated ovarian cancer samples showing no detectable P-glycoprotein [62] and overexpression of P-glycoprotein by immuno-histochemical analysis in 2 of 5 drug-resistant ovarian patients [63]. In a study of 50 ovarian cancer specimens, we also found undetectable levels of *MDR1* RNA in 35 untreated patient samples. However, of the 15 samples obtained at relapse after chemotherapy, 3 of 10 patients with ovarian cancer who had been treated with doxorubicin or doxorubicin plus vincristine expressed *MDR1* RNA [63]. These results strongly suggest that *MDR1* gene expression is one of the molecular determinants of acquired resistance in ovarian cancer.

Since verapamil was demonstrated to reverse adriamycin resistance in human drug-resistant ovarian cell lines [64], eight patients with refractory ovarian cancer were treated with verapamil and adriamycin [66]. There were no responses observed in these patients, and the dose of verapamil was limited by cardiac toxicity. The apparent absence of the modulation of adriamycin activity is not surprising due to the relatively low occurrence of *MDR1* expression in ovarian cancer, as well as the fact that the cardiotoxic-limiting doses of verapamil were too low to achieve adequate inhibitory concentrations, as determined in tissue culture. From the experience of serial clinical trials using such agents as adriamycin and vincristine, these drugs have been eliminated from the current active regimens for the treatment of ovarian cancer. Ovarian cancer is an example where *MDR1* gene expression parallels the clinical resistance of the tumor.

We have also studied neuroblastoma, which is a pediatric malignancy that is partially responsive to agents such as vincristine, doxorubicin, and VM26, in addition to other agents not included in the MDR group. The majority of patients with neuroblastoma develop progressive disease, either during or after chemotherapy. In a study of 49 neuroblastoma samples (Figure 2), 55% of the 31 untreated samples had low to moderate levels of *MDR1* RNA, whereas 83% of the 18 treated samples had elevated *MDR1* gene expression [50]. Bourhis et al. have found similar results in their study of neuroblastoma [51]. This group of malignancies is certainly worth investigating further. Intervention by inhibiting the multidrug transporter with MDR reversing agents in tumors with acquired drug resistance has been

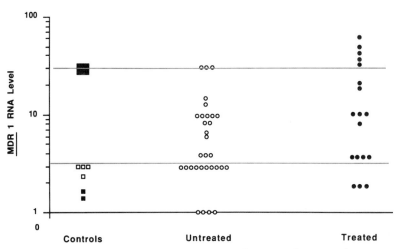

Figure 2. Quantitation of *MDR1* expression in neuroblastoma. Scattergraph representation of *MDR1* RNA levels in control samples and neuroblastoma samples obtained at diagnosis and from patients following chemotherapy. Controls with low *MDR1* RNA levels are acute lymphocytic leukemia at initial presentation (□), and normal bone marrow (■); drug-resistant KB-8-5 (■). (From J. Clin. Oncol., in press, with permission.)

initiated at the University of Arizona. In their pilot study, seven patients with multiple myeloma who failed therapy with vincristine, adriamycin, and dexamethasone (VAD) were evaluated for *MDR1* expression and then treated with verapamil, in addition to VAD. Of the five patients who expressed P-glycoprotein, two of these had a response to this regimen, while the two patients who did not express *MDR1* RNA had no response [67]. This information is now being incorporated into a cooperative group trial (see Chapter 9).

Factors affecting the variability of MDR1 gene expression

Within the group of cancers with high levels of *MDR1* RNA, there is a con-siderable amount of variability from sample to sample (Figure 3). Technical factors contributing to variable quality of RNA were not responsible for this variation, since all samples were analyzed by gels for intactness, and the quantity of RNA present on the nitrocellulose membranes was establihsed by hybridizing the blots with an actin probe. Other factors, however, may influence the variability of expression. First, many specimens may be com-posed of a heterogenous population of cells containing both cancer cells and stromal cells. Stromal cells, such as fibroblasts and inflammatory cells, tend to have very low *MDR1* RNA levels and therefore may contribute to an underestimation of *MDR1* gene expression. This is especially true for breast

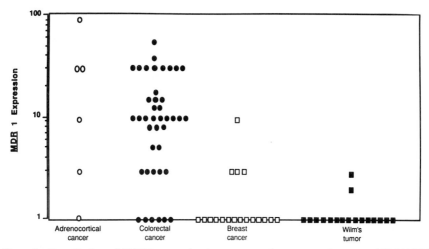

Figure 3. Quantitation of *MDR1* expression in representative untreated cancers. *MDR1* RNA levels are graphically displayed for adrenocortical carcinoma, colorectal cancer, breast cancer, and Wilm's tumor. Values of individual tumors were expressed relative to the expression of the multidrug-resistant KB-8-5 cell line, which was assigned a value of 30 units for the intensity of 10 μg of total RNA. (From J. Natl. Cancer Inst. 81:116–124, 1989, with permission.)

cancer specimens, where much of the tumor specimen is composed of stroma, and thus a low level of *MDR1* RNA may represent a population of cells with high *MDR1* content, which could grow during chemotherapy and eventually become the predominant cell type.

To examine the question of heterogeneity, evaluation of *MDR1* expression at the single-cell level will be important. Techniques such as using monoclonal antibodies for immunohistochemical analysis or in situ hybridization studies would be useful in detecting *MDR1* gene expression in tumors where only a small percentage of cells express the multidrug transporter at high levels.

A second influence on the level of *MDR1* expression is the cell type from which the tumor is derived. The localization of P-glycoprotein to the proximal tubules of the kidney where most renal cell carcinomas originate is an example of this. The state of differentiation of the tumor is a third factor that may affect the *MDR1* RNA level. As we have noted, in kidney cancer the less differentiated tumors tend to have lower *MDR1* RNA levels. In addition, retinoic acid and sodium butyrate have been used as differentiating agents on neuroblastoma cell lines and have produced an increase in *MDR1* expression [33].

From the above summary, some of the limitations of RNA slot blot analysis are obvious. In addition to establishing a reliable method of single-cell analysis of *MDR1* mRNA, the issue of sample size is important when we are dealing with clinical samples. At least 10^8 cells are required to prepare enough RNA by conventional methods for slot blot analysis. PCR after reverse transcription of RNA samples may overcome the problem of limited tumor size. Although this technology still needs to be refined with regard to its extreme sensitivity and the difficulty in quantification, it offers the possibility of detecting *MDR1* RNA from a single cell [68,69].

Strategies for applying information about *MDR1* gene expression in clinical studies

It is clear that the *MDR1* gene is responsible for multidrug resistance in both tissue culture and in the transgenic mouse model. The evaluation of over 600 human tumor specimens has revealed that the expression of *MDR1* gene is widespread and may be associated with both intrinsic and acquired multidrug resistance.

To determine if *MDR1* RNA levels are prognostic for tumor response to chemotherpay, serial samples pre- and post-treatment from the same patient must be evaluated and correlated with the clinical response in statistically significant numbers in the malignancy of interest. Once this correlation is established, information on the level of *MDR1* gene expression can be used in the selection of particular chemotherapeutic agents for a given tumor. If the *MDR1* RNA level is low, then one might choose to include drugs affected by the MDR phenotype and monitor *MDR1* expression during treatment to determine the possible development of multidrug resistance that would suggest eliminating the MDR drug and using an alternate agent to which P-glycoprotein does not confer resistance. If the *MDR1* RNA levels are high at diagnosis, one might eliminate these agents from the initial treatment regimen.

Another approach in which information about *MDR1* expression may be incorporated into clinical studies has been eluded to before — to inhibit the expression or function of P-glycoprotein. With this approach one could overcome the intrinsic resistance of a tumor or could prevent the development of resistance in a drug-sensitive cell. The most obvious method of accomplishing this is the utilization of reversing agents, such as verapamil, quinidine, amiodarone, phenothiazines, cyclosporins, and others (see Chapter 9). In addition, one can interfere with the function of P-glycoprotein by combining chemotherapy with antibodies or antibodies conjugated to toxins that would be directed against the antigenic determinants of P-glycoprotein. It has been demonstrated that *Pseudomonas* exotoxin can be conjugated with the anti-P-glycoprotein monoclonal antibody, MRK16, and that this fusion protein can kill multidrug-resistant cells in tissue culture [70]. Certainly, whether normal tissues that express *MDR1* would be injured is not known, but this does represent a potential toxicity. Preclinical animal models would be required to determine the safety and efficacy of such an approach.

The fact that expression of the human *MDR1* gene confers resistance on mouse bone marrow in transgenic mice suggests that is should be possible to introduce the *MDR1* gene into bone marrow to protect it from chemotherapy-induced myelosuppression. This could be accomplished using retroviral expression vectors. The feasibility of such an approach remains to be determined.

The *MDR1* gene encodes an energy-dependent drug efflux protein that may be responsible for at least one of the mechanisms of clinical multidrug resistance. Expression data for the *MDR1* gene in human malignancies suggest that there are many diseases that require further intense investigation to establish the role of *MDR1* as a prognostic molecular marker and to determine whether intervention in expression or function will have an impact on the ability to treat cancer.

Acknowledgments

We wish to thank Joyce Sharrar and Mary Lee Lanigan for their secretarial assistance in manuscript preparation and Steven Neal for photographic assistance.

References

1. DeVita, V.T. Principles of chemotherapy. In: Cancer Principles and Practice of Oncology, DeVita, V.T., Hellman, S., and Rosenberg, S.A. (eds). J.B. Lippincott, Philadelphia, pp. 276–298, 1989.
2. Hyrnink, W.M. The importance of dose intensity in the outcome of chemotherapy. In: Improved Advances in Oncology, DeVita, V.T., Hellman, S., and Rosenberg, S.A. (eds). J.B. Lippincott, Philadelphia, pp. 121–142, 1988.
3. Biedler, J.L. and Riehm, H. Cellular resistance to actinomycin D in Chinese hamster ovary cells *in vitro*: cross-resistance, radiographic and cytogenetic studies. Cancer Res. 30:1174–1184, 1970.
4. Ling, V. and Thompson, L.H. Reduced permeability in CHO cells as a mechanism of resistance to colchicine. J. Cell Physiol. 83:103–116, 1973.
5. Beck, W.T., Mueller, T.J., and Tanzer, L.R. Altered surface membrane glycoproteins in *Vinca* alkaloid-resistant human leukemic lymphoblasts. Cancer Res. 39:2070–2076, 1979.
6. Akiyama, S., Fojo, A., Hanover, J.A., Pastan, I., and Gottesman, M.M. Isolation and genetic characterization of human KB cell lines resistant to multiple drugs. Somat. Cell Mol. Genet. 11:117–126, 1985.
7. Shen, D.-W., Cardarelli, C., Hwang, J., Richert, N., Pastan, I., and Gottesman, M.M. Multiple drug resistant human KB carcinoma cells independently selected for high level resistance to colchicine, adriamycin or vinblastine show changes in expression of specific proteins. J. Biol. Chem. 261:7762–7770, 1986.
8. Fojo, A., Akiyama, S.I., Gottesman, M.M., and Pastan, I. Reduced drug accumulation in multiply drug-resistant human KB carcinoma cell lines. Cancer Res. 45:3002–3007, 1985.
9. Shen, D.-W., Fojo, A., Chin, J.E., Roninson, I.B., Richert, N., Pastan, I., and Gottesman, M.M. Human multidrug-resistant cell lines: increased mdr1 expression can precede gene amplification. Science 232:643–645, 1986.
10. Riordan, J.R., Deuchars, K., Kartner, N., et al. Amplification of P-glycoprotein genes in

multidrug resistant mammalian cell lines. Nature 316:817–819, 1985.

11. Van der Bliek, A.M., Van der Velde-Koerts, I., Ling, V., and Borst, P. Overexpression and amplification of five genes in a multidrug-resistant Chinese hamster ovary cell line. Mol. Cell Biol. 6:1671–1687, 1986.

12. Scotto, K.W., Biedler, J., and Melera, P.W. Amplification and expression of genes associated with multidrug resistance in mammalian cells. Science 232:751–755, 1986.

13. Gros, P., Croop, J., Roninson, I., Varshavsky, A., and Housman, D.E. Isolation and characterization of DNA sequences amplified in multidrug-resistant hamster cells. Proc. Natl. Acad. Sci. USA 83:337–341, 1986.

14. Roninson, I.B., Chin, J.E., Choi, K., Gros, P., Housman, D.E., Fojo, A., Shen, D.-W., Gottesman, M.M., and Pastan, I. Isolation of human *mdr* DNA sequences amplified in multidrug-resistant KB carcinoma cells. Proc. Natl. Acad. Sci. USA 83:4538–4542, 1986.

15. Horio, M., Gottesman, M.M., and Pastan, I. ATP-dependent transport of vinblastine in vesicles from human multidrug-resistant cells. Proc. Natl. Acad. Sci. USA 185:3580–3584, 1988.

16. Gottesman, M.M., and Pastan, I. The multidrug transporter: a double edged sword. J. Biol. Chem. 263:12163–12166, 1988.

17. Endicott, J. and Ling, V. The biochemistry of P-glycoprotein-mediated multidrug resistance. Annu Rev. Biochem. 58:137–171, 1989.

18. Croop, J.M., Gros, P., and Housman, D.E. Genetics of multidrug resistance. J. Clin. Invest. 81:1303–1309, 1988.

19. Ueda, K., Clark, D.P., Chen, C.J., Roninson, I.B., Gottesman, M.M., and Pastan, I. The human multidrug resistance (mdr1) gene, cDNA cloning and transcription initiation. J. Biol. Chem. 262:505–508, 1987.

20. Fojo, A., Ueda, K., Slamon, D.J., Poplack, D.G., Gottesman, M.M., and Pastan, I. Expression of a multidrug-resistance gene in human tumors and tissues. Proc. Natl. Acad. Sci. USA 84:265–269, 1987.

21. Thiebaut, F., Tsuruo, T., Hamada, H., Gottesman, M.M., and Pastan, I. Cellular localization of the multidrug-resistant gene product P-glycoprotein in normal human tissues. Proc. Natl. Acad. Sci. USA 84:7735–7738, 1987.

22. Cordon-Cardo, C., O'Brien, J.P., Casals, D., Rittman-Graner, L., Beidler, J.L., Melamed, M.R., and Bertino J.R. Multidrug-resistance gene (p-glycoprotein) is expressed by endothelial cells at blood-brain barrier sites. Proc. Natl. Acad. Sci. USA 86:695–698, 1989.

23. Thiebaut, F., Tsuruo, T., Hamada, H., Gottesman, M.M., Pastan, I., and Willingham, M.C. Immunohistochemical localization in normal tissues of different epitopes in the multidrug transport protein, P170: evidence for localization in brain capillaries and cross-reactivity of one antibody with a muscle protein. J. Histochem. Cytochem. 37:159–164, 1989.

24. Sugawara, I., Kataoka, I., Morishita, Y., Hamada, H., Tsuruo, T., Itayama, S., and Mori, S. Tissue distribution of P-glycoprotein encoded by a multidrug resistant gene as revealed by a monoclonal antibody, MRK16. Cancer Res. 48:4611–4614, 1988.

25. Gros, P., Ben Neriah, Y., Croop, J.M., and Housman, D.E. Isolation and expression of a complementary DNA that confers multidrug resistance. Nature 323:728–731, 1986.

26. Ueda, K., Cardarelli, C., Gottesman, M.M., and Pastan, I. Expression of a full-length cDNA for the human mdr1 gene confers resistance to colchicine, doxorubicin and vinblastine. Proc. Natl. Acad. Sci. USA 84:3004–3008, 1987.

27. Guild, B.C., Mulligan, R.C., Gros, P., and Housman, D.E. Retroviral transfer of a murine cDNA for multidrug resistance confers pleiotropic drug resistance to cells without prior drug selection. Proc. Natl. Acad. Sci. USA 85:1595–1599, 1988.

28. Pastan, I., Gottesman, M.M., Ueda, K., Lovelace, E., Rutherford, A.V., and Willingham, M.C. A retrovirus carrying an MDR1 cDNA confers multidrug resistance and polarized expression of P-glycoprotein in MDCK cells. Proc. Natl. Acad. Sci. USA 85:4486–4490, 1988.

116

29. Kakehi, Y., Kanamaru, H., Yoshida, O., Ohkubo, H., Nakanishi, S., Gottesman, M.M., and Pastan, I. Measurement of multidrug resistance messenger RNA in urogenital cancers; elevated expression in renal cell carcinoma is associated with intrinsic drug resistance. J. Urol. 139:862–865, 1988.

30. Fojo, A.T., Shen, D.-W., Mickley, L.A., Pastan, I., and Gottesman, M.M. Intrinsic drug resistance in human kidney cancer is associated with expression of a human multidrug resistance gene. J. Clin. Oncol. 5:1922–1927, 1987.

31. Galski, H., Sullivan, M., Willingham, M.C., Chin, K.V., Gottesman, M.M., Pastan, I., and Merlino, G. Expression of a human multidrug resistance cDNA (MDR1) in the bone marrow of transgenic mice: resistance to daunomycin-induced leukopenia. Mol. Cell Biol. 9:4357–4363, 1989.

32. Salmon, S.E., Grogan, T.M., Miller, T., Scheper, R., and Dalton, W.S. Prediction of doxorubicin-resistance in vitro in myeloma, lymphoma and breast cancer by P-glycoprotein staining. J. Natl. Cancer Inst. 81:696–701, 1989.

33. Bates, S.E., Mickley, L.A., Chen, Y.-N., Richert, N., Rudick, J., Biedler, J.L., and Fojo, A.T. Expression of a drug resistance gene in human neuroblastoma cell lines: modulation by retinoic acid induced differentiation. Mol. Cell. Biol. 9:4337–4344, 1989.

34. Chin, K.-V., Tanaka, S., Darlington, G., Pastan, I., and Gottesman, M.M. Heat shock and arsenite increase expression of the multidrug resistance (MDR1) gene in human renal carcinoma cells. J. Biol. Chem., in press.

35. Gottesman, M.M., Goldstein, L.J., Bruggemann, E., Currier, S., Galski, H., Cardarelli, C., Thiebaut, F., Willingham, M.C., and Pastan, I. Molecular diagnosis of multidrug resistance. In: Cancer Cells, Vol. 7; Molecular Diagnosis of Human Cancer, Furth, M. and Greaves, M. (eds). Cold Spring Harbor Laboratory, Cold Spring Harbor, NY, 1989.

36. Chirgwin, J., Przybyla, A., MacDonald, R., and Rutter, W.J. Isolation of biologically active ribonucleotide acid sources enriched in ribonuclease. Biochemistry 18:5294–5299, 1976.

37. Chomezynski, P. and Sacchi, N. Single step method of RNA isolation by acid quanidium thiocynate-phenolchloroform extracted. Anal. Biochem. 162:156–159, 1987.

38. Goldstein, L.J., Galski, H., Fojo, A., Willingham, M., Lai, S., Gazdar, A., Pirker, R., Green, A., Crist, W., Brodeur, G., Lieber, M., Cossman, J., Gottesman, M.M., and Pastan, I. Expression of a multidrug resistance gene in human cancers. J. Natl. Cancer Inst. 81:116–124, 1989.

39. Wallace, A.C. and Nairn, P.C. Renal tubular antigens in kidney tumors. Cancer 29: 977–981, 1972.

40. Mickley, F. and Fojo, A.T. In situ detection of MDR1 RNA in normal human tissues, submitted, 1989.

41. Kanamaru, H., Kakehi, Y., Yoshida, O., Nakanishi, S., Pastan, I., and Gottesman, M.M. MDR1 RNA levels in human renal cell carcinomas: correlation with grade and prediction of reversal of doxorubicin resistance by quinidine in tumor explants. J. Natl. Cancer Inst. 81:844–849, 1989.

42. Cancer Facts and Figures. American Cancer Society, 1988.

43. Grem, J.L. 5-fluorouracil plus leucovorin in cancer therapy. In: Principles and Practice of Oncology Update, Vol. 2, DeVita, V.T., Hellman, S., and Rosenberg, S.A. (eds). J.B. Lippincott, Philadelphia, p. 7, 1988.

44. Laurie, J.A., Moertel, C.G., Fleming, T.R., Wiend, H.S.M., Leigh, J.E., Rubin, J., McCormack, G.W., Gerstner, J.B., Krook, J.E., Malliard, J., Twito, D.T., Morton, R.F., Tschetter, L.K., and Barlow, J.F. Surgical adjuvant therapy of large bowel carcinoma: an evaluation of levamisole and the combination of levamisole and 5-fluorouracil. A study of the North Central Cancer Treatment Group and Mayo Clinic. J. Clin. Oncol. 7:1447–1456, 1989.

45. Carter, S.F. and Friedman, M. Integration of chemotherapy with combined modality treatment of solid tumors. II. Large bowel carcinoma. Cancer Treat. Rev. 1:111–129, 1974.

117

46. Van Sloten, K., Wiernik, P.H., Schiffer, C.A., and Schimpf, S.C. Evaluation of levamisole as an adjuvant to chemotherapy for treatment of ANLL. Cancer 51:1576, 1983.

47. Sato, H., Preisler, H., Day, R., Raza, A., Larson, R., Browman, A., Goldberg, J., Wagler, R., Grunwald, H., Gottlieb, A., Bennett, J., Gottesman, M.M., and Pastan, I. *MDR1* transcript levels as an indication of resistant disease in acute nonlymphocytic leukemia, B.J. Haematol. 75:340–345, 1990.

48. Sato, H., Gottesman, M.M., Goldstein, L.J., Pastan, I., Preisler, H.D., Block, A.M., and Sandberg, A.A. Expression of the multidrug resistance gene in myeloid leukemias. Leuk. Res., 14:11–22, 1990.

49. Pirker, R., Goldstein, L.J., Ludwig, H., Linkesch, W., Lechner, C., Gottesman, M.M., and Pastan, I. Expression of a multidrug resistance gene in blast crisis of chronic myelogenous leukemia. Cancer Commun. 1:141–144, 1989.

50. Goldstein, L.J., Fojo, A., Ueda, K., Crist, W., Green, A., Brodeur, A., Pastan, I., and Gottesman, M.M. Expression of the multidrug-resistance (MDR1) gene in neuroblastoma. J. Clin. Oncol., 8:128–136, 1989.

51. Bourhis, J., Bénard, J., Hartmann, O., Boccon-Gibod, L., Lemerle, J., and Riou, G. Correlation of *MDR1* gene expression with chemotherapy in neuroblastoma. J. Natl. Cancer Inst. 81:1401–1405, 1989.

52. Gerlach, J.H., Bell, D.R., Karakousis, Slocum, H.K., Kartner, N., Rustum, Y.M., Ling, V., and Baker, R.M. P-glycoprotein in human, sarcoma: evidence for multidrug resistance. J. Clin. Oncol. 5:1452–1460, 1987.

53. Lai, S.L., Goldstein, L.J., Gottesman, M.M., Pastan, I., Tsai, C.M., Johnson, B.E., Mulshine, J.L., Ihde, D.C., Kayser, K., and Gazdar, A. *MDR1* expression in lung cancer. J. Natl. Cancer Inst. 81:1144–1150, 1989.

54. Minna, J.P., Pass, H., Glatstein, E.J., and Ihde, D.C. Cancer of the lung. In Cancer: Principles and Practice of Oncology, DeVita, V.T., Hellman, S., and Rosenberg, S.A. (eds). J.B. Lippincott, Philadelphia, pp. 591–688, 1989.

55. Merkel, D.E., Fugua, S.A.W., Tandona, A.K., Hill, S.M., Buzdar, A.V., and MaGuire, W.L. Electrophoretic analysis of 248 clinical breast specimens for P-GP overexpression or gene amplification. J. Clin. Oncol. 7:1129–1136, 1989.

56. Keith, W.N., Stallard, S., and Brown, R. Expression of *mdr*1 and *gst*-pi in human breast tumors: comparison to *in vitro* chemosensitivity, submitted.

57. Ma, D.D., Davey, R.A., Harman, D.A., Isbister, J.P., Scurr, R.D., Mackertich, S.M., Dowden, C., and Bell, D.R. Detection of a multidrug resistant phenotype in acute non-lymphoblastic leukemia. Lancet 1:135–137, 1987.

58. Ito, Y., Tanimoto, M., Kumazawa, T., Okumura, M., Monshima, Y., Ohno, R., and Saito, H. Increased P-glycoprotein expression and multidrug-resistant gene (*mdr*1) amplification are infrequently found in fresh acute leukemia cells. Sequential analysis of 15 cases at initial presentation and relapsed stage. Cancer 63:1534–1538, 1989.

59. Salmon, S.E., Grogan, T.M., Miller, T., Scheper, K., and Dalton, W.S. Prediction of doxorubicin resistance *in vitro* in myeloma, lymphoma, and breast cancer by P-glycoprotein staining. J. Natl. Cancer Inst. 81:696–701, 1989.

60. Fojo, A., Cornwell, M., Cardarelli, C.O., Clark, D.P., Richert, N., Shen, D.-W., Ueda, K., Willingham, M.C., Gottesman, M.M., and Pastan, I. Molecular biology of drug resistance. Breast Cancer Res. Treat. 8:5–16, 1987.

61. Moscow, J.A., Fairchild, C.R., Madden, M.J., Ransom, D.T., Wieand, H.S., O'Brien, E.E., Poplack, D.G., Cossman, J., Myers, C.E., and Cowan, K.H. Expression in anionic glutathione S-transferase and P-glycoprotein genes in human tissues and tumors. Cancer Res. 49:1422–1428, 1989.

62. Fredericks, W., Murawski, H., Slocum, H., Gerlach, J., Ling, V., and Baker, R. Incidence of elevated P-glycoprotein in human tumors (abstr.). Proc. Am. Assoc. Cancer Res. 9:302, 1988.

63. Bell, D.R., Gerlach, J.H., Kartner, N., Buick, R.N., and Ling, V. Detection of

118

P-glycoprotein in ovarian cancer: a molecular marker associated with multidrug resistance. J. Clin. Oncol. 3:311–315, 1985.

64. Bourhis, J., Goldstein, L.J., Riou, G., Pastan, I., Gottesman, M.M., and Bénard, J. Expression of a human multidrug resistance gene in ovarian carcinomas. Cancer Res. 49:5062–5065, 1989.

65. Rogan, A.M., Hamilton, T.C., Young, R.C., Klecker, R.W., and Ozols, R.F. Reversal of adriamycin resistance by verapamil in human ovarian cancer. Science 224:994–996, 1984.

66. Ozols, R.F., Cunnion, R.E., Klecker, R.W., Hamilton, T.C., Ostchega, Y., Parrillo, J.C., and Young, R.C. Verapamil and adriamycin in the treatment of drug-resistant ovarian cancer patients. J. Clin. Oncol. 5:641–647, 1987.

67. Dalton, W.S., Grogan, T.M., Meltzer, P.S., Scheper, R.J., Durie, B.G., Taylor, C.W., Miller, T.P., and Salmon, S.E. Drug resistance in multiple myeloma and non-Hodgkins lymphoma: detection of P-glycoprotein and potential circumvention by addition of verapamil to chemotherapy. J. Clin. Oncol. 7:415–424, 1989.

68. Roninson, I.B., Patel, M.C., Lee, I., et al. Molecular mechanisms and diagnostics of multidrug resistance in human tumor cells. In: Cancer Cells, Vol. 7, Furth, M. and Greaves, M. (eds). Cold Spring Harbor Laboratory, Cold Spring Harbor, NY, 1989.

69. Rapollee, D.A., Marks, D., Branda, M.J., and Werb, Z. Wound macrophages express TGFa and other growth factors in vivo: analysis by mRNA phenotyping. Science 241: 708–711, 1988.

70. FitzGerald, D.J., Willingham, M.C., Cardarelli, C.O., Hamada, H., Tsuruo, T., Gottesman, M.M., and Pastan, I. A monoclonal Ab-Pseudomonas toxin conjugated that specifically kills multidrug-resistant cells. Proc. Natl. Acad. Sci. USA 84:4288–4297, 1987.

119

6. Immunoblot detection of P-glycoprotein in human tumors and cell lines

William J. Fredericks, YanFeng Chen, and Raymond M. Baker

Introduction

Significant progress has been made in elucidating the role of elevated expression of P-glycoprotein (Pgp), the *mdr1* gene product, as one mechanism underlying multidrug resistance (MDR) to cancer chemotherapeutic agents. Application of immunological and molecular biological techniques has enabled the derivation of a diversity of antibodies and nucleic acid probes suitable for detection of Pgp and its mRNAs. These probes have been used to characterize various genetic and biochemical aspects of Pgp-mediated MDR in human cell lines and tissues. A substantial research effort from numerous laboratories is currently extending studies to assess whether elevated expression of Pgp in particular human tumors can account for clinical resistance to treatment, and whether the Pgp marker may be used to predict for nonresponse to a spectrum of the important chemotherapeutic agents. The goal is to facilitate the tailoring of chemotherapeutic strategies and the development of new treatments directed toward circumventing resistance.

The reader is referred to a selection of recent reviews concerning the biochemistry and molecular biology of Pgp-mediated MDR [1–8]. The following few paragraphs are offered as a brief outline of the main features of Pgp in relation to "classic" pleiotropic MDR.

Pgp is a membrane glycoprotein with an approximate molecular weight (MW) of 170 kDa whose expression level in MDR cell lines generally correlates with the degree of pleiotropic drug resistance [9–12]. The term *pleiotropic* refers to the observed increased resistances to a broad range of unrelated drugs attributable to alterations affecting a single gene [13]. Important chemotherapeutic agents affected by MDR include the anthracyclines, *Vinca* alkaloids, actinomycin, epipodophyllotoxins, ellipticines, and a few alkylating agents [14–16]. Cells with increasing levels of MDR can be selected with increasing doses of these agents [14,17].

The *mdr1* gene encoding Pgp is expressed dominantly, so that relatively frequent single mutations could significantly affect cellular Pgp level and MDR phenotype [13,18,19]. Expression of transfected *mdr1* cDNAs or MDR genomic DNA suffice to elevate Pgp and confer the full MDR phenotype [3,20–22]. Both increased net transcription and/or *mdr1* gene amplification

Robert F. Ozols (ed.), MOLECULAR AND CLINICAL ADVANCES IN ANTICANCER DRUG RESISTANCE. Copyright © 1991.
Kluwer Academic Publishers, Boston. All rights reserved. ISBN 0-7923-1212-0

can account for elevation of Pgp in MDR cells [23–25]. Expression of Pgp may be induced in certain cells and tissues by various agents [26–29]. Regulation of Pgp levels at the level of *mdr1* mRNA stability has been demonstrated [30].

Sequence analysis of *mdr1* cDNAs predicts a molecular structure for Pgp consistent with a proposed function as an ATPase-dependent drug transporter with efflux capacity for multiple substrates [2,31–34]. Elevated *mdr1* gene expression occurs naturally within specific cell types in certain organs, including liver, adrenal, kidney, and colon [35–39]. Cellular detoxification is the presumed natural function. Although this could account for minimal drug toxicities to these tissues [38] and perhaps some intrinsic resistances to chemotherapy [40], it is uncertain whether important malignant cells typically retain this differentiated trait [41]. In addition to the *mdr1* gene encoding Pgp [10], human cells also contain another member of the gene family, designated *mdr3* (sometimes referred to as *mdr2*) [7,42–45]. It is unknown whether the more rarely expressed *mdr3* gene contributes to drug resistance [42,21].

This chapter will survey results from our laboratory's investigation of elevated Pgp expression in human solid tumors by western immunoblotting [46] with the well-characterized monoclonal antibodies (mAbs) C219 and C494 [15,47]. Emphasis is directed toward discussion of technical detail and rationale of the methodology in order that merits and constraints of this approach can be evaluated within the context of data from other laboratories derived by alternate approaches, such as immunohistochemical detection of Pgp and assays for *mdr1* mRNA. The western immunoblotting procedures are described in sufficient detail to be readily reproducible by other labs. Sensitivity and specificity of the immunoblot assays are illustrated with results for control calibrations of Pgp levels in a series of KB human MDR cell lines. Results to date for Pgp evaluations on 450 specimens of assorted solid tumors and for certain normal human tissues are summarized, with examples of immunoblot data. Characteristic features of the C219 and C494 mAb probes illustrated by these results are discussed, including possible cross-reactions.

The aim is to direct the reader's attention to salient aspects of the western immunoblotting approach and results to date in characterizing Pgp expression levels in different human tumors and tissues. Complementary features of alternate approaches, and reports of elevated *mdr1* mRNA or Pgp detected by these means, are indicated briefly where relevant. Further comparative and complementary studies will aid in understanding the role Pgp may play in clinical MDR and help to direct studies aimed at relating Pgp expression to clinical responses.

Immunoblot methodology

This section describes details of immunoblotting procedures. Results of immunoblotting and discussion are to be found in the next two sections. The actual immunoblot methodology described below is based on procedures originally implemented in the laboratory of Dr. V. Ling at the Ontario Cancer Institute, Toronto, by Drs. J. Gerlach, D. Bell, N. Kartner, and colleagues [9,15,48–50], and somewhat further adapted by ourselves. The collection of tumors at Roswell Park Cancer Institute was made possible by the collaboration of Drs. Y.M. Rustum and H.K. Slocum in procurement and disposition of specimens and by the cooperation of institute surgical staff, including Drs. C. Karakousis, M.S. Piver, A. Mittelman, D. Holyoke, and others.

Tumor sample acquisition and initial processing

Human tumor specimens assayed for Pgp were acquired from collaborating RPCI clinicians in accord with institutional review board guidlines. The specimens obtained represented a spectrum of primary and metastatic solid tumors from patients who had been staged and treated at RPCI. Clinical information concerning the course of disease would be available for correlative evaluations. Specimens from surgery were initially received by a pathologist for gross dissection of tumor tissue and standard histopathological evaluation. Excess tumor, and separated adjacent nontumor tissue if available, was received on ice in a core research facility, where it was sampled for additional histologic analyses, allocated with or without prior disaggregation, and cryopreserved.

Initial assays for Pgp overexpression in tumors were conducted using disaggregated tumor cell suspensions. These preparations were readily available to us and could be utilized concurrently in other projects for collateral results concerning the specimens (e.g., chemosensitivity and flow cytometric assays). The disaggregation process used in sample preparation enriches the yield for cellular material by removal of stroma and provides a sampling from throughout the tumor portion that is processed.

The two-step, mechanical and enzymatic disaggregation procedure has been described in detail by Dr. Slocum and colleagues [51]. The tissue is sliced and minced in culture medium and then strained through a 100 mesh (200 μ) screen to recover a "mechanically" derived cell suspension. A further "enzymatically" derived suspension is generated by subsequent incubations of the residual tissue material in culture medium with 0.8% (w/v) collagenase II (Worthington) and .002% (w/v) DNAse I (Sigma) for 2 hr, followed by filtration through the 100 mesh screen. After measurements of cell concentration and viability by trypan blue dye exclusion and preparation of slides for cytology, the disaggregated cell suspensions are stored frozen at $-90°C$ in medium containing 10% fetal bovine serum and 10% dimethyl sulfoxide. As previously described, the cell yields from disaggregation vary widely, even within a given tumor type. Median yields for various types average approximately 6×10^7 cells per gram wet weight of tissue [51]. For a number of solid tumor types (including colon, melanoma, ovarian, renal, and sarcoma), the average specimen size yields sufficient cells ($\geq 2 \times 10^7$) to process for immunoblotting. Cytological examination of the disaggregated specimens gives a direct estimate of the fraction of total cells that are tumor cells for each sample. This fraction ranges from 10% to 100%, with a median of 70%. Generalizing over all tumor types, median results for dye excluding cells are only 15% of cells from mechanically derived suspensions but >80% for cells from enzymatically derived preparations. To date we have not observed any differences in results of Pgp assays when the two types of suspensions are compared, and we have utilized them interchangeably [50].

A useful alternate methodology for processing tissue specimens is based on rapid freezing of solid (whole) specimen tissues by immersion in liquid nitrogen within 30 min after receipt from the pathologist. We have employed this alternate approach for recent specimens because it facilitates isolation of intact RNAs and minimizes the potential for damage to antigens. While maintained in the frozen state with the aid of liberal liquid nitrogen and a dry ice bed, 1–2 g of the solid specimen are pulverized quickly to small pieces (ca. 2 mm) with a hammer and ground to a fine powder with a chilled mortar and pestle, then aliquoted to prechilled containers for further processing or storage at −90°C. The grinding serves to homogenize the specimen, ensuring consistent and representative sampling.

For subsequent processing of pulverized solid specimens, the frozen powder is thawed at 4°C (1 g/5 ml) in PBS, pH 7.4, supplemented with protease inhibitors N p-tosyl-L-arginine methyl ester (0.38 mg/ml; TAME, Sigma) and aprotinin (1% v/v; Sigma). Coarse fragments are removed by passing this suspension through a 60 mesh stainless steel screen and then through a 150 mesh screen, using the PBS solution to rinse retained material.

For subsequent processing of frozen disaggregated cell suspensions, the samples are thawed and diluted into 25 ml cold PBS supplemented with protease inhibitors, as above. From this point, the same methodology is applied for the resuspensions of either pulverized solid tissue or disaggregated tumor cells, or cells from cultured lines. The samples are maintained at 0–4°C, and ice-cold reagents are used throughout, unless otherwise indicated.

Preparation of cell membrane fractions and solubilization of membrane proteins

Cells are pelleted by low-speed centifugation and resuspended to a concentration of 2×10^7 cells/ml in a hypotonic lysis buffer (10 mM KCl, 1.5 mM MgCl$_2$, 10 mM Tris-HCl, pH 7.4 at 4°C) supplemented with a freshly prepared cocktail of protease inhibitors: 2 mM phenylmethylsulfonyl fluoride (PMSF, Boeringer Mannheim), 3.2 μM (250 KIU/ml) aprotinin, and 1 mM TAME. Reproducible cell breakage is achieved using an air-driven Stansted cell-disrupting pump [52,53], model A0612, fitted with a no. 716 disrupting valve and operated according to manufacturer's specifications. The extent of disruption is monitored by phase contrast microscopy.

124

It is also possible to homogenize the samples using a conventional motor-driven Teflon® pestle with an ice-jacketed container, but this method can be arduous, as some samples are extremely refractory.

A plasma membrane enriched, microsomal membrane fraction is isolated by a simple series of differential centrifugations. The homogenate is first centrifuged at 400 xg for 10 min to pellet unbroken cells, nuclei, debris, etc.; then the supernatant is centrifuged at 4000 xg for 10 min to pellet a crude mitochondrial fraction. Immunoblot analyses of such 4000 xg pellets suggested that up to a third of total Pgp antigen in the sample can be lost or trapped in this fraction, but more refined separations have not seemed necessary or practical. A microsomal membrane fraction is collected by pelleting the postmitochondrial supernatant at 100,000 xg for 1 hr in a Beckman SW41 rotor. The pellet is resuspended in a minimum volume (10–100 μl) of filter-sterilized 8.6% (w/v) sucrose, 5 mM Tris, pH 7.4, containing protease inhibitors, as specified above for the lysis buffer, to obtain a protein concentration of 10–20 μg/μl, which is convenient for subsequent steps. Gentle vortexing with a Teflon micropestle facilitates homogeneous resuspension. An aliquot (typically ≤5 μl) is then taken for protein determination, and the sample is stored at −90°C in a tightly sealed microtube. Further enrichment for plasma membranes by fractionation on sucrose step gradients was found to be unnecessary, and also impractical, when assaying large numbers of samples. The banding patterns for different samples were quite variable and the procedure extremely labor intensive.

Determination of protein content in the resuspended microsomal membrane fraction is performed by a modified Lowry procedure [54] using trichloroacetic acid precipitation to remove interfering substances and detergent solubilization. Bovine serum albumin is used as a standard. Sampling errors can sometimes result from microheterogeneity (incomplete dispersion of particulate matter) in the membrane preparation. When protein determinations are repeated after solubilization of the membrane preparation with detergent (see below), there is generally good agreement with the assay prior to solubilization, but sometimes corrections of up to ±30% may be indicated. Therefore, we prefer protein readings from solubilized samples when comparing Pgp expression levels for samples of comparable type (e.g., cell lines).

Yields of membrane protein recovered in the crude membrane fraction vary extremely widely between different tumor specimens, even those of the same histopathologic type. The range for disaggregated specimens was 36–4500 μg (average = 540, n = 230) per 6×10^7 cells. Solid specimens processed by the alternate methodology yielded 25–5600 μg (average = 1300, n = 150) per gram frozen weight. The variation is presumably related to the heterogeneity of these diverse specimens and consequent differences in partitioning during fractionation.

Solubilization of membrane protein prior to sodium dodecyl sulfate (SDS) continuous polyacrylamide gel electrophoresis is performed using a modification [48] of the procedure of Fairbanks [55]. An aliquot of the crude membrane fraction is first diluted with water to a final protein concentration of 2.5 µg/µl, then 1/4 volume is added of a 5x solubilizing buffer consisting of 10% (w/v) SDS (BioRad, electrophoresis grade), 50% (w/v) sucrose (Boeringer Mannheim, ultrapure), 0.25 M dithiothreitol (BioRad), 5 mM di-sodium EDTA (Kodak), 12.5 mg/ml Pyronin Y (BioRad), and 50 mM Tris base, pH 8.0. The sample in a tightly capped 0.5 ml microtube is heated for 5 min in a boiling water bath and then rapidly cooled to room temperature. This suspension is then mixed with an equal volume of a 2× urea buffer comprised of 9.0 M urea (BioRad, electrophoresis grade) in 1× solubilizing buffer. Unsolubilized material can be removed by centrifugation at 100,000 ×g at 20°C for 1 hr. Solubilized samples can be stored frozen prior to electrophoresis. Repeated freezing and thawing can cause aggregation and damage to membrane proteins, however [56].

Electrophoresis and electroblotting

Polyacrylamide gels are prepared in Fairbanks electrophoresis buffer (final concentrations: 1% (w/v) SDS, 2 mM di-sodium EDTA, 20 mM sodium acetate, 40 mM Tris base adjusted to pH 7.4 with glacial acetic acid) containing 9.0 M urea, 5.6% (w/v) acrylamide, and 0.21% (w/v) bis-acrylamide polymerized by the addition of 0.25% v/v TEMED and 0.15% (w/v) ammonium persulfate (electrophoresis grade reagents from BioRad). Duplicate 0.15 × 14 × 16 cm slab gels are cast (with 12-well combs) and run using the Hoeffer SE600 apparatus. Each sample well is flushed repeatedly with buffer to ensure removal of any diffused urea and then samples are loaded by underlayering. Electrophoresis is carried out at 5 W per slab (constant power) for 4.0–4.5 hr (with gentle magnetic stirring but without cooling) until the Pyronin Y dye front is 1 cm from the bottom of the gel.

For testing tumors, we routinely load 100 µg protein for each sample if possible. Control membrane samples from the drug-sensitive KB-31 (100 µg) and MDR KB-8 (25 or 50 µg) or KB-85 (25 µg) cell lines are included on each gel. Sample volumes are ≤50 µl (if possible) to obtain reasonable band resolution, since the Fairbanks continuous gel system does not incorporate a stacking gel. To enable comparisons of immunoblotting with C219 and C494 mAbs under nearly identical experimental conditions, if possible, twin gels are run concurrently for subsequent probing with the different mAbs. High-range ^{14}C-labeled MW standard proteins (BRL) included on each gel allow direct size calibration on autoradiograms.

At the conclusion of electrophoresis, in preparation for electroblotting, gels are trimmed to remove projecting well partitions and removed from the glass plates. The gels are submerged for 10 min in deionized water and then equilibrated for 20 min at room temperature in transfer buffer (described below). Gels are handled in solutions that are above 18°C to prevent precipitation of urea. Nitrocellulose (0.45 µ, BioRad), cut 1 cm longer than the gel, is similarly prepared by soaking in water for 10 min and then in transfer buffer for 15 min.

Gel proteins are electroblotted to nitrocellulose in a Hoeffer TE46 Transphor apparatus by Towbin's procedure [46], except use of a lower ionic strength transfer buffer [10.3 mM Tris base, 79.25 mM glycine (BioRad), 20% (v/v) methanol (Baker reagent grade)] permits higher voltages at equivalent current levels while retaining sufficient buffering capacity. Transfer buffer is degassed for 15 min. Methanol in the transfer buffer prevents swelling of the gel in the low ionic strength buffer. This helps to avoid distortions and to increase the binding capacity of nitrocellulose for protein (although it may bias somewhat against elution of larger proteins from the gel). The transfer cassette is assembled while its components are submerged in a tray of transfer buffer. For optimal quality of the blots, care is taken that no bubbles reside between the gel and nitrocellulose. Fiber pads employed to maintain uniform pressure on the gel during transfer are replaced (3 mm Scotchbrite fiber pad, BioRad) before deforming from repeated use. During electroblotting, the buffer in the transfer chamber is mixed by magnetic stirring.

Electroblotting is carried out at a constant voltage of ~130 V (16.25 V/cm) for 4.5 hr. The current is initially 400 mAmp, approaching 1 Amp during the course of the transfer. Temperature in the transfer chamber is monitored. After approximately 3 hr, cold water is passed slowly through a cooling coil to keep the temperature $\leq 50°C$. After transfer the western blots are gently rinsed in PBS. The imprint of the lane origins at the top of the blot and the transferred Pyronin Y dye front at the bottom serve to indicate the positions of the gel lanes and the orientation of the transferred proteins. To quench nonspecific protein-binding sites, blots are submerged in a tray of blocking solution consisting of 5% bovine serum albumin (BSA, Sigma #A7906 throughout these procedures) and 15 mM sodium azide in PBS pH 7.4 (filtered through a 0.45 μ membrane). In our experience, blots can be stored for several months at 4°C in air-tight containers without detrimental effect. We routinely stain the gels themselves with Coomassie blue R-250 after electroblotting to confirm that nearly all of the high MW protein has been successfully transferred.

Radio-iodination of monoclonal antibodies

C219 and C494 mAbs (see Properties of C219 and C494 monoclonal antibody probes) purified by protein-A sepharose chromatography from ascites were obtained either from Dr. V. Ling or, for C219, subsequently from Centocor (Malvern, PA). In our experience, markedly superior results from immuno-blotting are obtained by utilizing C219 directly labelled with ^{125}I, rather than relying on labelled secondary antibodies. We have employed a chloramine-T procedure for ^{125}I-labelling of antibodies, which has reproducibly yielded immunoreagent at $3-10 \times 10^7$ cpm/ml and corresponding specific activities of 3–10 mCi/mg. This method, provided by Dr. J. Gerlach of Kingston

Regional Cancer Center [adapted from 57], employs less chloramine-T per µg of protein than those usually described. This presumably biases for monoiodination of antibody and results in less damage and improved stability of the antibody during storage [58].

Our standard procedure is to iodinate 50 µg of antibody, previously aliquoted and stored frozen in PBS at 1–3.3 µg protein/µl. First, two Sephadex G-25 chromatographic columns are prepared. For the first column, G-25 m beads (Pharmacia) are swollen overnight at room temperature with 5 ml/g of PBS, pH 7.4, with 0.02% (w/v) sodium azide, degassed, and 9.5 ml are used to pack a Kontes disposable 19 cm column unit. The second column is a PD-10 disposable 10 ml Sephadex G-25 unit available from Pharmacia. Each column is washed, in turn, with 25 ml of PBS, 1 ml of 0.45 µ-filtered 10% (w/v) BSA in PBS, pH 7.4 (to block nonspecific protein-binding sites within the column), 10 ml of filtered 3% (w/v) BSA in 0.9% (w/v) NaCl, 10 mM Tris, pH 7.4, and then 25 ml of PBS. Just before the iodination, fresh solutions of 0.5 mg/ml chloramine-T (Baker), 1.0 mg/ml Na metabisulfite (Baker), and 1.0% (w/v) Na azide in PBS are prepared. Na [125]I (carrier-free, IMS 30, 0.1 N NaOH solution, pH 7–11) is obtained from Amersham. The volume used to react 500 µCi with 50 µg antibody will vary with the specific activity, but is typically ≤5 µl.

For a typical labelling reaction, 50 µg of antibody in 15–50 µl of PBS, 2.5 µl of dimethyl sulphoxide (Fisher), 500 µCi Na ^{125}I, and 2.5 µl of 0.5 mg/ml chloramine T in PBS are mixed gently in a 1.5 ml polypropylene microtube and incubated for 20 minutes at room temperature with gentle agitation every few minutes. Then 5 µl of 1.0 mg/ml sodium metabisufite is added to halt the reaction. The reaction mixture is diluted to 500 µl with PBS and loaded onto the Kontes column. When the reaction mixture has passed into the beads, 10 ml of PBS is loaded on the column and 30 sequential 5-drop (~0.25 ml) fractions are collected. Duplicate 2 µl aliquots are taken from each fraction for gamma counting. Typically the peak of labelled antibody is contained between fractions 5 and 12, while the beginning of the free iodine peak is observed after fraction 15. The first peak fractions containing labelled antibody are pooled, brought to 2.5 ml volume with PBS, and loaded on the PD-10 column. The run-through is discarded and the ^{125}I-labelled antibody is collected as a single 3.5 ml fraction obtained by eluting the column with 3.5 ml of PBS. This preparation is supplemented with 0.5 ml of 10% (w/v) BSA, 0.5 ml of 1% (w/v) sodium azide, and PBS to a final volume of 5 ml, and stored at 4°C.

The average yield is 6×10^7 cpm/ml, approximately 6 mCi/mg. This radiolabelled probe is useful for a period of 2 months or more and is sufficient for assaying at least 50 western blots. For each radio-iodination, control blots of well-characterized cell lines are tested to assess sensitivity, specificity, optimal dilution of immunoprobe activity, signal intensity and background noise levels, and film exposure times, so that different aspects of the immunoprobing technique can be tuned to achieve optimal results.

Immunoprobing of western blots

Western blots to be immunoprobed are first submerged in 500 ml blocking solution, incubated at 37°C for 12–24 hr with gentle rocking, and then rinsed in blocking solution at 4°C. Each blot is then overlaid in an individual tray with 75–100 ml of ^{125}I-C219 or ^{125}I-C494 diluted in fresh blocking solution to a concentration of $1-5 \times 10^5$ cpm/ml, and shaken very gently for 20–30 hr at 4°C.

After immunoprobing, at room temperature, each blot is rinsed twice for a few minutes in 500 ml of PBS, pH 7.4, then washed five consecutive times for 30 minutes in 1 l of PBS each time, air dried on blotter paper for approximately 1 hr, and enclosed in Saran Wrap®.

The probed blots are autoradiographed using Kodak X-Omat R film in cassettes fitted with Dupont Cronex Lightening-Plus intensifying screens. Exposure is for 1–5 days at −90°C. Bound antibody is visualized in autoradiograms exposed for a range of times to obtain the optimal signal to background contrast at ~170 kDa and to confirm that signals are evaluated within the linear range of the film response.

(We have also utilized a procedure [59] that enables one to strip bound antibody from the nitrocellulose without significant elution of blotted proteins and to reprobe the same blot with a second radiolabelled antibody.)

Properties of C219 and C494 monoclonal antibody probes

The murine anti-Pgp mAbs C219 and C494 were developed by Kartner and Ling [15]. The epitopes on Pgp for these antibodies have been mapped by Georges and Ling to different continuous peptide sites near the evolutionarily conserved intracellular ATP-binding domains of Pgp [47]. The C219 epitopes have been found in the deduced amino acid sequences of all known cDNA cloned members of the *mdr* gene family, which in humans is limited to *mdr1* and *mdr3*. The epitope for C494 has only been detected in the *mdr1* gene product. Based on these specificities, it has been proposed that coordinate use of these two antibodies allows for discrimination between the different human Pgp isoforms [47].

Detection of P-glycoprotein overexpression in human cell lines and tumors

Calibration of C219 immunoblot assay with multidrug-resistant cell lines

Application of the immunoblot assay for detection of Pgp using ^{125}I-labelled C219 mAb is illustrated by the autoradiograms in Figure 1, which show results for a series of human KB cell lines that display the classic MDR phenotype. These cell lines were isolated by Akiyama et al. [14] from the KB-31 parental (drug-sensitive) line by sequential selections for resistance to colchicine. For

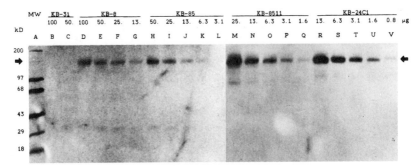

Figure 1. Calibration immunoblots illustrating detection by ^{125}I-labelled C219 monoclonal antibody of P-glycoprotein (Pgp) in the KB series of multidrug-resistant human cell lines [14] (Table 1). The labels above the reproductions indicate the cell lines and microgram amounts of membrane protein loaded in the lanes B–V of the two gels. Note that different ranges of sample amounts were assayed for the different cell lines. The arrows point to the prominent autoradiographic signals indicating detected Pgp. Approximate molecular weight (MW) in kDa of the ^{14}C-labelled markers in lane A are shown to the left. Procedures for this and the other immunoblots shown below were as described in the text.

Table 1. P-glycoprotein gene expression by C219 western immunoblotting and *mdr* RNA slot analyses

Cell Line	KB-31	KB-8	KB-85	KB-8511	KB-24C1
Relative resistance[a]					
Colchicine	1.0	2.1	3.8	40.	260.
Adriamycin	1.0	1.1	3.2	23.	160.
Vinblastine	1.0	1.2	6.3	51.	96.
Relative level					
mdr gene[b]	1.0	1.0	1.0	7.0	10.
mdr mRNA[c]	1.0	10.	30.	800.	3000.
P-glycoprotein[d]	1.0	9.5	16.	150.	250.

[a] Data from ref. 14.
[b] Data from ref. 16.
[c] Data from ref. 61.
[d] Data from Figure 3 and unpublished results, Fredericks, Chen, and Baker.

the initial-step MDR mutant KB-8 and the progressively more drug-resistant multistep isolates — KB-85, KB-8511, and KB-24C1 — increasing levels of MDR correlate with elevations in *mdr1* transcripts [12] and Pgp expression. Serial dilutions of membrane protein preparations from the various cell lines were loaded for the immunoblots in Figure 1. Detected Pgp is indicated by the prominent autoradiographic signals at ~170 kDa, resulting from bound antibody. Relative Pgp levels in the different cell lines can be estimated by comparing signal intensities per unit sample size (see Table 1 and Figure 3 below).

The same data provide an indication of the assay's potential sensitivity for detecting overexpression of Pgp within heterogeneous samples using the C219 probe, which is very important because it is expected that Pgp may be elevated in only a subpopulation of cells within tumor specimens analyzed. For a mixed cell population containing both MDR and sensitive cells, the intensity of signal detected on the immunoblot will depend on both the level of Pgp in the MDR cells and the proportion of MDR cells in the total population. The higher the level of Pgp expressed by the resistant cells, the smaller will be the subpopulation of such resistant cells that can be detected among a population of sensitive cells that do not express elevated Pgp. For the first step KB-8 MDR mutant, which displays only twofold or less drug resistance relative to the sensitive KB-31 line [14] (Table 1), the signal from a sample of 25 µg (and sometimes 13 µg, as in Figure 1) is clearly elevated over that for 100 µg from KB-31 (which is usually below the limit of detection). For a mixed sample, then, the threshold requirement for detection could be a subpopulation that overexpresses Pgp at the relatively low KB-8 level and that constitutes 25% or less of the total cells. For cells exhibiting progressively increased levels of Pgp (KB-85, KB-8511, and KB-24C1; Figure 1), resulting in signal for correspondingly smaller amounts of membrane protein, correspondingly smaller subpopulations of the resistant variants could be detected in a heterogeneous specimen.

C494 immunoblot assay with multidrug-resistant cell lines

The immunoblots in Figure 2 show results for the C494 mAb probe with the drug-sensitive KB-31 and the resistant KB-8 and KB-24C1 cell lines. The differences here are less marked than observed with C219, yet comparison of signals at ca. 170 kDa indicates that C494 does distinguish elevated Pgp levels, even for KB-8 compared to KB-31. Signal intensities for Pgp with C494 are reduced compared to C219 on comparable immunoblots, presumably reflecting the fact that there is only one C494 epitope per Pgp molecule, as opposed to two different C219 epitopes per Pgp molecule [47].

The immunoblot in Figure 2 shows bands other than Pgp that are detected by C494 mAb probe. The most prominent of these are at high apparent MW, ~200 kDa, and their intensity varies with amount of sample, but not with resistance level of the source cell line. We consider these bands, also observed for CHO cell lines and for human tumor specimens, to represent a cross-reacting antigen unrelated to MDR. (This ~200 kDa antigen appears rather labile [60], and on blots of samples processed with only PMSF to protect against proteolysis, C494 detects presumed fragments of ~70 kDa instead.) In addition to the cross-reaction at ~200 kDa, minor bands are evident for the KB-31 sample (lane A) just above and below the position for Pgp and also at lower apparent MW. We interpret these also as due to cross-reactions of the probe (conceivably involving degradation products). Analogous signals are sometimes observed for tumor specimens. In our experience the presence of

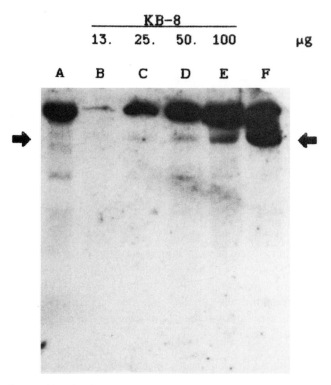

KB-8

13.   25.   50.   100   µg

A   B   C   D   E   F

Figure 2. An immunoblot showing samples of the KB series of multidrug-resistant human cell lines [14] (Table 1) probed with ^{125}I-labelled monoclonal antibody C494. Lane A was loaded with 100 µg membrane protein from drug-sensitive KB-31 cells, and lane F was loaded with 25 µg membrane protein from highly resistant KB-24C1 cells. Lanes B through E were loaded with membrane protein from the initial step mutant KB-8, as indicated above the photograph. The arrows indicate the migration position for detected P-glycoprotein, progressively more visible in lances C–F. The prominent bands at very high apparent MW (ca. 200 kDa), and the faint bands for the KB-31 sample (lane A) bracketing the position for Pgp, and also at lower apparent MW, represent cross-reactions of the antibody probe that do not correlate with multidrug resistance.

these cross-reactive bands generally does not interfere with the use of C494 to confirm a C219 signal for Pgp at ca. 150–170 kDa, but they do argue against the usefulness of C494 as a primary screening probe or for any but the most carefully controlled immunohistochemical analyses. A merit of C494, nonetheless, is its predicted lack of reactivity for the polypeptide encoded by the human *mdr3* gene, in contrast to C219, which is expected to react with all known members of *mdr* gene families, so that in theory the C219 and C494 probes can be applied in concert to discriminate products of the *mdr1* and *mdr3* genes [47].

Quantitation of P-glycoprotein in multidrug-resistant cell lines

The approach shown above for endpoint dilutions of samples to compare signal intensities on immunoblots can be useful for semiquantitative evaluations of Pgp content. Two more detailed methods for numerical quantitation of the Pgp signals on immunoblots are densitometric scanning of the auto-radiograms and direct gamma counting of bound ^{125}I-labelled mAb.

The C219 autoradiograms in Figure 1 for the KB cell line series were analyzed using a computing densitometer (Molecular Dynamics, Sunnyvale, CA, model 301) to obtain the results shown in Figure 3. For these plots of

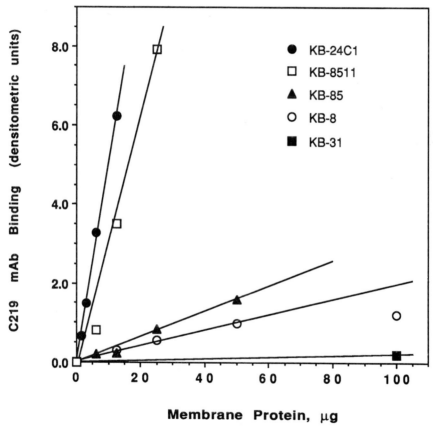

Membrane Protein, μg

Figure 3. The dependence of P-glycoprotein signal intensity from immunoblots probed with ^{125}I-labelled C219 antibody for the KB series of multidrug-resistant human cell lines [14]. The plots were derived from the data shown in Figure 1, using a computing densitometer to quantify the entire Pgp signal for each sample and cross-calibrating between the two blots comprising Figure 1 on the basis of common positive samples (not shown). The lines were fitted by regression analysis, disregarding a few aberrant points. The slopes of the lines, increasing with increasing resistance of the cell lines, furnish relative measures of Pgp content, as summarized in Table 1.

densitometric units versus micrograms of membrane protein assayed, the relative slopes of the lines obtained for the different cell lines reflect the differences in apparent "specific activity" of antigen, or Pgp content. The increases in Pgp content with increasing MDR measured from this plot are indicated in Table 1, which summarizes relevant characteristics of these KB cells. Other data have been reported concerning the KB series for Pgp determinations [61] and for *mdr1* determinations by polymerase chain reaction (PCR) [45]. Together these serve to elaborate the earlier conclusion that the *mdr1* gene encodes P-glycoprotein [10].

An alternative method for exact quantitation of bound ^{125}I-mAb is to excise size-normalized segments from the nitrocellulose blot (defined by reference to an autoradiogram as a map for location of signals and lanes). Each excised segment can then be assayed for bound label directly in a gamma counter. Compared to autoradiography, an advantage of direct gamma counting is avoidance of nonlinear biases inherent in the use of x-ray film at both low and high levels of specific activity per unit area. Satisfactory results were obtained when this method was applied for describing differences in Pgp content between cell lines [62].

All of these methods for quantitation are subject to blot-to-blot variations in background binding of labelled probe, as well as variations in specific activities of the probe and autoradiographic exposures. Therefore they can be readily applied only for comparison of samples assayed on the same immunoblot. However, blots suitable for quantitative interblot comparisons may be judged (and cross-calibrated) on the basis of standard control samples assayed on each blot. As a practical matter, we have reserved application of detailed quantitations to instances where the different samples are comprised of relatively homogeneous cell types, as in comparisons of cell lines.

Immunoblot detection of elevated P-glycoprotein in human tumors

Figure 4 and Table 2 show results from application of western immunoblotting assays to assess the incidence pattern of detectable Pgp overexpression in human solid tumor specimens from patients treated at RPCI. The principal malignancies examined have been soft tissue sarcoma, melanoma, ovarian, colorectal, gastric, and renal carcinomas. Figure 4 is a composite of autoradiographs that illustrate representative results with ^{125}I-labelled C219 mAb for assays of membrane preparations derived from preserved whole tumor tissues. Table 2 summarizes cumulative data for assays of membrane preparations, both from disaggregated specimens and from solid (whole) specimen tissues, according to the methodologies described above.

The majority of tumor specimens (exemplified in Figure 4 by lanes E, M, and N) do not yield detectable signals in the region expected for Pgp, nor does the negative control KB-31 drug-sensitive cell line (lane A, Figure 4) on most blots. Specimens that give a signal that is unambiguous and/or

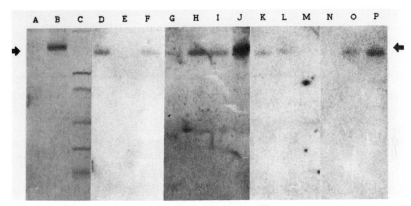

Figure 4. Composite immunoblot illustrating detection by ^{125}I-C219 monoclonal antibody of P-glycoprotein in various human tumor specimens. Except as indicated, all sample lanes were loaded with 100 µg protein of membrane preparation derived from whole tissue. The arrows at the sides of the blot mark the migration position for Pgp from the control KB-8 cell line: Lane A, drug-sensitive KB-31 cells (negative control); lane B, low-level MDR mutant KB-8 cells, 25 µg (positive control); lane C, ^{14}C-labelled MW markers (as in Figure 1); lanes D–F, three sarcoma specimens; lanes G, H, a colon tumor (G) and corresponding normal tissue (H) from the same patient; lanes I, J, another colon tumor (I) and corresponding normal tissue (J) from the same patient; lanes K–M, three melanoma specimens; lanes N–P, three renal tumor specimens.

Table 2. Immunoblot detection of P-glycoprotein

Tumor Type	Disaggregated Specimens			Solid Tissue Specimens		
	Tested	Positive[a]	(%)	Tested	Positive[a]	(%)
Sarcoma[b]						
No. of specimens	153	24	(16%)	78	18	(23%)
No. of patients	107	19	(18%)	64	14	(22%)
Colorectal	39	5	(13%)	17	12	(71%)
Gastric	13	0	(0%)	4	0	(0%)
Melanoma	19	3	(16%)	15	5	(33%)
Ovarian	54	3	(6%)	15	0	(0%)
Renal	14	4	(29%)	9	6	(67%)
Other	14	1	(7%)	6	1	(17%)
Total specimens	306	40		144	42	

[a] Elevated Pgp detected with both C219 and C494 monoclonal antibodies.
[b] Includes 65 disaggregated specimens from 52 patients analyzed at Ontario Cancer Institute.
(From Gerlach et al. [50] and unpublished data of Gerlach et al., with permission.)

exceeds that for KB-31 are scored positive. The strength of the signal can be noted on a "+1 to +5" scale. In most cases the signal intensity does not exceed the "+2" level typically obtained for a positive control sample of 25 or 50 µg KB-8 (lane B, Figure 4). Because of the heterogeneity inherent within and between the tumor specimens, as well as unavoidable intensity variations between blots, we have not considered it meaningful to further quantify the positive signals numerically.

For many of the specimens shown in Figure 4, the Pgp evidenced by the ^{125}I-C219 signals migrates at positions corresponding to somewhat lower apparent MWs than for the KB-8 positive control. This could reflect tissue-specific glycosylation heterogeneity, as discussed further below. On immuno-blots of most tumor specimens, C219 recognizes no more than a single major band, at an apparent MW consonant with Pgp. Occasionally apparent cross-reactions are encountered, however, usually at apparent MW ≤ 100 kDa; such antigens do not react with C494 mAb [63].

The results in Figure 4 and Table 2 all refer to specimens that have been tested with both C219 and C494 mAb probes. Only specimens that showed immunoreactive bands at 150–180 kDa with both mAbs are scored positive. We consider this a conservative standard; it was adopted with a view to minimizing false positives. It also ensures that only Pgp product of the *mdr1* gene, detected by both mAbs, is reported as positive. The C219 mAb, but not C494, could detect a product of the *mdr3* gene [47].

Lanes D–F in Figure 4 show results for three sarcoma specimens, two of which are positive for elevated Pgp (D and F). Cumulative data for sarcoma are shown in Table 2 (including specimens from RPCI analyzed at the Ontario Cancer Institute in a collaborative effort with Drs. V. Ling, J. Gerlach, D. Bell, and colleagues). These elaborate our earlier findings [50] of elevated Pgp expression in a significant fraction of these tumors, consistent with reports based on alternate approaches [36,64].

Pgp signals obtained from melanoma specimens scored positive for Pgp are illustrated in lanes K and L of Figure 4, while a melanoma specimen negative for Pgp is shown in lane M. To our knowledge there is no other published report of Pgp detection in melanoma at present. The reports of nondetection of Pgp in melanoma with mAbs HYB-241, HYB-612, and C219 in an immunohistochemical assay [39] and absence of *mdr* mRNA expression in another study [65] may be due to the small number of samples examined.

Lanes G–J in Figure 4 illustrate examples of Pgp detection from two colon carcinoma specimens (G and I) and from corresponding normal colon adjacent to each tumor (H and J). For most matched preparations of colon and normal colon prepared from solid samples, as here, we have observed the Pgp signals for the normal to be perceptibly more intense than for the corresponding tumor. This difference could be attributable to higher levels of Pgp expression by the normal differentiated colon cells than by less differ-entiated tumor cells. In view of cellular heterogeneity in such samples, however, substantiation of this interpretation requires further analyses at the level of individual cells [66,67].

For renal carcinoma there are numerous reports of either immunohisto-chemical detection of Pgp [38,68,39] or *mdr1* mRNA [65,40,69–71]. The results exemplified in Figure 4 are consistent with these. Lanes O and P show two Pgp-positive renal specimens, while a negative specimen is shown in lane N.

136

While tumors that arise from tissues such as colon and kidney that are normally capable of expressing high levels of Pgp or its mRNA are prominent candidates for detection of Pgp by immunoblotting, the data in Table 2 imply that such tumors may not always express elevated Pgp. Of course, the tumor phenotype would be expected to depend on the cell type of origin and progression of the tumor cells. Heterogeneous *mdr1* expression has been observed in colon and renal carcinoma, suggesting considerable clonal diversity [66,69,70].

It is quite noticeable in Table 2 that for some of the tumor types, the frequencies of specimens scored positive are substantially greater for samples from solid tissue than for disaggregated specimens. The effect is dramatic for colorectal samples (a fivefold increase in Pgp detection) and might also be significant for melanoma and renal samples. For sarcoma, however, the difference in detection of Pgp-positives for the two sample types is relatively small. It appears that the disaggregation methodology may bias more strongly against Pgp-containing cells or stroma in some types of specimens (e.g., colorectal) than in others (e.g., sarcoma). Detection of Pgp in samples prepared from solid specimens could have been aided by improved protection of the antigens from degradation, as a consequence of bypassing trauma of disaggregation procedures and cryopreserving them more immediately. On the other hand, the fact that epitopes recognized by C219 and C494 mAbs are located intracellularly would favor their survival, and in some types of disaggregated tumors (e.g., sarcoma) they are preserved sufficiently for detection.

While the incidences of detectable Pgp elevation summarized in Table 2 are appreciable for sarcoma, melanoma, renal, and especially colon tumor specimens, elevated Pgp is observed infrequently for ovarian (3/69) and gastric (0/17) tumors. Our results indicating only 3/69 positive ovarian tumors compare with recent assessments by others based on *mdr1* RNA levels [67,72–74], immunohistochemical assays [74,75], or immunoblotting [49,74]. Although we did not detect Pgp in gastric cancers, few specimens were studied (Table 2). Others have described detection of Pgp in gastric tumors based on immunohistochemical [38,39,76] or *mdr* RNA assays [77,78]. High intrinsic proteolytic activity of gastric tumor tissue might account for our negative result. Additional precautions against proteolysis might be appropriate for certain tumor and tissue types (e.g., those harboring exceptional degradative capacity). Of the tumor types grouped in the "other" category, 1 of 9 lung and 1 of 5 breast scored positive for elevated Pgp, consistent with other reports based on *mdr1* mRNA expression [65,79,80] or Pgp detected immunocytochemically [38,39,81,82].

Results for normal tissues and P-glycoprotein heterogeneity

The immunoblots shown in Figure 5 illustrate C219 mAb detection of Pgp in normal human adrenal, kidney, liver, and muscle tissues derived from an autopsy. These results, together with those for normal colon shown in Figure

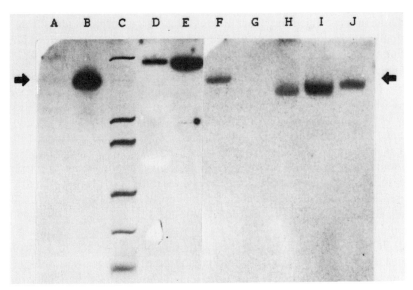

Figure 5. Immunoblots showing detection by ^{125}I-C219 antibody of P-glycoprotein in membrane preparations from various normal human tissues. Except as indicated, all sample lanes were loaded with 100 μg protein of membrane preparation derived from whole tissue. A, KB-31 cells, 50 μg (negative control); B, MDR mutant KB-24C1 cells, 10 μg (very positive control); C, ^{14}C-labelled MW markers (as in Figure 1); D, skeletal muscle; E, cardiac muscle, 56 μg; F, MDR mutant KB-8 cells, 50 μg (positive control); G, KB-31 cells (negative control) again; H, liver; I, adrenal; J, kidney. All tissues shown here were derived from autopsy of the same individual.

4, are consistent with a number of reports of Pgp detection in such normal tissues based on immunohistochemical studies with various mAbs [37–39,83], C219 immunoblotting [84], and *mdr* mRNA expression assayed by slot blots [36,40,69], sections in situ [66], or PCR [45].

The results in both Figure 4 and 5 show significant variation in the apparent MW of Pgp bands for different tissue and tumor specimens relative to migration of Pgp from control cell lines. For example, in Figure 5 Pgp from kidney (lane J) migrates with an apparent MW of 160–170 kDa, but for adrenal and liver (lanes I and H) the Pgp bands are at slightly lower apparent MW (ca. 155 kDa and 150 kDa, respectively). Observed differences in migration may be due to different Pgp glycosylation [85,86], and perhaps in some cases to resolution of distinct precursors and products of the *mdr* gene family [87,88]. On the other hand, some of the broad variation in apparent MW for Pgp reported in the literature (ranging from 120 to 180 kDa) may be ascribed to technical factors in electrophoresis [88,89]. Membrane glycoproteins display anomalous migration in SDS-PAGE systems [90–92]. For specimens with abundant Pgp, overloading in the high-MW region of the gel affects resolution. The MW of the nonglycosylated peptide backbone of Pgp has been estimated to be approximately 140 kDa, based on deduction from its cDNA sequence [31], from resolution of Pgp from N-glycosylation-deficient MDR mutants [93], and from experiments that enzymatically remove Pgp's N-glycosylated carbohydrate moiety prior to gel electrophoresis [85,86,88].

An important point illustrated in Figure 5 (lanes D and E) is the C219 immunoreactive band at just below ~200 kDa that is observed for human skeletal and cardiac muscle samples processed from frozen solid tissue. Parallel C494 immunoblots of such muscle also show a ~200 kDa immunoreactive band (unpublished data). However, it is impossible to discriminate whether the latter includes a signal distinct to these specimens or simply represents the 200 kDa C494 cross-reaction observed for control samples, whether or not there is a C219 band denoting elevated Pgp. We previously described the occurrence of this C219-reactive antigen at ~170 kDa in 11 of 13 disaggregated normal muscle specimens trimmed from adjacent sarcoma specimens [94]. The reactivity of disaggregated normal muscle was distinguishable from that observed for Pgp-positive disaggregated sarcomas in that normal muscle showed no reaction on immunoblots probed with C494. The pattern of reactivity with C219 but not with C494 is consistent with detection of an *mdr3* isoform [47]. However, this pattern has been reproducible only for samples of disaggregated muscle tissues, which evidently were subject to some proteolysis. The identity of this high MW antigen in normal muscle warrants further investigation to establish whether it represents a member of the Pgp family [35,45,47] or a cross-reaction [38,83]. Our current practice is to disregard these ~200 kDa immunoreactive bands when scoring for Pgp associated with MDR.

Relationship of elevated P-glycoprotein to course of disease

To assess possible relationships between elevated Pgp expression and clinical course of disease and response to chemotherapy, we have studied medical records of patients from whom specimens for Pgp analysis were obtained, focusing on extension of our earlier observations concerning (adult) sarcoma patients [50]. Analyses have been completed for 89 patients to date, including 15 patients whose tumors were scored Pgp-positive (unpublished data). Nine of these 15 patients had not received prior chemotherapy, confirming that elevated Pgp can occur as an innate property of tumors, even from tissues that do not normally express high levels of the marker [40,50,65,69,82]. Analyses for 51 longitudinal specimens from 21 sarcoma patients, representing recurrences and/or different tumor sites, revealed no consistent trends with tumor site, progression, or metastasis.

Our initial observations on longitudinal sarcoma specimens have indicated that for nearly all patients the Pgp phenotype does not change when consecutive specimens are tested, even in cases in which there was intermittent chemotherapy between specimens. This suggests that chemoresistance in recurrent sarcoma may not often result from tumor repopulation by cells expressing higher levels of Pgp. However, the bulk tissue immunoblotting assay could miss small foci of low-level Pgp-positive cells in a heterogeneous tumor. In this regard, a recent immunohistochemical study of childhood soft tissue sarcoma, also employing C219 and C494 mAbs, has presented evidence of progressive Pgp expression in longitudinal specimens that correlated with progressive clinical MDR [64]. This was evidenced by a change from a focal distribution of low-level expression prior to chemotherapy to a more diffuse pattern with higher levels of Pgp after multiple chemotherapy. This study concluded that any level of positive detection of Pgp expression might be clinically relevant.

A number of other recent reports in the literature that related Pgp [76,81,95] or *mdr1* mRNA [72,79,96] determinations in other tumor types to clinical responses generally support the role of Pgp as a marker for clinical MDR, but are based on insufficient data for firm conclusions. Similarly, in our own studies no clinical responses were observed for 6 Pgp-positive sarcoma patients treated with chemotherapeutic drugs to which Pgp-mediated MDR confers resistance in model systems. At this point the available data are consistent with Pgp as a mechanism involved in chemotheraputic failure, but much more extensive sampling will be required to test its utility as a marker for clinical MDR with adequate statistical analyses.

Discussion: immunoblot results in relation to other assay approaches

Frequencies of protein or mRNA elevations in tumors estimated by different approaches are not always concordant. Such discrepancies may reflect actual in vivo differences in expression of the molecular species assayed, or may have a technical or a statistical basis. In comparing evaluations of *mdr1* gene expression, it may be useful to consider that methodologies share common approaches in either characterizing fractions derived from bulk tissue (immunoblotting, Northern and RNA slot blots) or in determining properties at the cellular level (immunohistochemistry and in situ mRNA hybridization). Naturally there are inherent technical biases in each approach. Bulk tissue approaches that homogenize the specimen are subject to inclusion of tumor cell subpopulations that differ in level of Pgp expression, as well as normal tissue and other components. For tumors derived from tissues that do not naturally express Pgp, the extent of Pgp expression in resistant tumor cells of interest is likely to be greater than the weighted average measured by these assays. On the other hand, "in situ" assays at the cellular level may not be representative of the entire tumor, and cannot distinguish cross-reactions by confirming specificity on the basis of molecular size detected. The reliability of any of these evaluations will, of course, be profoundly dependent on specificity of the probes.

A difference between results from immunoblot assays and from *mdr1* mRNA slot assay data reported to date is that there has been a generally lower incidence of elevated Pgp detected by immunoblotting, even though the assays appear to be of comparable sensitivity with control cell lines.

Relevant to this point, we have recently obtained data from both immuno-blotting and RNA slot blotting assays on the same specimens of 13 ovarian, 8 renal, 12 melanoma, and 59 sarcoma tumors [97]. The instances of detected elevation of *mdr1* RNA and of Pgp gene product are concordant for the cases of renal and ovarian tumors. For sarcoma specimens, on the other hand, although 12 of 13 specimens that were positive for Pgp by immunoblotting were also positive for elevated *mdr1* mRNA, an additional 27 tumors were positive only by RNA slot blot and negative by immunoblot assay. For melanoma, conversely, only 1 of 5 specimens positive for Pgp by immunoblot also showed elevated *mdr1* mRNA by slot blot assay. One obvious possibility to explain these differences is post-transcriptional regulation of *mdr1* gene expression, but there is no direct evidence on this matter yet.

Several other factors may help to explain or qualify the findings from immunoblot analyses in comparison to *mdr1* mRNA slot assays. First, a significant issue implicit in applying these bulk assays is that measurements on tissue specimens yield data on the tissue properties that may or may not be representative of the characteristics of the actual tumor cells of interest. Thus one would expect that stroma would contribute disproportionate amounts of protein compared to RNA to the respective sample fractions assayed from tumor specimens [98]. This could result in dilution of signals from tumor cells on immunoblots compared to RNA blots. On the other hand, for either immunoblots or RNA blots one could also encounter signal enhancement due to the presence in specimen tumor tissue of specialized normal cells expressing elevated Pgp. (Yet a further dimension is encountered if one considers possible origins of differences between results for disaggregated and whole tissue specimens.) Clearly, caution is warranted in extrapolating from measurements on tumor tissue to draw conclusions concerning tumor cell properties. At present it remains uncertain which assay approach for Pgp expression would provide the most informative data for judging drug-resistance phenotypes of relevant tumor cells.

Second, a technical factor worth noting is that the cDNA probes used in some *mdr* RNA slot blotting studies do not effectively discriminate *mdr1* from *mdr3* [8]. This is not expected to be a serious source of error in assessments of *mdr1* expression, since the conclusions are supported by specific RNAse protection assays [65,70,71,79], and the available evidence suggests that *mdr3* expression in humans may be limited [42,45,97].

In situ immunohistochemical methodologies for Pgp detection at the single-cell level have provided valuable infomation concerning specific sites of Pgp expression within the complex architecture of tissues and tumors. Provided that the specimen is thoroughly sampled, incidences of Pgp expression observed in situ might be greater than for bulk assays, since it seems that the signal contribution by a small proportion of positive cells would more likely be missed in the latter case. A drawback of immunohistochemical assays applied to heterogeneous tumor or tissue specimens is that MW of the mAb-bound species is not documented.

C219 and C494 mAbs can be utilized in both immunoblotting and immuno-histochemical assays for comparative results, as they recognize both denatured and native Pgp. In addition to C219 and C494, there are several other apparently high-quality mAbs currently being utilized in Pgp assays — including MRK-16 [99], HYB-612 and HYB-341 [100], JSB-1 [101], and 265/F4 [102]. JSB-1 and 265/F4, reported to react with intracellular and extracellular epitopes, respectively, also may be useful for both immuno-blotting and immunohistochemistry. MRK-16, HYB-612, and HYB-341 are applicable for immunohistochemistry but do not react with denatured Pgp on immunoblots, perhaps because they detect discontinuous epitopes.

Except for C219, C494, and C32 [47] (see Properties of C219 and C494 monoclonal antibody probes), the epitope and family member specificities of these antibodies have not been thoroughly characterized. Specificity is inferred in studies that use a panel of at least two antibodies on the same specimen and find concordant immunostaining [8,38,39,64,81]. Although there is general agreement, there are also discrepancies between different mAbs [38,83], and cross-reactions have been inferred for each probe. Concern over heterospecific cross-reactions is well justified, albeit unpopular, as they are often observed in immunochemical studies [103–105]. For C219 and C494, application of epitope-specific competing peptides can aid in discriminating instances of nonspecific cross-reactions [47]. Recently developed antisera against peptide fragments of Pgp [88,106,107] should aid in evaluating the merits of other mAbs, as well as furnishing additional useful probes. Ultimately, immunoaffinity approaches coupled with microsequencing could confirm specificities. Most of these mAbs can be used in immunoprecipitation assays, which allow subsequent gel resolution of precipitated proteins. Certainly it is important that the molecular specificity of immunodetection be proven if the data are to serve as a basis for clinical decisions.

Summary and concluding remarks

The results discussed in this chapter illustrate detection of P-glycoprotein by immunoblotting with C219 and C494 mAbs in human cell lines, solid tumors, and normal tissues. The value of this methodological approach derives from its sensitivity and its reliable measurement of the *final mdr1* gene product, based on partial enrichment of a subcellular fraction known to be enriched in Pgp, specificity of the mAb probes, and confirmation of apparent MW of reacting antigens. The threshold sensitivity for detection of Pgp elevations is illustrated by resolution of Pgp in small samples from the least resistant of human MDR cell lines. Quantitative determinations demonstrate the increased levels of Pgp with increasing expression of the *mdr1* gene in progressively more resistant cells.

Overall, approximately 20% of the solid tumor specimens that we have analyzed exhibit elevated Pgp levels. The criterion applied for scoring elevated Pgp is coordinate immunodetection with both C219 and C494 mAbs. Evaluation of C494 binding at ~170 kDa is useful, notwithstanding cross-reactions at other apparent MWs, for confirmation that a C219 signal represents the *mdr1* gene product. Results for particular tumor types assayed from both disaggregated and solid (whole) tissue specimens are summarized in Table 2. Immunoblotting results for Pgp expression in normal kidney, adrenal, liver, and colon accord with the consensus from other studies that these tissues exhibit natural Pgp elevation, and tissue-specific heterogeneities in apparent MW of Pgp are observed. Pgp elevation is not always observed in tumors derived from such tissues.

The association of Pgp phenotype with the clinical course of disease has been examined for 89 sarcoma patients so far, of whom 15 (17%) showed elevated Pgp, and 21 furnished longitudinal specimens. Occurrence of elevated Pgp did not depend on prior chemotherapy, and our analyses show no appreciable trends to preferential association of elevated Pgp with tumor site, progression, or metastasis. No clinical responses were observed for the relatively few Pgp-positive patients who were subsequently treated with relevant chemotherapy, consistent with the hypothesis that a Pgp-mediated mechanism may confer clinical resistance.

Although the immunoblotting approach enhances specificity of Pgp determinations relative to single-cell analysis, as with all bulk tissue approaches, it obscures the perception of heterogeneity at the cellular level. We expect that future avenues of development will include and emphasize the application of multiple characterizations on the same specimen to obtain complementary information and to clarify the specific merits of each methodology. Precise definition of the histologic type and differentiation status of cells expressing Pgp by coordinate analysis of appropriate markers will aid in identifying tumor cell populations that pose an obstacle to therapy. Studies that determine chemosensitivity, MDR reversability, and drug accumulation of clinical material, together with molecular characterization of Pgp expression and regulation, will help determine the extent to which the Pgp detected is functional and relevant to clinical MDR [69,70,78,81,108].

Acknowledgements

We appreciate the collaboration and assistance of Drs. V. Ling and J. Gerlach in establishing the analytical system described here. Drs. Y.M. Rustum and H.K. Slocum made key contributions to our work through their efforts in tumor procurement and their continuous encouragement. The studies described here were made possible by unstinting cooperation of a number of clinical staff at Roswell Park Cancer Institute. We are grateful to M.J. Murawski and R.L. Meegan for valued technical assistance, and to Dr. M. Gottesman for making the KB cell lines available to ms.

Our research has been supported by grants from the U.S. National Cancer

Institute, in various aspects, CA21071, CA13038, CA40553, CA28853, Core CA16056, and Training Grant CA09072.

References

1. Beck, W.T. The cell biology of multiple drug resistance. Biochem. Pharmacol. 36: 2879–2887, 1987.
2. Bradley, G., Juranka, P.F., and Ling, V. Mechanism of multidrug resistance. Biochim. Biophys. Acta 948:87–128, 1988.
3. Croop, J.M., Gros, P., and Housman, D.E. Genetics of multidrug resistance. J. Clin Invest. 81:1303–1309, 1988.
4. Roninson, I.B. Molecular mechanism of multidrug resistance in tumor cells. Clin. Physiol. Biochem. 5:140–151, 1987.
5. Endicott, J.A. and Ling, V. The biochemistry of P-glycoprotein mediated multidrug resistance. Annu. Rev. Biochem. 58:137–171, 1989.
6. Gottesman, M.M. and Pastan, I. The multidrug transporter, a double-edged sword. J. Biol. Chem. 263:12163–12166, 1988.
7. Van der Bliek, A.M. and Borst, P. Multidrug resistance. Adv. Cancer Res. 52:165–203, 1989.
8. Weinstein, R.S., Kuszak, J.R., Kluskens, L.F., and Coon, J.S. P-glycoproteins in pathology: the multidrug resistance gene family in humans. Hum. Pathol. 21:34–48, 1990.
9. Kartner, N., Riordan, J.R., and Ling, V. Cell surface P-glycoprotein associated with multidrug resistance in mammalian cell lines. Science 221:1285–1288, 1983.
10. Ueda. K., Cornwell, M.M., Gottesman, M.M., Pastan, I., Roninson, I.B., Ling, V., and Riordan, J.R. The mdr-1 gene, responsible for multidrug-resistance, codes for P-glycoprotein. Biochem. Biophys. Res. Commun. 141:956–962, 1986.
11. Gerlach, J., Kartner, N., Bell, D., and Ling, V. Multidrug resistance. Cancer Sur. 5:25–46, 1986.
12. Richert, N.D., Aldwin, L., Nitecki, D., Gottesman, M.M., and Pastan, I. Stability and covalent modification of P-glycoprotein in multidrug resistant KB cells. Biochemistry 27:7607–7613, 1989.
13. Baker, R.M. and Ling, V. Membrane mutants of mammalian cells in culture. In: Methods in Membrane Biology, Vol. 9. Korn, E.D. (ed). Plenum Press, New York, pp. 337–384, 1978.
14. Akiyama, S., Fojo, A., Hanover, J.A., Pastan, I., and Gottesman, M.M. Isolation and characterization of human KB cell lines resistant to multiple drugs. Somat. Cell Mol. Genet. 11:117–126, 1985.
15. Kartner, N., Evernden-Porelle, D., Bradley, G., and Ling, V. Detection of P-glycoprotein in multidrug-resistant cell lines by monoclonal antibodies. Nature 316:820–823, 1985.
16. Pastan, I. and Gottesman, M.M. Multiple drug resistance in human cancer. N. Engl. J. Med. 316:1388–1393, 1987.
17. Ling, V. and Thompson, L.H. Reduced permeability in CHO cells as a mechanism of resistance to colchicine. J. Cell. Physiol. 83:103–116, 1974.
18. Ling, V. and Baker, R.M. Dominance of colchicine resistance in hybrid CHO cells. Somat. Cell Genet. 4:193–200, 1978.
19. Choi, K., Chen, C., Kreigler, M., and Roninson, I.B. An altered pattern of cross resistance in multidrug resistant human cells results from spontaneous mutations in the mdr-1 (P-glycoprotein) gene. Cell 53:519–529, 1988.
20. Ueda, K., Cardarelli, C., Gottesman, M.M., and Pastan, I. Expression of a full-length cDNA for the human "mdr1" gene confers resistance to colchicine, doxorubicin, and vinblastine. Proc. Natl. Acad. Sci. USA 84:3004–3008, 1987.

144

21. Van der Bliek, A.M., Kooiman, P.M., Schneider, C., and Borst, P. Sequence of *mdr3* cDNA encoding a human P-glycoprotein. Gene 71:401–411, 1988.

22. Shen, D.W., Fojo, A., Roninson, I.B., Chin, J.E., Soffir, I., Pastan, I., and Gottesman, M.M. Multidrug resistance of DMA mediated transformants is linked to transfer of the human *mdr1* gene. Mol. Cell Biol. 6:4039–4044, 1986.

23. Riordan, J.R., Deuchars, K., Kartner, N., Alon, N., Trent, J., and Ling, V. Amplification of P-glycoprotein genes in multidrug-resistant mammalian cell lines. Nature 316:817–819, 1985.

24. Scotto, K.W., Biedler, J.L., and Melera, P.W. Amplification and expression of genes associated with multidrug resistance in mammlian cells. Science 232:751–755, 1986.

25. Shen, D.W., Fojo, A., Chin, J.E., Roninson, I.B., Richert, N., Pastan, I., and Gottesman, M.M. Human multidrug-resistant cell lines: increased *mdr1* expression can precede gene amplification. Science 232:643–645, 1986.

26. Mickley, L.A., Bates, S.E., Richert, N.D., Currier, S., Tanaka, S., Foss, F., Rosen, N., and Fojo, A.T. Modulation of the expression of a multidrug resistance gene (mdr-1/P-glycoprotein) by differentiating agents. J. Biol. Chem. 264:18031–18040, 1989.

27. Kohno, K., Sato, S., Takano, H., Matsuo, K., and Kuwano, M. The direct activation of human multidrug resistance (MDR1) gene by anticancer agents Biochem. Biophys. Res. Comm. 165:1415–1421, 1989.

28. Chin, K.-V., Tanaka, S., Darlington, G., Pastan, I., and Gottesman, M.M. Heat shock and arsenite increase expression of the multidrug resistance (MDR1) gene in human renal carcinoma cells. J. Biol. Chem. 265:221–226, 1990.

29. Gottesman, M.M. Multidrug resistance during chemical carcinogenesis: a mechanism revealed? J. Natl. Cancer Inst. 80:1352–1353, 1988.

30. Marino, P.A., Gottesman, M.M., and Pastan, I. Regulation of the multidrug resistance gene in regenerating rat liver. Cell Growth Differen. 1:57–62, 1990.

31. Chen, C., Chin, J.E., Ueda, K., Clark, D.P., Pastan, I., Gottesman, M.M., and Roninson, I.B. Internal duplication and homology with bacterial transport proteins in the *mdr1* (P-glycoprotein) gene from multidrug-resistant human cells. Cell 47:381–389, 1986.

32. Gerlach, J.H., Endicott, J.A., Juranka, P.F., Henderson, G., Sarangi, F., Deuchars, K.L., and Ling, V. Homology between P-glycoprotein and a bacterial haemolysin transport protein suggests a model for multidrug resistance. Nature 324:485–489, 1986.

33. Hamada, H. and Tsuruo, T. Characterization of the ATPase activity of the Mr 170,000 to 180,000 membrane glycoprotein (P-glycoprotein) associated with multidrug resistance in K562/ADM cells. Cancer Res. 48:4926–4932, 1988.

34. Horio, M., Gottesman, M.M., and Pastan, I. ATP-dependent transport of vinblastine in vesicles from multidrug-resistant cells. Proc. Natl. Acad. Sci. USA 85:3580–3584, 1988.

35. Croop, J.M., Raymond, M., Haber, D., Devault, A., Arceci, R.J., Gros, P., and Housman, D.E. The three mouse multidrug resistance (*mdr*) genes are expressed in a tissue-specific manner in normal mouse tissues. Mol. Cell. Biol. 9:1346–1350, 1989.

36. Fojo, A.T., Ueda, K., Slamon, D.J., Poplack, D.G., Gottesman, M.M., and Pastan, I. Expression of a multidrug-resistance gene in human tumors and tissues. Proc. Natl. Acad. Sci. USA 84:265–269, 1987.

37. Thiebaut, F., Tsuruo, T., Hamada, H., Gottesman, M.M., Pastan, I., and Willingham, M.C. Cellular localization of the multidrug resistance gene product in normal human tissues. Proc. Natl. Acad. Sci. USA 84:7735–7738, 1987.

38. van der Valk, P., van Kalken, C.K., Ketelaars, H., Broxterman, H.J., Scheffer, G., Kuiper, C.M., Tsuruo, T., Lankelma, J., Meijer, C.J.L.M. Pinedo, H.M., and Scheper, R.J. Distribution of multi-drug resistance-associated P-glycoprotein in normal and neoplastic human tissues. Analysis with 3 monoclonal antibodies recognizing different epitopes of the P-glycoprotein molecule. Ann. Oncol. 1:56–64, 1990.

39. Cordon-Cardo, C., O'Brien, J.P., Casals, D., Boccia, J., and Bertino, J.R. Immuno-anatomic and immunopathologic expression of the multidrug resistance gene product. In

Cancer Cells, Vol. 7, Furth, M. and Greaves, M. (eds). Cold Spring Harbor Laboratory, Cold Spring Harbor, NY, pp. 87–93, 1989.

40. Kakehi, Y., Kanamaru, H., Yoshida, O., Ohkubo, H., Nakanishi, S., Gottesman, M.M., and Pastan, I. Measurement of multidrug-resistance messenger RNA in urogenital cancers; elevated expression in renal cell carcinoma is associated with intrinsio drug resistance. J. Urol. 139:862–865, 1988.

41. Ling, V. Does P-glycoprotein predict response to chemotherapy? J. Natl. Cancer Inst. 81:84–85, 1989.

42. Van der Bliek, A.M., Baas, F., Ten Houte de Lange, T., Kooiman, P.M., Van der Velde-Koerts, T., and Borst, P. The human *mdr3* gene encodes a novel P-glycoprotein homologue and gives rise to alternatively spliced mRNAs in liver. EMBO J. 6:3325–3331, 1987.

43. Juranka, P.F., Zastawny, R.L., and Ling, V. P-glycoprotein: multidrug-resistance and a superfamily of membrane-associated transport proteins. FASEB J. 3:2583–2592, 1989.

44. Chang-jie, C., Clark, D., Ueda, K., Pastan, I., Gottesman, M.M., and Roninson, I.B. Genomic organization of the human multidrug resistance (MDR1) gene and origin of P-glycoproteins. J. Biol. Chem. 265:506–514, 1990.

45. Chin, J.E., Soffir, R., Noonan, K.E., Choi, K., and Roninson, I.B. Structure and expression of the human MDR (p-glycoprotein) gene family. Mol. Cell Biol. 9:3808–3820, 1989.

46. Towbin, H., Staehelin, T., and Gordon, J. Electrophoretic transfer of proteins from polyacrylamide gels to nitrocellulose sheets: procedures and some applications. Proc. Natl. Acad. Sci. USA 76:4350–4354, 1979.

47. Georges, E., Bradley, G., Gariepy, J., and Ling, V. Detection of P-glycoprotein isoforms by gene specific monoclonal antibodies. Proc. Natl. Acad. Sci. USA 87:152–156, 1990.

48. Debenham, P.G., Kartner, N., Siminovitch, L., Riordan, J.R., and Ling, V. DNA-mediated transfer of multiple drug resistance and plasma membrane glycoprotein expresion. Mol. Cell. Biol. 2:881–889, 1982.

49. Bell, D.R., Gerlach, J.H., Kartner, N., Buick, R.N., and Ling, V. Detection of P-glycoprotein in ovarian cancer: a molecular marker associated with multidrug resistance. J. Clin. Oncol. 3:311–315, 1985.

50. Gerlach, J.H., Bell, D.R., Karakousis, C., Slocum, H.K., Kartner, N., Rustum, Y.M., Ling, V., and Baker, R.M. P-glycoprotein in human sarcoma: evidence for multidrug resistance. J. Clin. Oncol. 5:1452–1460, 1987.

51. Slocum, H.K., Pavelic, Z.P., Creaven, P.J., Karakousis, C., Takita, H., and Greco, W.R. Characterization of cells obtained by mechanical and enzymatic means from human myeloma, sarcoma and lung tumors. Cancer Res. 41:1428–1434, 1981.

52. Riordan, J.R. and Ling, V. Purification of P-glycoprotein from plasma membrane vesicles of Chinese hamster ovary cell mutants with reduced colchicine permeability. J. Biol. Chem. 254:12701–12705., 1979.

53. Crumpton, M.J. and Snary, D. In: Contemporary Topics in Moleculor Immunology, Vol. 3, Ada, G.L. (ed). pp. 27–56. 1974.

54. Peterson, G.L. A simplification of the protein assay method of Lowry et al. which is more generally applicable. Anal. Biochem. 83:346–356, 1977.

55. Fairbanks, G., Steck, T.L., and Wallach, D.F.H. Electrophoretic analysis of the major polypeptides of the human erythrocyte membrane. Biochemistry 10:2606–2617, 1971.

56. Evans, W.H., Preparation and characterization of mammalian plasma membranes. In: Laboratory Techniques in Biochemistry and Molecular Biology, Work, T.S. (ed). Elsevier, Amsterdam, 1978.

57. Sonoda, S. and Schlamowitz, M. Studies of ^{125}I trace labeling of immunoglobulin G by chloramine-T. Immunochemistry 7:885–898, 1970.

58. Chard, T. An introduction to radioimmunoassay and related techniques. In: Laboratory Techniques in Biochemistry and Molecular Biology, Work, T.S. (ed). Elsevier, Amsterdam, 1982.

59. Kaufmann, S.H., Ewing, C.M., and Shaper, J.H. The erasable western blot. Anal.

Biochem. 161:89–95, 1987.

60. Juliano, R.L. and Ling, V., A surface glycoprotein modulating drug permeability in Chinese hamster cell mutants. Biochim. Biophys. Acta 455:152–162, 1976.

61. Gottesman, M.M., Goldstein, L.J., Bruggemann, E., Currier, S.J., Galski, H., Cardarelli, C.O., Thiebaut, F., Willingham, M., and Pastan, I. Molecular diagnosis of multidrug resistance. In: Furth, M. and Greaves, M. (eds). Cancer Cells, Vol. 7, Cold Spring Harbor Laboratory, Cold Spring Harbor, NY, CSH pp. 75–80, 1989.

62. Ujhazy, P., Chen, Y.F., Fredericks, W.J., Mihich, E., Baker, R.M., and Ehrke, M.J. The relationship between multidrug resistance and tumor necrosis factor resistance in an EL4 cell line model. Submitted for publication.

63. Baker, R.M., Fredericks, W.J., Chen, Y., Murawski, M.J., Meegan, R.L., Rustum, Y.M., Karakousis, C., and Piver, M.S. Detection of P-glycoportein in human tumors by immunoblot analyses. In: Pezcoller Foundation Symposium "Drug Resistance: Mechanisms and Reversal," Trento, Italy, in press, 1989.

64. Chan, H.S.L., Thorner, P.S., Haddad, G., and Ling, V. Immunohistochemical detection of P-glycoprotein. Prognostic correlation in soft tissue sarcoma of childhood. J. Clin. Oncol., in press.

65. Goldstein, L.J., Galski, H., Fojo, A., Willingham, M., Lai, S.-L., Gazdar, A., Pirker, R., Green, A., Crist, W., Brodeur, G.M., Grant, C., Lieber, M., Cossman, J., Gottesman, M.M., and Pastan, I. Expression of a multidrug-resistance gene in human tumors. J. Natl. Cancer Inst. 81:116–124, 1989.

66. Mickley, L.A., Rothenberg, M.L., Hamilton, T.C., Ozols, R.F., and Fojo, A.T. Expression of a multidrug resistance gene in normal tissue and human tumors. Proc. Ann. Assoc. Cancer Res. 29:297, 1988.

67. Roninson, I.B., Patel, M.C., Lee, I., Noonan, K.E., Chen, C.-J., Choi, K., Chin, J.E., Kaplan, R., and Tsuruo, T. Molecular mechanism and diagnostics of multidrug resistance in human tumor cells. In: (eds). Cancer Cells, Vol. 7, Furth, M. and Greaves, M. Cold Spring Harbor Laborabory, Spring Harbor, NY. pp. 81–86, 1989.

68. Bak, M., Effreth, T., Mattern, J., and Volm, M. Detection of drug resistance and P-glycoprotein in human renal cell carcinomas. Eur. Urol. 17:72–75, 1990.

69. Fojo, A.T., Shen, D.W., Mickley, Pastan, I., and Gottesman, M.M. Intrinsic drug resistance in human kidney cancer is associated with expression of a human multidrug-resistance gene. J. Clin. Oncol. 5:1922–1927, 1987.

70. Kanamaru, H., Kakehi, Y., Yoshida, O., Nakanishi, S., Pastan, I., and Gottesman, M.M. MDR1 RNA levels in human renal cell carcinomas: correlation with grade and prediction of reversal of doxorubicin resistance by quinidine in tumor explants. J. Natl. Cancer Inst. 81:844–849, 1989.

71. Ueda, K., Yamano, Y., Kioka, N., Kakehi, Y., Yoshida, O., Gottesman, M.M., Pastan, I., and Komano, T. Detection of multidrug resistance (MDR1) gene RNA expression in human tumors by a sensitive ribonuclease protection assay. Jpn. J. Cancer Res. 80:1127–1132, 1989.

72. Bourhis, J., Goldstein, L.J., Riou, G., Pastan, I., Gottesman, M.M., and Benard, J. Expression of a human multidrug resistance gene in ovarian carcinomas. Cancer Res. 49:5062–5065, 1989.

73. Brophy, N.A., Berry, J.M., Marie, J.P., Smith, S.D., Swensen, R.E., Soudder, S.A., Ehsan, M.N., Warnke, R.A., and Sikic, B.I., Selection in vivo for high expression of the multidrug Resistance gene mdr1 by chemotherapy of human ovarian cancers, leukemias, and lymphomas (abstr. 50). In: Conference on Multidrug resistance: Molecular Biology and Clinical Relevance. National Cancer Institute, April 1989.

74. Volm, M., Efferth, T., Bak, M., Ho, A.D., and Mattern, J. Detection of the multidrug resistant phenotype in human tumors by monoclonal antibodies and the streptavidin-biotinylated phycoerythrin complex method. Eur. J. Cancer Clin. Oncol. 25:743–749, 1989.

75. Volm, M., Efferth, T., Bak, M., and Mattern, J. Detection of drug resistance in human

ovarian carcinoma. Arch. Gynecol. Obstet. 244:123–128, 1989.

76. Robey-Cafferty, S.S., Rutledge, M.L., and Bruner, J.M. Expression of a multidrug resistance gene in esophageal adenocarcinoma. Correlation with response to chemotherapy and comparison with gastric adenocarcinoma. Am. J. Clin. Pathol. 93:1–7, 1990.

77. Moscow, J.A., Fairchild, C.R., Madden, M.J., Ransom, D.T., Wieland, H.S., O'Brien, E.E., Poplack, D.G., Cossman, J., Myers, C.E., and Cowan, K.H. Expression of anionic glutathione-S-transferase and P-glycoprotein genes in human tissues and tissues. Cancer Res. 49:1422–1428, 1989.

78. Sugimoto, Y., Asami, N., and Tsuruo, T. Expression of P-glycoprotein mRNA in human gastric tumors. Jpn. J. Cancer Res. 80:993–999, 1989.

79. Lai, S.L., Goldstein, L.J., Gottesman, M.M., and Pastan, I., Tsai, C.M., Johnson, B.E., Mulshine, J.L., Ihde, D.C., Kayser, K., and Gazdar, A.F. MDR1 gene expression in lung cancer. J. Natl. Cancer Inst. 81:1144–1150, 1989.

80. Kacinski, B.M., Yee, L.D., Carter, D., Li, D., and Kuo, M.T. Human breast carcinoma cell levels of MDR-1 (P-glycoprotein) transcripts correlate in vivo inversely and reciprocally with tumor progesterone receptor content. Cancer Commun. 1:1–6, 1989.

81. Salmon, S.E., Grogan, T.M., Miller, T., Scheper, R., and Dalton, W.S. Prediction of doxorubicin resistance in vitro in myeloma, lymphoma, and breast cancer by P-glycoprotein staining. J. Natl. Cancer Inst. 81:696–701, 1989.

82. Radosevich, J.A., Robinson, P.G., Rittmann-Grauer, L.S., Wilson, B., Leung, J.P., Maminta, M.L., Warren, W., Rosen, S.T., and Gould, V.E. Immunohistochemical analysis of pulmonary and pleural tumors with the monoclonal antibody HYB-612 directed against the multidrug resistance (MDR-1) gene product, P-glycoprotein. Tumor Biol. 10:252–257, 1989.

83. Willingham, M.C., Richert, N.D., Cornwell, M.M., Tsuruo, T., Hamada, H., Gottesman, M.M., and Pastan, I. Immunohistochemical localization in normal tissues of different epitopes in the multidrug transport protein P170: evidence for localization in brain capillaries and crossreactivity of one antibody with a muscle protein. J. Histochem. Cytochem. 37:159–164, 1989.

84. Hitchins, R.N., Harman, D.H., Davey, R.A., and Bell, D.R. Identification of a multidrug resistance associated antigen (P-glycoprotein) in normal human tissues. Eur. J. Cancer Res. 24:449–453, 1987.

85. Greenberger, L., Williams, S.S., and Horowitz, S. Biosynthesis of heterogeneous forms of multidrug resistance-associated glycoproteins J. Biol. Chem. 262:13685–13689, 1988.

86. Greenberger, L., Croop, J.M., Horowitz, S.B., and Arceci, R.J. P-glycoproteins encoded by mdr1 in murine gravid uterus and multidrug resistant cell lines are differently glycosylated. FEBS Lett. 257:419–421, 1989.

87. Greenberger, L., Lothstein, L., Williams, S.S., and Horowitz, S.B. Distinct P-glycoprotein precursors are overproduced in independently isolated drug-resistant cell lines. Proc. Natl. Acad. Sci. USA 85:3762–3766, 1988.

88. Yoshimura, A., Kuwazuru, T., Ikeda, S., Ichikawa, M., Usagawa, T., and Akiyama, S. Biosynthesis, processing and half life of P-glycoprotein in a human multidrug resistant KB cell. Bioch. Biophys. Acta 992:307–314, 1989.

89. Greenberger, L., Williams, S.S., Georges, E., Ling, V., and Horowitz, S. Electrophoretic analysis of P-glycoproteins produced by mouse J774.2 and Chinese hamster ovary multidrug-resistant cells. J. Natl. Cancer Inst. 80:506–510, 1988.

90. Banker, G.A., and Cotman, C.W. Measurement of free electrophoretic mobility and retardation coefficient of protein-sodium dodecyl sulfate complexes by gel electrophoresis. A method to validate moleucular weight estimates. J. Biol. Chem. 247:5856–5861, 1972.

91. Glossman, H. and Neville, D.M., Jr. Glycoproteins of cell surfaces, A comparative study of three different cell surfaces of the rat. J. Biol. Chem. 246:6339–6346, 1971.

92. Leach, B.S., Collawn, J.F., and Fish, W.W. Behaviour of glycopeptides with empirical molecular weight estimation methods. 1. In sodium dodecyl sulfate. Biochemistry 19: 5734–5741, 1980.

148

93. Ling, V., Kartner, N., Siminovitch, L., and Riordan, J.R. Multidrug-resistance phenotype in Chinese hamster ovary cells. Cancer Treat. Rep. 67:869–874, 1983.
94. Gerlach, J.H., Bell, D.R., Karakousis, C., Slocum, H.K., Kartner, N., Rustum, Y.M., Ling, V., and Baker, R.M. Detection of P-glycoprotein in human sarcoma by two monoclonal antibodies. Proc. Am. Assoc. Cancer Res. 28:912, 1987.
95. Kuwazuru, T., Yoshimura, A., Hanada, S., Ichikawa, M., Saito, T., Uozomi, K., Utsonomia. A., Arima, T., and Akiyama, S. Expression of the multidrug transporter, P-glycoprotein in chronic myelogenous leukemia cells in blast crisis. Br. J. Hematol. 74:24–29, 1990.
96. Goldstein, L.J., Fojo, A., Ueda, K., Crist, W., Green, A., Brodeur, G.M., Pastan, I., and Gottesman, M.M. Expression of the multidrug resistance, MDR1, gene in neuroblastomas. J. Clin. Oncol. 8:128–136, 1990.
97. Chen, Y.F., Murawski, M.J., Fredericks, W.J., Karakousis, C., and Baker, R.M. Comparison of western blot and RNA slot blot detection of *mdr1* gene expression in human tumors. Proc. Am. Assoc. Cancer Res. 31:537, 1990.
98. Slamon, D.J., Godolphin, W., Jones, L.A., Holt, J.A., Wong, S.G., Keith, D.E., Levin, W.J., Stuart, S.G., Udove, J., Ullrich, A., and Press, M.F. Studies of the HER-2/neu proto-oncogene in human breast and ovarian cancer. Science 244:707–712, 1989.
99. Hamada, H. and Tsuruo, T. Functional role for the 170- to 180-kDa glycoprotein specific to drug-resistant tumor cells as revealed by monoclonal antibodies. Proc. Natl. Acad. Sci. USA 83:7785–7789, 1986.
100. Meyers, M.B., Rittmann-Grauer, L., O'Brien, J.B., and Safa, A.R. Characterization of monoclonal antibodies recognizing a Mr 180,000 P-glycoprotein: differential expression of the Mr 180,000 and Mr 170,000 P-glycoproteins in multidrug resistant human tumor cells. Cancer Res. 49:3209–3214, 1989.
101. Scheper, R.J., Bulte, J.W.M., Brakke, J.G.P., Quak, J.J., Van der Schoot, E., Balm, A.J.M., Meijer, C.J.L.M., Broxterman, H.J., Kuiper, C.M., Lankelma, J., and Pinedo, H.M. Monoclonal antibody JSB-1 detects a highly conserved epiotope on the P-glycoprotein associated with mult-drug-resistance. Int. J. Cancer 42:389–394, 1988.
102. Lathan, B., Edwards, D.P., Dressler, L.G., Von Hoff, D.D., and McGuire, W.L. Immunological detection of Chinese hamster ovary cells expressing a multidrug resistance phenotype. Cancer Res. 45:5064–5069, 1985.
103. Lane, D. and Koprowski, H. Molecular recognition and the future of monoclonal antibodies. Nature 296:200–202, 1982.
104. Van Regenmortel, M.H.V. Which structural features determine protein antigenicity? Trends Biochem. Sci. 11:36–39, 1986.
105. Van Regenmortel M.H.V. Antigenic cross-reactivity between proteins and peptides: new insights and applications. Trends Biochem. Sci. 12:237–240, 1987.
106. Tanaka, S., Currier, S.J., Bruggemann, E.P., Ueda, K., Germann, U.A., Pastan, I., and Gottesman, M.M. Use of recombinant P-glycoprotein fragments to produce antibodies to the multidrug transporter. Bioch. Biophys. Res. Commun. 166:180–186, 1990.
107. Marquardt, D., McCrone, S., and Center, M.S., Mechanisms of multidrug resistance in HL60 cells: Detection of resistance associated proteins with antibodies against synthetic peptides that correspond to the deduced sequence of P-glycoprotein. Cancer Res. 50: 1426–1430, 1990.
108. Dalton, W.S., Grogan, T.M., Rybski, J.A., Scheper, R.J., Richter, L., Kailey, J., Broxterman, H.J., Pinedo, H.M., and Salmon, S.E. Immunohistochemical detection and quantitation of P-glycoprotein in multiple drug-resistant human myeloma cells: association with level of drug resistance and drug accumulation. Blood 73:747–752, 1989.

7. Modulators of P-glycoprotein-associated multidrug resistance

William T. Beck

Introduction

Multidrug resistance associated with overexpression of P-glycoprotein (Pgp-MDR) is a well-documented experimental phenomenon whose pharma-cologic, biochemical, and molecular basis is known. Its importance resides in the fact that it appears to have clinical correlates, so attempts to reverse or circumvent Pgp-MDR clearly assume high priority. There is a considerable body of experimental work showing that certain classes of membrane-active drugs are capable of circumventing MDR to varying degrees, but it remains to be seen whether these agents will be useful clinically. The goal in this chapter is to discuss the actions of these modulators. The general features of Pgp-MDR will be briefly outlined and its and differences from other forms of MDR recently described will be highlighted. The main focus will be on compounds that can modulate Pgp-MDR. Our current understanding of the mechanism(s) by which these agents work in MDR cells will be summarized, current models for modulator design will be discussed, and some of the ongoing clinical studies with these agents, as well as their attendant prob-lems will be outlined. The conclusion offers some thoughts about future directions of modulator studies.

General features of P-glycoprotein-associated multidrug resistance

Pgp-MDR has been the subject of several recent reviews [1–7]. Briefly, cells expressing Pgp-MDR display a broad cross-resistance to a variety of "natural product" anticancer drugs of dissimilar structure and mechanism of action. This is due to decreased drug accumulation and retention, apparently mediated by the action of an ATP-dependent integral membrane protein, P-glycoprotein (Pgp). Pgp and its mRNA are overexpressed in cells displaying Pgp-MDR. The cDNA encoding the *mdr1* gene has been cloned [8–10], and when inserted into an expression vector and transfected into drug-sensitive cells, confers on these cells the complete phenotype of multidrug resist-ance. Of considerable interest, transfectants expressing abundant amounts

Robert F. Ozols (ed.), *MOLECULAR AND CLINICAL ADVANCES IN ANTICANCER DRUG RESISTANCE.* Copyright © 1991.
Kluwer Academic Publishers, Boston. All rights reserved. ISBN 0-7923-1212-0

of Pgp bearing point mutations in the nucleotide (ATP) binding site are drug sensitive [11 I.B. Roninson, personal communication]. Finally, as will be detailed below, certain classes of membrane-active agents, such as verapamil, have the ability to overcome Pgp-MDR, in part or completely.

Recent studies have demonstrated that other forms of natural product MDR are expressed in cultured mammalian tumor cells. For example, some human tumor cell lines selected for resistance to the anthracycline, doxorubicin (DOX; adriamycin), display broad cross-resistance, decreased drug accumulation and retention, and verapamil responsiveness, but do *not* overexpress Pgp and its mRNA (but see below) [12,13]. Other cell lines, selected for resistance to either epipodophyllotoxins [14] or mitoxantrone [15], are also broadly cross-resistant to many natural product anticancer drugs and do not overexpress *mdr1* or Pgp, have no alteration in drug accumulation or retention, and are unaffected by the actions of such modulators of MDR as verapamil. Where it has been studied, it appears that this form of MDR is due to *a*lterations in amount or activity of *t*opoisomerase II; accordingly, we have termed this type of natural product MDR *at-MDR* [16]. Finally, it should be noted that some MDR cell lines, notably those selected for resistance to DOX, frequently express several biochemical lesions, including overexpression of *mdr1* and Pgp, decreased activities of topoisomerase II [17–22], and in some cases, disorders of glutathione metabolism [17,21,22]. It is likely that the multitude of lesions in these DOX-selected MDR cell lines reflects the many cellular targets of the drug, including the cell membrane, topoisomerase II, and the ability to form free radicals [23].

Although these other mechanisms of MDR are not the subject of this chapter, their existence has cautionary implications for those studies in patients whose tumors do not or no longer respond to chemotherapy with natural product anticancer drugs. Because of the relative ease in selecting cell lines for these alternate, non-Pgp forms of MDR (especially at-MDR), and also because of the clinical use of the drugs employed to select such cell lines, many of the negative results seen in clinical studies attempting to detect Pgp-MDR [24] may be related to non-Pgp-based MDR, especially at-MDR. Efforts are currently underway in this laboratory, as well as others, to determine whether these other types of MDR to occur in patients' tumors, and other efforts are focused on developing new therapeutic agents to circumvent or overcome these kinds of resistance.

P-glycoprotein is the target of drugs and modulators of MDR

The evidence that Pgp functions as an efflux pump has been summarized recently [1–5,25]. Also clear is the fact that drugs to which Pgp-MDR cells are resistant and cross-resistant bind to Pgp, albeit to varying degrees

Table 1. Agents shown to modulate Pgp-MDR

Type/Chemical Class	Example	Reference
Detergents	Tween 80, Triton X-100	32
Calcium channel blockers	Phenylalkylamines, e.g., verapamil	34
	Dihydropyridines	35–37
Calmodulin inhibitors	Phenothiazines	38
Coronary vasodilators	Dipyridamole	39,40
	Perhexiline	41
	Amiodarone	42
Indole alkaloids	Reserpine; vindoline	43–45
Quinolines	Chloroquine, quinine	44,45
Acridines	Quinacrine	44
Lysosomotropic agents	Monensin, nigericin, chloroquine	44,46
		47,48
Bisbenzylisoquinoline (biscoclaurine) alkaloids	Cepharanthines	49
Isoprenoids (polyprenoids)	N-(p-methylbenzyl) decaprenylamine	50
Steroids	Progesterone	51
Triparanol analogs	Tamoxifen, clomiphene	52
Cephalosporins	Cefoperazone, ceftriaxone	53
Anthracycline analogs	N-acetyl daunorubicin	33
	Cyanomorpholino doxorubicin	54
	N-benzyladriamycin-14-valerate (AD-198)	55
Cyclosporins	Cyclosporins A, C, G, others	56,57

[26–28]. Importantly, modulators of Pgp-MDR also appear to bind to Pgp [29–31], providing a biochemical basis for their action, as will be discussed.

Modulators of Pgp-MDR

Compounds shown to "reverse" Pgp-MDR

The compounds that modulate or circumvent Pgp-MDR represent a wide range of chemical structures and different classes of drugs, including detergents, anthracycline analogs, progestational and antiestrogenic agents, antibiotics, antihypertensives, antimalarials, and immunosuppressives. Most of these agents are listed in Table 1, and their structures are shown in Figure 1. Some of the first compounds shown to reverse Pgp-MDR were Tween 80 [32] and N-acetyldaunorubicin [33], but the major developments in the field came after the seminal observation by Tsuruo et al. [34] that verapamil, a membrane-active drug used in cardiology, could sensitize VCR-resistant cells to the cytotoxic actions of VCR and VLB, both in vitro and in mice bearing VCR-resistant Ehrlich ascites tumors. Since verapamil

153

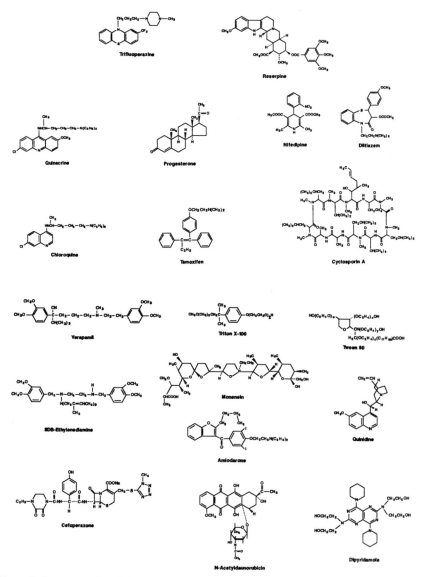

Figure 1. Structures of modulators of P-glycoprotein-associated multidrug resistance.

blocks the voltage-gated Ca^{2+} current in excitable tissues, other calcium channel blockers and calmodulin antagonists were quickly studied for their ability to circumvent Pgp-MDR, and many, if not most, of these agents were found to have varying degrees of activity [reviewed in 25]. Worth noting is the fact that the morpholino analogs of anthracyclines, originally demonstrated with cyanomorpholino doxorubicin [54], apparently do not act as

154

anthracyclines, but may behave as highly lipophilic alkylating agents [54]. Also of interest is the fact that cyclosporins exert their modulatory action through some mechanism independent of their immunosuppressive activity [57]. These compounds are also highly lipophilic. Finally, cepharanthine [49] and N-(p-methylbenzyl) decaprenylamine [50], while bearing some structural similarity to verapamil, are also both highly lipophilic agents.

Are there "rules" for Pgp-MDR modulators? Are there exceptions?
If so, what do they tell us?

Because there did not appear to be any common chemical basis for the modulating action of some of the agents shown in Table 1 and Figure 1, we studied a series of indole alkaloids for their ability to reverse Pgp-MDR [44]. Based on these studies, we developed "rules" for the design of the "ideal" modulator of Pgp-MDR [44], namely, the compound should be hydrophobic, have two planar aromatic rings, and a tertiary nitrogen that would be charged at physiological pH. In fact, looking at the compounds and classes of modulators in Table 1 and Figure 1, it is clear that many would likely conform to these rules. There are, however, possible exceptions, notably cyclosporin and N-acetyldaunorubicin. The cyclosporins are highly hydrophobic cyclic peptides and do not appear to resemble the alkaloids, but molecular comparisons of these compounds have not yet been performed. The anthracycline analog is also highly lipophilic, but it is not charged. So the question remains whether there are basic physical-chemical requirements for a modulator of Pgp-MDR or whether the property of lipophilicity is sufficient for an agent to circumvent this form of resistance.

Structure-activity studies of Pgp-MDR modulators

To date, there have been but few studies devoted to elucidating structure-activity relationships among the modulators of Pgp-MDR [35–37,39,58,59]. Based on our observation that reserpine was one of the most potent modulators of MDR in our system [44] and that it produced the strongest inhibition of NASV binding to Pgp [60], Pearce et al. [58] developed several analogs of reserpine in order to test our hypothesis about the requirements for a modulator of MDR. We found in that study that the pendant aromatic ring of the reserpine and yohimbine backbones was absolutely essential for activity. We also found that while the aromatic ring was in a spatially defined conformation in the effective reserpine analogs, the best structures resembled verapamil in three dimensions. Other structure-activity studies with dihydropyridine [35–37,39], phenothiazine [59], and dipyridamole [39,40] analogs have revealed that a wide range of compounds can effectively modulate MDR, but since many of the ineffective compounds in these series are closely related to the active ones, it suggests that subtle three-dimensional structural variations are important for this action. While the MDR "pharmacophore" has not yet been defined, these structure-activity studies have revealed a more striking degree of structural specificity for agents to "reverse" Pgp-MDR and bind to Pgp than had been anticipated.

Are all modulators equally effective against all the drugs to which a cell line is resistant?

An interesting feature of these compounds relates to the fact that a given modulator, e.g., verapamil, will enhance the cytotoxicity of different drugs differently in an MDR cell line. For example, we showed that verapamil was most effective in enhancing the cytotoxicity of vinblastine and vincristine in CEM MDR cell lines selected for primary resistance to either vinblastine or doxorubicin [61]. That there may be some unique physical or chemical features of vinblastine or verapamil in terms of interacting with Pgp is seen most dramatically in a recent study from my laboratory [62]. We found that [^{3}H] progesterone could directly photoaffinity label Pgp, and the most effective agents to block this labelling were (in addition to un-labelled progesterone) vinblastine and verapamil. Paradoxically, several other steroids, including estradiol, testosterone, dexamethasone, and aldosterone, were either ineffective or minimally effective in blocking the covalent binding of [^{3}H]-progesterone to Pgp [62]. Finally, in other studies, verapamil appears to be most effective against cell lines of greatest resistance [31]. Despite this effect, verapamil cannot completely reverse the resistance of the two most resistant cell lines, whereas it can completely abrogate the VLB resistance of the two cell lines of lowest resistance ($\approx$18- and 70-fold resistant).

Enhancement of drug cytotoxicity by MDR modulators in drug-sensitive cells

There have been reports that some of the agents shown in Table 1 are able to enhance drug cytotoxicity in drug-sensitive cells. For example, Yalowich and Ross showed that a variety of calcium-channel blocking drugs, including verapamil, enhanced the strand-breaking activity of VP-16 in L1210 cells [63]. As Pgp levels were not measured in these cells, the mechanism by which this potentiation occurred is not clear, but it is possible that the "modulators" were able to block the activity of very low levels of Pgp that may be expressed in these cells. This may also be the basis for very early reports of local anesthetic enhancement of DOX cytotoxicity in some cell lines [64]. Howell et al. [65] recently showed that dipyridamole enhanced the cytotoxicity of VP-16, doxorubicin, and vinblastine in the drug-sensitive human ovarian carcinoma cell line, 2008, which was not selected for MDR. This line does not express *mdr1*, nor does it react with anti-Pgp antibodies

156

[S.B. Howell, personal communication]. Similar enhancement of drug cytotoxicity by dipyridamole in drug-sensitive cells was reported by Asoh et al. [40]. Further, verapamil apparently enhances the cytotoxicity of cisplatinum [66], a drug that is not known to bind to Pgp or to which Pgp-MDR cells are cross-resistant. The basis for this effect of verapamil is unclear, but it suggests that other actions of verapamil may be important and raises a question about the apparent relationship between verapamil binding to Pgp and its effect on the cytotoxicity of natural product drugs to which Pgp-MDR cells express cross-resistance. For example, it has been shown that at sufficiently high concentration, verapamil can inhibit Na^+ transport [67] and also has lysosomotropic actions [68]. While it is unlikely that reversal of Pgp-MDR by verapamil, dipyridamole, and other agents is due to actions other than inhibition of the efflux function of Pgp, studies with drug-sensitive cells suggest that some of the actions of these modulators are mediated through non-Pgp mechanisms.

Mechanisms of action of modulators of Pgp-MDR

Cell pharmacology

Early studies by Tsuruo and colleagues revealed that verapamil and other phenylalkylamines, dihydropyridines, and phenothiazines that enhanced anticancer drug cytotoxicity in Pgp-MDR cells were capable of increasing the accumulation and retention of anticancer drugs, notably vinblastine and doxorubicin, in these cells [38,39], and this is believed to be the basis for the action of these agents in modulating Pgp-MDR, notwithstanding the cautions mentioned above.

Only recently has the cellular pharmacology of the modulators themselves been studied in drug-sensitive and -resistant tumor cells. Tsuruo and colleagues have shown that the accumulation of verapamil by Pgp-MDR cells appears to be similar to that seen with the anticancer drugs [30]. It is also clear that the anticancer drugs that bind to Pgp are capable of competing with verapamil or a photoaffinity analog of verapamil for binding to Pgp [29–31]. This raises some questions, however. Is the modulator itself bound and effluxed from the MDR cell in the same manner as the anticancer drug? If so, how does it exert its modulatory action? Why are the cells not cross-resistant to the modulator? One possibility is that the modulator (e.g., verapamil) binds to sites on Pgp that are different than those to which the anticancer drug (e.g., vinblastine) binds. Another is that relative Pgp-binding affinities of the modulator and anticancer drug differ. Further, the relative cytotoxic concentrations of modulators are considerably higher than those of the anticancer drugs (e.g., non-specific versus specific cellular targets).

Finally, recent studies examining cyclosporin A accumulation in drug-sensitive and -resistant cells have produced conflicting results: one showed that there was no difference in accumulation of this agent by either cell line [70], whereas another showed that cyclosporin A accumulation was decreased in the MDR cells, compared to the drug-sensitive cell line [71]. Clearly, more work needs to be done in this area to understand the cellular pharmacology of this potentially important class of Pgp-MDR reversing agents.

The binding of modulators to membranes of Pgp-MDR cells and to Pgp itself

Anticancer drugs such as vinblastine [72] and vincristine [73], and modulators such as verapamil [73,74], bind to plasma membranes from Pgp-MDR cells, and this binding is greater than in membranes from the drug-sensitive cells. Further, the binding of these agents was inhibited by other anticancer drugs and modulators, suggesting that the plasma membrane was a target for these agents. Significant progress in our understanding of the action of Pgp, natural product anticancer drug resistance, and modulator action came from the development by Safa of a photoaffinity analog of vinblastine, N (p-azido-[3-^{125}I]salicyl)-N'-β-aminoethylvindesine (NASV) [27]. Safa and colleagues showed that NASV bound to a protein specifically immuno-precipitated by anti-Pgp antibodies, indicating that Pgp is a drug-binding target of NASV [27]. NASV labelling of Pgp was shown to be specific and inhibited by drugs to which the cells express cross-resistance, as well as by such modulators of MDR as verapamil [26]. However, it is also clear that some drugs, notably the *Vinca* alkaloids, are more effective in competing for binding to Pgp than are others, such as doxorubicin, colchicine, and dactinomycin [26], suggesting that either the drugs have different binding affinities for Pgp or they bind to different sites on the protein. More recently, several studies with photoaffinity analogs of verapamil showed clearly that this agent binds directly to Pgp, and that this binding can be inhibited to different degrees by anticancer drugs whose cytotoxic action is enhanced in MDR by modulators [29–31], thereby offering a biochemical basis for its action in reversing MDR.

Where it has been studied, compounds that modulate Pgp-MDR all compete with NASV or [^{3}H]azidopine for binding to Pgp [36,37,58,60, 71,75] and suggests a basis for their action in Pgp-MDR cells. That these agents all appear to work by inhibiting the efflux function of Pgp has implications for clinical studies, as will be discussed below. What is unclear from these studies is the nature of the binding sites on Pgp for the anticancer drugs and modulators. Efforts in several laboratories, including this one, are focused on identifying the peptides and amino acids in Pgp that bind these agents. Several azidopine-binding peptides have been reported [76–78]. The identity of these binding sites will be important to our understanding of drug and modulator interactions with Pgp, and will be of immeasurable aid in the development of the MDR pharmacophore.

Verapamil effects on subcellular drug distribution

The subcellular distribution of drugs such as doxorubicin differ in drug-sensitive and Pgp-MDR cells. Specifically, while flourescence from doxorubicin is evenly distributed throughout drug-sensitive cells, it is seen to be localized in discrete, punctate cytoplasmic regions in MDR cells [79–81]. While these areas of drug accumulation have not been identified biochemically, it has been suggested that they are acid compartments [4]. Verapamil appears to affect the subcellular disposition of anticancer drugs. For example, Chauffert et al. showed that doxorubicin is accumulated into the nucleus of drug-resistant cells, and then with time, redistributes to the cytoplasm; verapamil blocks this redistribution [82]. Whether this is related to the lysosomal effect of verapamil [68] is unknown.

Effect of verapamil on ATP consumption and pH in Pgp-MDR cells

Verapamil clearly has many actions in the cell [reviewed in 67], mostly documented in excitable tissues. As discussed above, it is unlikely that these other actions play important roles in the ability of verapamil to circumvent Pgp-MDR. Of potential relevance, however, is the observation that verapamil increases the consumption of ATP [83] and the production of lactate [84] in Pgp-MDR cells. Under these conditions, verapamil is known to increase anticancer drug accumulation. The paradigm for this effect is in the decrease of ATP levels produced by metabolic inhibitors, which also causes increased drug accumulation in the Pgp-MDR cells [85].

Keiser and Joenje showed that the cytoplasmic pH of Pgp-MDR cells increased in proportion to their degree of resistance [86]. Of considerable interest is the observation that verapamil caused a decrease in this pH toward levels seen in drug-sensitive cells [86]. Whether this effect is related to the increased ATP consumption mediated by this compound [83] is not known. It will be important to determine whether these changes in pH and ATP consumption can be mediated by other Pgp-MDR modulators, such as cyclosporin A, or whether they are uniquely restricted to verapamil.

The effects of Pgp-MDR modulators on plasma membrane potentials

Using cationic fluorescent dyes, Hasmann et al. [87] have shown that the plasma membrane potential of Pgp-MDR cells is decreased in the Pgp-MDR cells compared to the drug-sensitive counterparts. Of interest are the observations that both verapamil and cyclosporin A [88] "correct" the the decreased membrane potentials of the Pgp-MDR cells back to levels seen in the drug-sensitive cells. Whether these effects on membrane potential are related to the actions of verapamil on cytoplasmic pH [86] and/or ATP consumption [83] is unknown. However, caution in interpreting these studies is warranted: the cationic dyes used to measure membrane potential are likely to be substrates for Pgp efflux themselves [89], thus complicating the interpretation of the results. Accordingly, some assessment of membrane potential independent of dye accumulation is needed.

Collateral sensitivity of Pgp-MDR cells to verapamil

A few reports indicated that Pgp-MDR cells were collaterally sensitive to the cytotoxic actions of verapamil [90,91]. These are intriguing observations whose mechanism is unclear and that need to be examined with other MDR modulators (such as cyclosporin A) and other cell lines, especially cells transfected with the *mdr1* cDNA that express Pgp. If confirmed, it could add a new therapeutic dimension to efforts to circumvent Pgp-MDR.

Is there a role for Ca^{2+} in modulator action?

Because some of the first effective agents to reverse Pgp-MDR were Ca^{2+} channel blockers and calmodulin inhibitors, there was speculation that Ca^{2+} played some role in Pgp-MDR. Indeed, Tsuruo subsequently presented data indicating that Ca^{2+} levels were elevated in Pgp-MDR cells, compared to controls [92]. However, several studies have demonstrated either indirectly by measuring Ca^{2+} levels or fluxes [93,94] or directly by patch-clamp techniques [95,96], that there were no differences in voltage-gated Ca^{2+} channels between drug-sensitive and -resistant cells. It should also be noted that some Pgp-MDR cells overexpress a low molecular weight Ca^{2+} binding protein, sorcin [97], and this added to the suggestion that Ca^{2+} is involved in this form of resistance. However, the sorcin gene is one of several that appear to be coamplified with the *mdr1* gene in some, but not all [98], Pgp-MDR cell lines. While a role for Ca^{2+} in Pgp-MDR cannot be completely excluded, it should be recalled that transfection of drug-sensitive cells with the cDNA encoding the *mdr1* gene will confer complete multidrug resistance on the cells [8–10]. Why, then, are Ca^{2+} channel blockers so effective in modulating Pgp-MDR? The cloning of the bovine adenylyl cyclase gene has revealed that the predicted protein structure shares a remarkable degree of topological similarity with P-glycoprotein [99a]. I would suggest that the structures or binding pockets to which drugs like verapamil bind are similar in each protein. Additionally, CA^{2+} channels themselves appear to share topological similarities with Pgp [99b].

In vivo and clinical studies with modulators of Pgp-MDR

General findings

Several studies with verapamil and other modulators in animals are listed in Table 2. The general finding was that these agents had some effect in

160

Table 2. Some evidence for reversal of Pgp-MDR in vivo

Tumor	Drug/Effect	Investigator	Reference
EHR 2/DNR+	N-Acetyl-DNR + DNR/53% ILS	Skovsgaard	33
P388/VCR (mouse)	Verapamil + VCR/145% ILS	Tsuruo	34
	Verapamil + VLB/150% ILS		34
	Clomipramine + VCR/138% ILS		100
EAC/DR (mouse)	Verapamil + DNR/220% ILS	Slater	101
P388/ADR (mouse)	Verapamil + ADR/~25% ILS	Radel	102
HXL (human lung xenograft)	Verapamil + VCR/63, 39% T/C (only 6-day measurement)	Mattern	103

Table 3. Clinical studies of modulators of Pgp-MDR

Investigator	Study Type/Modulator	Result	Reference
Benson	Phase I: VLB + verap	Cardiotoxic	104
Ozols	Ovarian carcinoma: ADR + verap	Cardiotoxic	105
Bessho	Refract. ped. ALL: VCR + diltiazem	Cytolysis; reversible AV block	106
Miller	Phase I/II: DOX + trifluoperazine	7/36 responses; extrapyramidal side effects limiting	107
Presant	Pilot Phase I/II: solid tumors, primarily carcinomas; ADR + verap	Some moderate but transient responses; no palliation; cardiotoxic	108
Cairo	Refractory pediatric leukemia: verap. infusion followed by VLB + VP-16	Cardiotoxic (6/11 courses); 8/11 PR cytoreduction of peripheral blasts	109
Dalton	Pilot multiple myeloma, non-Hodgkins lymphoma; verapamil + VAD (VCR + ADR + DEX)	3/8 responders, all Pgp-positive; cardiotoxic	110
Fojo	Colon carcinoma: ADR + quinidine	Ongoing	

overcoming drug resistance in vivo, but close inspection of the data reveals that the effect was for the most part a modest one. Nevertheless, several clinical studies have attempted to exploit the marked therapeutic potential of verapamil seen in vitro, and these studies are summarized in Table 3. It has been shown that for verapamil to be an effective modulator in vitro, concentrations of $1-10\,\mu M$ must be used [e.g., 34,61]. In the initial clinical studies [104,105], verapamil proved to be too toxic, as these plasma levels could not be achieved safely; the limiting toxicity was heart block. Further, there was no attempt in the earlier studies to determine whether P-glycoprotein was expressed in the patients' tumor cells. More recently, however, Dalton and colleagues achieved some success in inducing a remission in patients with refractory multiple myeloma after adding verapamil to the treatment regimen [110]. In addition to this very encouraging result, these investigators were able to examine the patients' tumor cells for expression of Pgp and show a relationship between Pgp expression and verapamil effect.

Clinical problems with Pgp modulators and their circumvention

Several problems are attendent with these clinical studies. As mentioned above, Pgp needs to be measured in the tumors of these patients. Importantly, the high concentrations of verapamil that are needed to reverse Pgp-MDR in vitro cannot be achieved in vivo. However, verapamil as given clinically and as used in most in vitro studies is a racemic mixture. It is known that R-verapamil is about 10 times less cardioactive than is the S-form [111], but both isomers are equally effective in reversing Pgp-MDR [112] and in competing with anticancer drugs and modulators for binding to P-glycoprotein [31]. Accordingly, it may be possible to enhance clinical anticancer drug cytotoxicity with less cardiotoxicity by using the R-isomer of verapamil.

Horton et al. have recently highlighted another problem [113]. These investigators were able to achieve high steady-state plasma levels of verapamil in mice bearing human tumor xenografts through the use of implanted minipumps. Under these conditions, they showed that verapamil significantly enhanced the levels of vincristine in liver, small intestine, and kidney, and the combination proved to be toxic to the animals. Likewise, Merriman et al. have found that the potent modulator of Pgp-MDR, trimethoxy-benzoylyohimbine [114], was very toxic in mice by itself. The significance of these studies is that inhibition of normal tissue Pgp is potentially a major impediment to the use of these agents to reverse clinical Pgp-MDR, and highlight the need for pharmacokinetic modelling of these agents in order to achieve a positive clinical response. These studies also emphasize the need to examine the patients' tumor cells for expression of *mdr1*/Pgp; treatments with modulators of Pgp-MDR are likely to be without effect if the tumors do not express the protein [115]. Clearly more studies like those of Dalton et al. [110] are warranted.

These studies indicate the need to develop new strategies to circumvent Pgp-MDR. For example, since the various compounds that are clinically available, such as verapamil, chlorpromazine, reserpine, etc., have different dose-limiting toxicities, it may be possible to combine modulators at lower doses to achieve effective concentrations that will block the function of tumor cell Pgp in vivo. I have suggested elsewhere other possibilities for alternate strategies to circumvent Pgp-MDR [116]. To summarize, some lipophilic anthracycline analogs are as cytotoxic in Pgp-MDR (and at-MDR) cells, as they are in drug-sensitive cells [54,55], suggesting that drugs can be designed that will not be recognized by Pgp. Antisense oligonucleotides appear to be able to inhibit the synthesis of Pgp [117] and may afford a new approach to the circumvention of Pgp-MDR. That our CEM/VLB_{100} cells are collaterally sensitive to tumor necrosis factor [118] suggests that certain cytotoxic biologicals may be effective "modulators." Likewise, immuno-toxins are equally effective against drug-sensitive and -resistant cells [119] and immunotoxins made with an antibody against Pgp are in fact more toxic against the Pgp-MDR cells than against the drug-sensitive cells [120]. Finally, some anti-Pgp antibodies appear to be tumor inhibitory [121]. Although the mechanism by which these antibodies work is far from clear, it suggests that appropriately directed immunotherapy might have some value in eliminating residual drug-resistant tumor.

Conclusions and future directions

It is now evident that P-glycoprotein is responsible for a major form of multidrug resistance. The *mdr1* gene and Pgp are expressed not only in a variety of tumors, but also in normal tissues as well. Also clear is the fact that many different drugs and chemicals can bind to Pgp and prevent the efflux of certain natural product anticancer drugs from the cell. It appears that many of these compounds share properties of lipophilicity and also have certain structural features in common, namely, at least two planar aromatic rings and a basic nitrogen atom. When the drug and modulator binding sites on Pgp are identified, it may be possible to design highly effective and specific chemicals — "MDR pharmacophores" — that will inhibit the apparent efflux function of Pgp. However, it remains to be determined whether distinctions can be made between tumor and normal tissue Pgp, and inhibition of Pgp in normal tissues may restrict the use of these types of modulators. Most clinical studies designed to circumvent MDR have not been highly successful to date because of the toxicities of the modulators, suggesting that other strategies to circumvent Pgp-MDR are warranted. Clearly, one problem with most of the clinical studies of modulators is the lack of data about Pgp expression in the individual tumors, although most colon carcinomas express the protein. Thus, in addition to identifying the drug/modulator binding site on Pgp in order to design the MDR phar-macophore, new strategies to circumvent Pgp-MDR should be considered, and include new drug design, antisense oligonucleotides, cytotoxic bio-logicals, and inhibitory antibodies.

Acknowledgments

I wish to thank Bob Ozols for the opportunity to contribute this chapter and I am grateful to him for his cheerful patience while I was preparing it. I am indebted to Linda Rawlinson for the artwork and to Vicki Gray and Fabrienne Holloway for excellent preparation of the manuscript. My work in the area of circumvention of multidrug resistance has been funded in part by research grant CA 40570 and cancer center support (CORE) grant CA 21765, both from the National Cancer Institute, DHHS, Bethesda, Maryland, and in part by American Lebanese Syrian Associated Charities.

References

1. Endicott, J.A., and Ling, V. The biochemistry of P-glycoprotein-mediated multidrug resistance. Annu. Rev. Biochem. 58:137–171, 1989.
2. van der Bliek, A.M., and Borst P. Multidrug resistance. Adv. Cancer Res. 52:165–203, 1989.
3. Moscow, J.A., and Cowan, K.H. Multidrug resistance. J. Natl. Cancer Inst. 80:14–20, 1988.
4. Beck, W.T. The cell biology of multiple drug resistance. Biochem. Pharmacol. 36: 2879–2887, 1987.
5. Roninson, I.B. (ed). Molecular and Cellular Biology of Multidrug Resistance in Tumor Cells. Plenum Publishing, New York, in press, 1990.
6. Beck, W.T. Multidrug resistance and its circumvention. Eur. J. Cancer 26:513–515, 1990.
7. Friche, E., Skovsgaard, T., and Danø, K. Multidrug resistance: drug extrusion and its counteraction by chemosensitizers. Eur. J. Haematol. 42(Suppl 48):59–67, 1989.
8. Chen, C.-J., Chin, J.E., Ueda, K., Clark, D.P., Pastan, I., Gottesman, M.M., and Roninson, I.B. Internal duplication and homology with bacterial transport proteins in the mdr1 (P-glycoprotein) gene from multidrug-resistant human cells. Cell 47:381–389, 1986.
9. Gros, P., Croop, J., and Housman, D. Mammalian multidrug resistance gene: complete cDNA sequence indicates strong homology to bacterial transport proteins. Cell 47: 371–380, 1986.
10. Gerlach, J.H., Endicott, J.A., Juranka, P.F., Henderson, G., Sarangi, F., Deuchars, K.L., and Ling, V. Homology between P-glycoprotein and a bacterial haemolysin transport protein suggests a model for multidrug resistance. Nature 324:485–489, 1986.
11. Azzaria, M., Schurr, E., and Gros, P. Discrete mutations introduced in the predicted nucleotide-binding sites of the mdr1 gene abolish its ability to confer multidrug resistance. Mol. Cell. Biol. 9:5289–5297, 1989.
12. Bhalla, K., Hindenburg, A., Taub, R.N., Grant, S. Isolation and characterization of an anthracyline-resistant human leukemic cell line. Cancer Res. 45:3657–3662, 1985.
13. McGrath, T., and Center, M.S. Adriamycin resistance in HL60 cells in the absence of detectable P-glycoprotein. Biochem. Biophys. Res. Commun. 145:1171–1176, 1987.
14. Danks, M.K., Yalowich, J.C., and Beck, W.T. Atypical multiple drug resistance in a human leukemic cell line selected for resistance to teniposide (VM-26). Cancer Res. 47:1297–1301, 1987.
15. Harker, W.G., Slade, D.L., Dalton, W.S., Meltzer, P.S., and Trent, J.M. Multidrug resistance in mitoxantrone-selected HL-60 leukemia cells in the absence of P-glycoprotein overexpression. Cancer Res. 49:4542–4549, 1989.
16. Danks, M.K., Schmidt, C.A., Cirtain, M.C., Suttle, D.P., and Beck, W.T. Altered catalytic activity of and DNA cleavage by DNA topoisomerase II from human leukemic cells selected for resistance to VM-26. Biochemistry 27:8861–8869, 1988.
17. Fairchild, C.R., Ivy, S.P., Kao-Shan, C.-S., Whang-Peng, J., Rosen, N., Israel, M.A., Melera, P.W., Cowan, K.H., and Goldsmith, M.E. Isolation of amplified and over-expressed DNA sequences from adriamycin-resistant human breast cancer cells. Cancer Res. 47:5141–5148, 1987.
18. Sinha, B.K., Haim, N., Dusre, L., Kerrigan, D., and Pommier, Y. DNA strand breaks produced by etoposide (VP-16,213) in sensitive and resistant human breast tumor cells: implications for the mechanism of action. Cancer Res. 48:5096–5100, 1988.

164

19. Deffie, A.M., Batra, J.K., and Goldenberg, G.J. Direct correlation between DNA topoisomerase II activity and cytotoxicity in adriamycin-sensitive and -resistant P388 leukemia cell lines. Cancer Res. 49:58–62, 1989.

20. Cowan, K.H., Batist, G., Tulpule, A., Sinha, B.K., and Myers, C.E. Similar biochemical changes associated with multidrug resistance in human breast cancer cells and carcinogen-induced resistance to xenobiotics in rats. Proc. Natl. Acad. Sci. USA 83:9328–9332, 1986.

21. Bellamy, W.T., Dalton, W.S., Meltzer, P., and Dorr, R.T. Role of glutathione and its associated enzymes in multidrug-resistant human myeloma cells. Biochem. Pharmacol. 38:787–793, 1989.

22. Yusa, K., Hamada, H., and Tsuruo, T. Comparison of glutathione S-transferase activity between drug-resistant and -sensitive human tumor cells: is glutathione S-transferase associated with multidrug resistance? Cancer Chemother. Pharmacol. 22:17–20, 1988.

23. Myers, C. Anthracyclines. In: Cancer Chemotherapy 8, Pinedo, H.M., and Chabner, B.A. (eds). Elsevier Science, Amsterdam, pp. 52–64, 1986.

24. Goldstein, L.J., Galski, H., Fojo, A., Willingham, M., Lai S.-I., Gazdar, A., Pirker, R., Green, A., Crist, W., Brodeur, G.M., Lieber, M., Cossman, J., Gottesman, M.M., and Pastan, I. Expression of a multidrug resistance gene in human cancers. J. Natl. Cancer Inst. 81:116–124, 1989.

25. Beck, W.T. Drug accumulation and binding in P-glycoprotein-associated multidrug resistance. In: Molecular and Cellular Biology of Multidrug Resistance in Tumor Cells, Roninson, I.B. (ed) Plenum Publishing, New York, pp. 215–227, 1991.

26. Cornwell, M.M., Safa, A.R., Felsted, R.L., Gottesman, M.M., and Pastan, I. Membrane vesicles from multidrug-resistant human cancer cells contain a specific 150- to 170-kDa protein detected by photoaffinity labeling. Proc. Natl. Acad. Sci. USA 83:3847–3850, 1986.

27. Safa, A.R., Glover, C.J., Meyers, M.B., Biedler, J.L., and Felsted, R.L. Vinblastine photoaffinity labeling of a high molecular weight surface membrane glycoprotein specific for multidrug-resistant cells. J. Biol. Chem. 261:6137–6140, 1986.

28. Safa, A.R., Mehta, N.D., and Agresti, M. Photoaffinity labeling of P-glycoprotein in multidrug resistant cells with photoactive analogs of colchicine. Biochem. Biophys. Res. Commun. 162:1402–1408, 1989.

29. Safa, A.R. Photoaffinity labeling of the multidrug-resistance-related P-glycoprotein with photoactive analogs of verapamil. Proc. Natl. Acad. Sci. USA 85:7187–7191, 1988.

30. Yusa, K., and Tsuruo, T. Reversal mechanism of multidrug resistance by verapamil: direct binding of verapamil to P-glycoprotein on specific sites and transport of verapamil outward across the plasma membrane of K562/ADM cells. Cancer Res. 49:5002–5006, 1989.

31. Qian, X., and Beck, W.T. Binding of an optically pure photoaffinity analog of verapamil, LU-49888, to P-glycoprotein from multidrug-resistant human leukemic cell lines. Cancer Res. 50:1132–1137, 1990.

32. Riehm, H., and Biedler, J.L. Potentiation of drug effect by Tween 80 in Chinese hamster cells resistant to actinomycin D and daunomycin. Cancer Res. 32:1195–1200, 1972.

33. Skovsgaard T. Circumvention of resistance to daunorubicin by N-acetyldaunorubicin in Ehrlich ascites tumor. Cancer Res. 40:1077–1083, 1980.

34. Tsuruo, T., Iida, H., Tsukagoshi, S., and Sakurai, Y. Overcoming of vincristine resistance in P388 leukemia *in vivo* and *in vitro* through enhanced cytotoxicity of vincristine and vinblastine by verapamil. Cancer Res. 41:1967–1972, 1981.

35. Kamiwatari, M., Nagata, Y., Kikuchi, H., Yoshimura, A., Sumizawa, T., Shudo, N., Sakoda, R., Seto, K., and Akiyama, S.-I. Correlation between reversing of multidrug resistance and inhibiting of [^{3}H]azidopine photolabeling of P-glycoprotein by newly synthesized dihydropyridine analogues in a human cell line. Cancer Res. 49:3190–3195, 1989.

36. Nogae, I., Kohno, K., Kikuchi, J., Kuwano, M., Akiyama, S.-I., Kiue, A., Suzuki, K.-I., Yoshida, Y., Cornwell, M.M., Pastan, I., and Gottesman, M.M. Analysis of structural

165

features of dihydropyridine analogs needed to reverse multidrug resistance and to inhibit photoaffinity labeling of P-glycoprotein. Biochem. Pharmacol. 38:519–527, 1989.

37. Yoshinari, T., Iwasawa, Y., Miura, K., Takahashi, I.S., Fukuroda, T., Suzuki, K., and Okura, A. Reversal of multidrug resistance by new dihydropyridines with lower calcium antagonistic activity. Cancer Chemother. Pharmacol. 24:367–370, 1989.

38. Tsuruo, T., Iida, H., Tsukagoshi, S., and Sakurai, Y. Increased accumulation of vincristine and adriamycin in drug-resistant P388 tumor cells following incubation with calcium antagonists and calmodulin inhibitors. Cancer Res. 42:4730–4733, 1982.

39. Ramu, N., and Ramu, A. Circumvention of adriamycin resistance by dipyridamole analogues: a structure-activity relationship study. Int. J. Cancer 43:487–491, 1989.

40. Asoh, K.-I., Saburi, Y., Sato, S.-I., Nogae, I., Kohno, K., and Kuwano, M. Potentiation of some anticancer agents by dipyridamole against drug-sensitive and drug-resistant cancer cell lines, Jpn. J. Cancer Res. 80:475–481, 1989.

41. Ramu, A., Fuks, Z., Gatt, S., and Glaubiger, D. Reversal of acquired resistance to doxorubicin in P388 murine leukemia cells by perhexiline maleate. Cancer Res, 44: 144–148, 1984.

42. Chauffert, B., Martin, M.S., Hammann, A., Michel, M.F., and Martin, F. Amiodarone-induced enhancement of doxorubicin and 4'deoxydoxorubicin cytotoxicity to rat colon cancer cells *in vitro* and *in vivo*. Cancer Res. 46:825–830, 1986.

43. Wakusawa, S., Miyamoto, K., and Koshiura, R. Increase of sensitivity and uptake of vinblastine by reserpine in rat ascites hepatoma. Jpn. J. Pharmacol. 36:187–195, 1984.

44. Zamora, J.M., Pearce, H.L., and Beck, W.T. Physical-chemical properties shared by compounds that modulate multidrug resistance in human leukemic cells. Mol. Pharmacol. 33:454–462, 1988.

45. Inaba, M., and Nagashima, K. Non-antitumor vinca alkaloids reverse multidrug resistance in P388 leukemia cells *in vitro*. Jpn. J. Cancer Res. 77:197–204, 1986.

46. Klohs, W.D., and Steinkampf, R.W. The effect of lysosomotropic agents and secretory inhibitors on anthracycline retention and activity in multiple drug-resistant cells. Mol. Pharmacol. 34:180–185, 1989.

47. Zamora, J.M., and Beck, W.T. Chloroquine enhancement of anticancer drug cytotoxicity in multiple drug resistant human leukemic cells. Biochem. Pharmacol. 35:4303–4310, 1986.

48. Shiraishi, N., Akiyama, S.-I., Kobayashi, M., and Kuwano, M. Lysosomotropic agents reverse multiple drug resistance in human cancer cells. Cancer Lett. 30:251–259, 1986.

49. Shiraishi, N., Akiyama, S.-I., Nakagawa, M., Kobayashi, M., and Kuwano, M. Effect of bisbenzylisoquinoline (biscoclaurine) alkaloids on multidrug resistance in KB human cancer cells. Cancer Res. 47:2413–2416, 1987.

50. Nakagawa, M., Akiyama, S.-I., Yamaguchi, T., Shiraishi, N., Ogata, J., and Kuwano, M. Reversal of multidrug resistance by synthetic isoprenoids in the KB human cancer cell line. Cancer Res. 46:4453–4457, 1986.

51. Yang, C.-P.H., DePinho, S.G., Greenberger, L.M., Areci, R.J., and Horwitz, S.B. Progesterone interacts with P-glycoprotein in multidrug-resistant cells and in the endo-metrium of gravid uterus. J. Biol. Chem. 264:782–788, 1989.

52. Ramu, A. Glaubiger, D., and Fuks, Z. Reversal of acquired resistance to doxorubicin in P388 murine leukemia cells by tamoxifen and other triparanol analogues. Cancer Res. 44:4392–4395, 1984.

53. Goslan, M.P., Lum, B.L., and Sikic B.I. Reversal by cefoperazone of resistance to etoposide, doxorubicin, and vinblastine in multidrug resistant human sarcoma cells. Cancer Res. 49:6901–6905, 1989.

54. Scudder, S.A., Brown, J.M., and Sikic, B.I. DNA cross-linking and cytotoxicity of the alkylating cyanomorpholino derivative of doxorubicin in multidrug-resistant cells. J. Natl. Cancer Inst. 80:1294–1298, 1988.

55. Ganapathi, R., Grabowski, D., Sweatman, T.W., Seshadri, R., and Israel, M. N-Benzyladriamycin-14-valerate *versus* progressively doxorubicin resistant murine tumors:

166

cellular pharmacology and characterization of cross resistance *in vitro* and *in vivo*. Br. J. Cancer 60:819–826, 1989.

56. Slater, L.M., Sweet, P., Stupecky, M., and Gupta, S. Cyclosporin A reverses vincristine and daunorubicin resistance in acute lymphatic leukemia in vivo. J. Clin. Invest. 77:1405–1408, 1986.

57. Twentyman, P.R., Fox, N.E., and White, D.J.G. Cyclosporin A and its analogues as modifiers of adriamycin and vincristine resistance in a multidrug resistant human lung cancer cell line. Br. J. Cancer 56:55–57, 1987.

58. Pearce, H.L., Safa, A.R., Bach, N.J., Winter, M.A., Cirtain, M.C., and Beck, W.T. Essential features of the P-glycoprotein pharmacophore as defined by a series of reserpine analogs that modulate multidrug resistance. Proc. Natl. Acad. Sci. USA 86:5128–5132, 1989.

59. Ford, J.M., Prozialeck, W.C., and Hait, W.N. Structural features determining activity of phenothiazines and related drugs for inhibition of cell growth and reversal of multidrug resistance. Mol. Pharmacol. 35:105–115, 1989.

60. Beck, W.T., Cirtain, M.C., Glover, C.J., Felsted, R.L., and Safa, A.R. Effects of indole alkaloids on multidrug resistance and labeling of P-glycoprotein by a photoaffinity analog of vinblastine. Biochem. Biophys. Res. Commun. 153:959–966, 1988.

61. Beck, W.T., Cirtain, M.C., Look, A.T., and Ashmun, R.A. Reversal of *Vinca* alkaloid resistance but not multiple drug resistance in human leukemic cells by verapamil. Cancer Res. 46:778–784, 1986.

62. Qian, X.-D. and Beck, W.T. Progesterone photoaffinity labels P-glycoprotein in multi-drug resistant human leukemic lymphoblasts. J. Biol. Chem. 265:18753–18756, 1990.

63. Yalowich, J.C. and Ross, W.E. Potentiation of etoposide induced DNA damage by calcium antagonists in L1210 cells *in vitro*. Cancer Res. 44:3360–3365, 1984.

64. Chlebowski, R.T., Block, J.B., Cundiff, D., and Dietrich, M.F. Doxorubicin cytotoxicity enhanced by local anesthetics in a human melanoma cell line. Cancer Treat. Rep. 66: 121–125, 1982.

65. Howell, S.B., Hom, D., Sanga, R., Vick, J.S., and Abramson, I.S. Comparison of the synergistic potentiation of etoposide, doxorubicin, and vinblastine cytotoxicity by dipyridamole. Cancer Res. 49:3178–3183, 1989.

66. Simmonds, A.P., Moyes, P., Nicol, A., Davidson, K.G., and Faichney, A. Enhancement of cytotoxicity of vindesine and *cis*-platinum for human lung tumours by the use of verapamil *in vitro*. Br. J. Cancer 54:1015–1018, 1986.

67. Janis, R.A. and Scriabine, A. Sites of action of Ca^{2+} channel inhibitors. Biochem. Pharmacol. 32:3499–3507, 1983.

68. Ranganathan, S. and Jackson, R.L. Effect of calcium-channel-blocking drugs on lysosomal function in human skin fibroblasts. Biochem. Pharmacol 33:2377–2382, 1984.

69. Tsuruo, T., Iida, H., Yamashiro, M., Tsukagoshi, S., and Sakurai, Y. Enhancement of vincristine- and adriamycin-induced cytotoxicity by verapamil in P388 leukemia and its sublines resistant to vincristine and adriamycin. Biochem. Pharmacol. 31:3138–3140, 1982.

70. Hait, W.N., Stein, J.M., Koletsky, A.J., Harding, M.W., and Handschumacher, R.E. Activity of cyclosporin A and a non-immunosuppressive cyclosporin against multidrug resistant leukemic cell lines. Cancer Commun. 1:35–43, 1989.

71. Goldberg, H., Ling, V., Wong, P.Y., and Skorecki, K. Reduced cyclosporin accumulation in multidrug-resistant cells. Biochem. Biophys. Res. Commun. 152:552–558, 1988.

72. Cornwell, M.M., Gottesman, M.M., and Pastan, I.H. Increased vinblastine binding to membrane vesicles from multidrug-resistant KB cells. J. Biol. Chem. 281:7921–7928, 1986.

73. Naito, M. and Tsuruo, T. Competitive inhibition by verapamil of ATP-dependent high affinity vincristine binding to the plasma membrane of multidrug-resistant K562 cells without calcium ion involvement. Cancer Res. 49:1452–1455, 1989.

74. Naito, M., Hamada, H., and Tsuruo, T. ATP/Mg^{2+}-dependent binding of vincristine to

167

the plasma membrane of multidrug-resistant K562 cells. J. Biol. Chem. 263:11887–11891, 1988.

75. Akiyama S.-I., Yoshimura, A., Kikichi, H., Sumizawa, T., Kuwano, M., and Tahara, Y. Synthetic isoprenoid photoaffinity labeling of P-glycoprotein specific to multidrug-resistant cells. Mol. Pharmacol. 36:730–735, 1989.

76. Yang, C.P., Mellado, W., and Horwitz, S.B. Azidopine photoaffinity labeling of multidrug resistance-associated glycoproteins. Biochem. Pharmacol. 37:1417–1421, 1988.

77. Bruggemann, E.P., Germann, U.A., Gottesman, M.M., and Pastan, I. Two different regions of phosphoglycoprotein are photoaffinity-labeled by azidopine. J. Biol. Chem. 264:15483–15488, 1989.

78. Yoshimura, A., Kuwazuru, Y., Sumizawa, T., Ichikawa, M., Ikeda, S.-I., Uda, T., and Akiyama, S.-I. Cytoplasmic orientation and two-domain structure of the multidrug transporter, P-glycoprotein, demonstrated with sequence-specific antibodies. J. Biol. Chem. 264:16282–16291, 1989.

79. Beck, W.T., Danks, M.K., Yalowich, J.C., Zamora, J.M., and Cirtain, M.C. Different mechanisms of multiple drug resistance in two human leukemic cell lines. In: Mechanisms of Drug Resistance in Neoplastic Cells, Wooley, P. and Tew, K. (eds). Academic Press, New York, pp. 211–222, 1988.

80. Willingham, M.C., Cornwell, M.M., Cardarelli, C.O., Gottesman, M.M., and Pastan, I. Single cell analysis of daunomycin uptake and efflux in multidrug-resistant and -sensitive KB cells: effects of verapamil and other drugs. Cancer Res. 46:5941–5946, 1986.

81. Hindenburg, A.A., Gervasoni, J.E. Jr., Krishna, S., Stewart, V.J., Rosado, M., Lutzky, J., Bhalla, K., Baker, M.A., and Taub, R.N. Intracellular distribution and pharmacokinetics of daunorubicin in anthracycline-sensitive and -resistant HL-60 cells. Cancer Res. 49:4607–4614, 1989.

82. Chauffert, B., Martin, F., Caignard, A., Jeannin, J.-F., and Leclerc, A. Cytofluorescence localization of adriamycin in resistant colon cancer cells. Cancer Chemother. Pharmacol. 13:14–18, 1984.

83. Broxterman, H.J., Pinedo, H.M., Kuiper, C.M., Kaptein, L.C.M, Schuurhuis, G.J., and Lankelma, J. Induction by verapamil of a rapid increase in ATP consumption in multidrug-resistant tumor cells. FASEB J. 2:2278–2282, 1988.

84. Broxterman, H.J., Pinedo, H.M., Kuiper, C.M., Schuurhuis, G.J., and Lankelma, J. Glycolysis in P-glycoprotein-overexpressing human tumor cell lines. Effects of resistance-modifying agents. FEBS Lett. 247:405–410, 1989.

85. Beck, W.T., Cirtain, M.C., and Lefko, J.L. Energy-dependent reduced drug binding as a mechanism of Vinca alkaloid resistance in human leukemic lymphoblasts. Mol. Pharmacol. 24:485–492, 1983.

86. Keizer, H.G. and Joenje, H. Increased cytosolic pH in multidrug-resistant human lung tumor cells: effect of verapamil. J. Natl Cancer Inst. 81:706–709, 1989.

87. Hasmann, M., Valet, G.K., Tapiero, H., Trevorrow, K., and Lampidis, T. Membrane potential differences between adriamycin-sensitive and -resistant cells as measured by flow cytometry. Biochem. Pharmacol. 38:305–312, 1989.

88. Vayuvegula, B., Slater, L., Meador, J., and Gupta, S. Correction of altered plasma membrane potentials. A possible mechanism of cyclosporin A and verapamil reversal of pleiotropic drug resistance in neoplasia. Cancer Chemother. Pharmacol. 22:163–168, 1988.

89. Tapiero, H., Munck, J.-N., Fourcade, A. and Lampidis, T.J. Cross-resistance to rhodamine 123 in adriamycin- and daunorubicin-resistant Friend leukemia cell variants. Cancer Res. 44:5544–5549, 1984.

90. Warr, J.R., Brewer, F., Anderson, M., and Fergusson, J. Verapamil hypersensitivity of vincristine resistant Chinese hamster ovary cell lines. Cell Biol. Intl. Rep. 10:389–399, 1986.

91. Cano-Gauci, D.F. and Riordan, J.R. Action of calcium antagonists on multidrug resistant cells. Biochem. Pharmacol. 36:2115–2123, 1987.

168

92. Tsuruo, T., Iida, H., Kawabata, H., Tsukagoshi, S., and Sakurai, Y. High calcium content of pleiotropic drug-resistant P388 and K562 leukemia and Chinese hamster ovary cells. Cancer Res 44:5095–5099, 1984.

93. Huet, S. and Robert, J. The reversal of doxorubicin resistance by verapamil is not due to an effect on calcium channels. Int. J. Cancer 41:283–286, 1988.

94. Kessel, D. and Wilberding, C. Interactions between calcium antagonists, calcium fluxes and anthracycline transport. Cancer Lett. 25:97–101, 1984.

95. Yamashita, N., Hamada, H., Tsuruo, T., and Ogata, E. Enhancement of voltage-gated Na^+ channel current associated with multidrug resistant in human leukemia cells. Cancer Res. 47:3736, 3741, 1987.

96. Lee, S.C., Deutsch, C., and Beck, W.T. Comparison of ion channels in multidrug-resistant and -sensitive human leukemic cells. Proc. Natl. Acad. Sci. USA 85:2019–2023, 1988.

97. Meyers, M.B., Schneider, K.A., Spengler, B.A., Chang, T.D., and Biedler, J.L. Sorcin (V19), a soluble acidic calcium-binding protein overproduced in multidrug-resistant cells. Identification of the protein by anti-sorcin antibody. Biochem. Pharmacol. 36:2373–2380, 1987.

98. Van der Bliek, A.M., Meyers, M.B., Biedler, J.L., Hes, E., and Borst, P. A 22-kd protein (sorcin/V19) encoded by an amplified gene in multidrug-resistant cells, is homologous to the calcium-binding light chain of calpain. EMBO J 5:3201–3208, 1986.

99a. Krupinski, J., Coussen, F., Bakalyar, H.A., Tang, W.-J., Feinstein, P.G., Orth, K., Slaughter, C., Reed, R.R., and Gilman, A.G. Adenylyl cyclase amino acid sequence: possible channel- or transporter-like structure. Science 244:1558–1564, 1989.

99b. Catterall, W.B. Structure and function of voltage-sensitive ion channels. Science 242: 50–61, 1988.

100. Tsuruo, T., Iida, H., Nojiri, M., Tsukagoshi, S., and Sakurai, Y. Potentiation of chemotherapeutic effect of vincristine in vincristine resistant tumor bearing mice by calmodulin inhibitor clomipramine. J. Pharm. Dyn. 6:145–147, 1983.

101. Slater, L.M., Murray, S.L., and Weitzer, M.W. Verapamil restoration of daunorubicin responsiveness in daunorubicin-resistant Ehrlich ascites carcinoma. J. Clin. Invest. 70:1131–1134, 1982.

102. Radel, S., Bankusli, I., Mayhew, E., and Rustum, Y.M. The effects of verapamil and a tiapamil analogue, DMDP, on adriamycin-induced cytotoxicity in P388 adriamycin-resistant and -sensitive leukemia *in vitro* and *in vivo*. Cancer Chemother. Pharmacol. 21:25–30, 1988.

103. Mattern, J., Bak, M., and Volm, M. Occurrence of a multidrug-resistant phenotype in human lung xenografts. Br. J. Cancer 56:407–411, 1987.

104. Benson, A.B. III, Trump, D.L., Koeller, J.M., Egorin, M.I., Olman, E.A., White, R.S., Davis, T.E., and Tormey, D.C. Phase I study of vinblastine and verapamil given by concurrent IV infusion. Cancer Treat Rep. 69:795–799, 1985.

105. Ozols, R.F., Cunnion, R.E., Klecker, R.W. Jr., Hamilton, T.C., Ostchega, Y., Parrillo, J.E., and Young, R.C. Verapamil and adriamycin in the treatment of drug-resistant ovarian cancer patients. J. Clin. Oncol. 5:641–647, 1985.

106. Bessho, F., Kinumaki, H., Kobayashi, M., Habu, H., Nakamura, K., Yokota, S., Tsuruo, T., and Kobayashi, N. Treatment of children with refractory acute lymphocytic leukemia with vincristine and diltiazem. Med. Pediatr. Oncol. 13:199–202, 1985.

107. Miller, R.L., Bukowski, R.M., Budd, G.T., Purvis, J., Weick, J.K., Shepard, K., Midha, K.K., and Ganapathi, R. Clinical modulation of doxorubicin resistance by the calmodulin-inhibitor, trifluoperazine: a phase I/II trial. J. Clin. Oncol. 6:880–888, 1988.

108. Presant, G.A., Kennedy, P.S., Wiseman, C., Gala, K., Bouzaglou, S., Wyres, M., and Naessig, V. Verapamil reversal of clinical doxorubicin resistance in human cancer. A Wilshire Oncology Medical Group pilot phase I-II study. Am. J. Clin. Oncol. 9:355–357, 1986.

109. Cairo, M.S., Siegel, S., Anas, N., and Sender, L. Clinical trial of continuous infusion

verapamil, bolus vinblastine, and continous infusion VP-16 in drug-resistant pediatric tumors. Cancer Res. 49:1063–1066, 1989.

110. Dalton, W.S., Grogan, T.M., Meltzer, P.S., Scheper, R.J., Durie, B.G.M., Taylor, C.W., Miller, T.P., and Salmon, S.E. Drug-resistance in mulptiple myeloma and non-Hodgkin's lymphoma: detection of P-glycoprotein and potential circumvention by addition of verapamil to chemotherapy. J. Clin. Oncol. 7:415–424, 1989.

111. Echizen, H., Brecht, T., Neidergesass, S., Vogelgesang, B., and Eichelbaum, M. The effect of dextro-, levo-, and racemic verapamil on atrioventricular conduction in humans. Am. Heart J. 109:210–217, 1985.

112. Keilhauer, G., Emling, F., Raschack, M., Gries, J., and Schlick, E. The use of R-verapamil (R-VPM) is superior to racemic VPM in breaking multidrug resistance (MDR) of malignant cells. Proc. Am. Assoc. Cancer Res. 30:503, 1989.

113. Horton, J.K., Thimmaiah, K.N., Houghton, J.A., Horowitz, M.E., and Houghton, P.J. Modulation by verapamil of vincristine pharmacokinetics and toxicity in mice bearing human tumor xenografts. Biochem. Pharmacol. 38:1727–1736, 1989.

114. Merriman, R.L., Dantzig, A.H., Engelhardt, J., Minor, P.L., Poore, G.A., Shackelford, K.A., Tanzer, L.R., VanPelt, C., Winter, M.A., Beck, W.T., and Pearce, H.L. Increased toxicity of vincristine (VCR) when combined with the multidrug resistance (MDR) modulator, trimethoxybenzoylyohimbine (TMBY). Proc. Am. Assoc. Cancer Res. 31, 361, 1990.

115. Beck, W.T., Cirtain, M.C., Danks, M.K., Felsted, R.L., Safa, A.R., Wolverton, J.S., Suttle, D.P., and Trent, J.M. Pharmacological, molecular, and cytogenetic analysis of "atypical" multidrug-resistant human leukemic cells. Cancer Res. 47:5455–5460, 1987.

116. Beck, W.T. Strategies to circumvent multidrug resistance due to P-glycoprotein or to altered DNA topoisomerase II. Bull. Cancer 77:1131–1141, 1990.

117. Vasanthakumar, G. and Ahmed, N.K. Modulation of drug resistance in a daunorubicin resistant subline with oligonucleoside methylphosphonates. Cancer Commun. 1:225–232, 1989.

118. Salmon, S.E., Soehnlen, B., Dalton, W.S., Meltzer, P., and Scuderi, P. Effects of tumor necrosis factor on sensitive and multidrug resistant human leukemia and myeloma cell lines. Blood 74:1723–1727, 1989.

119. Lyall, R.M., Hwang, J., Cardarelli, C., Fitzgerald, D., Akiyama, S.-I., Gottesman, M.M., and Pastan, I. Isolation of human KB cell lines resistant to epidermal growth factor-Pseudomonas exotoxin conjugates. Cancer Res. 47:2962–2966, 1987.

120. Fizgerald, D.J., Willingham, M.C., Cardarelli, C.O., Hamada, H., Tsuruo, T., Gottesman, M.M., and Pastan, I. A monoclonal antibody-Pseudomonas toxin conjugate that specifically kills multidrug-resistant cells. Proc. Natl. Acad. Sci. USA 84:4288–4292, 1987.

121. Tsuruo, T., Hamada, H., Sato, S., and Heike, Y. Inhibition of multidrug-resistant human tumor growth in athymic mice by anti-P-glycoprotein monoclonal antibodies. Jpn. J. Cancer Res. 80:627–631, 1989.

170

8. Clinical implications of multidrug resistance to chemotherapy

E.G.E. de Vries and H.M. Pinedo

Introduction

One of the major problems in clinical oncology is the existence or development of drug resistance. Improvement of therapeutic modalities will only be possible with better understanding of mechanisms of drug resistance and identification of resistant tumor cells in human tumors. With this knowledge special treatments in case of drug resistance should be developed. Tumors with intrinsic (de novo) resistance, known to be refractory to chemotherapy at initial diagnosis are, for example, colon carcinomas, adenocarcinomas of the lung, and melanomas. Other tumors respond initially, but later on show acquired resistance. This is illustrated by the clinical course of small-cell lung carcinomas and acute myeloid leukemias. Initially, a high remission percentage is found, but often relapses occur within 1–2 years. Subsequent attempts to obtain remission induction either fail, or the results are incomplete and remissions are nearly always of shorter duration.

Over the last years extensive laboratory research has been directed to different types of drug resistance, in particular, the multidrug resistant (MDR) phenotype. Cells that exhibit the MDR phenotype show cross-resistance to a variety of natural products, such as *Vinca* alkaloids, anthracyclines, colchicine, actinomycin D, epipodophyllotoxins, and other cytostatic drugs, which have in common that they are derived from natural toxins. The MDR cells often show a reduced drug accumulation, due to an enhanced efflux of the drug. This enhanced efflux has been attributed to (the so-called) P-glycoprotein, a 170 kDa membrane glycoprotein. This drug carrier is the product of the *mdr1* gene. This type of resistance is found in de novo as well as in acquired resistance.

In cells with the MDR phenotype also other mechanisms for drug resistance may play a role. Altered topoisomerase II and protein kinase C activity, elevated intracellular glutathione levels, and enhanced detoxifying enzyme activities, including raised glutathione peroxidase, glutathione S-transferase (GST), and catalase have been reported [1–7].

Robert F. Ozols (ed.), MOLECULAR AND CLINICAL ADVANCES IN ANTICANCER DRUG RESISTANCE. Copyright © 1991.
Kluwer Academic Publishers, Boston. All rights reserved. ISBN 0-7923-1212-0

P-glycoprotein mediated multidrug resistance in cell lines and human tumors

The most extensive knowledge of drug resistance at the molecular level has been gathered about MDR. The first studies of *mdr1* gene amplification, mRNA, and P-glycoprotein expression were performed in resistant tumor cell lines. It is known that *mdr1* mRNA overexpression can occur in human MDR cell lines without gene amplification [8]. An increase in P-glycoprotein can also occur without a change in *mdr1* mRNA and gene amplification. Bradley et al. recently observed this in the cell line SK VCR2, selected for a high level of vincristine resistance [9]. The P-glycoprotein is expressed in a number of normal human tissues, including kidney, liver, pancreas, and gastrointestinal tract [10–12]. In the liver, P-glycoprotein was found on the biliary canalicular front of the hepatocytes and on the apical surface of epithelial cells in small biliary ducts. In the kidney, the expression is seen in the proximal tubule and in the gastrointestinal tract in the surface epithelium. The location of the P-glycoprotein on the apical surfaces of these cells suggests that in the physiological situation it is also involved in outwards-directed transport mechanisms (most probably of toxic substances).

Goldstein et al. measured *mdr1* RNA in over 400 human cancers. These levels were usually elevated in a high percentage of untreated, intrinsically drug-resistant tumors, including colon carcinomas, renal cell carcinomas, carcinoid tumors, and hepatomas [13]. P-glycoprotein expression has recently been detected in a wide variety of other cancers, such as ovarian cancer, soft tissue sarcoma, acute lymphoblastic leukemia, acute myelocytic leukemia, myeloma, and non-Hodgkin's lymphoma [13–18]. There is a low occurrence of *mdr1* expression in patients with ovarian cancer, and the occurrence seems to be related to pretreatment with doxorubicin or vincristine [17]. Gerlach studied, with an immunoblot assay, tumor samples of 25 sarcoma patients. Six, three of whom were previously untreated, had elevated levels of P-glycoprotein [19]. Ma et al. described two patients with drug-resistant AML and elevated P-glycoprotein. During follow-up, together with disease progression, the intensity of staining and the proportion of tumor cells that reacted with P-glycoprotein antibody increased [20]. An increase in *mdr1* mRNA with disease progression is also described in the tumor of a patient with pheochromocytoma [10]. Goldstein et al. found *mdr1* RNA levels increased in some cancers at relapse after chemotherapy, including ALL, ANLL, breast cancer, neuroblastoma, pheochromocytoma, and nodular poorly differentiated lymphoma [13]. In 22 patients with DNA-aneuploid myeloma, the tumor cells were studied with indirect immunofluorescence with the P-glycoprotein antibody C-219 in a flow cytometric assay. The tumor cells were recognized by analyzing the DNA content with propidium iodide. High levels of P-glycoprotein were associated with clinically acquired resistance for the combination vincristine, doxorubicin, and dexamethason [16]. In most lung cancers (non small-cell and small-cell lung carcinoma), low or no P-glycoprotein expression is detected [13,21]. In 248 breast carcinoma specimens of patients with primary or refractory relapsing disease, no P-glycoprotein overexpression or gene amplification was detected with southern, northern, and western blotting techniques [22]. In a smaller study with immunohistochemical detection of P-glycoprotein, 1 out of 4 primary breast tumors and 4 out of 9 tumors obtained from patients with recurrent metastatic breast carcinoma were positive [23].

The optimal design of cancer chemotherapy for the individual patient with a resistant tumor probably requires a fair estimate of the proportion of P-glycoprotein-positive cells and the degree of P-glycoprotein expression within the tumor. In addition, information on other mechanisms of resistance in the same tumor may be of equal importance. Refinement of techniques, such as in situ hybridization and immunohistochemical staining, should make it possible to study both the cellular localization and quantitation of tumor cell expression of *mdr1* and other gene products related to resistance in individual cells in tumor specimens [24–26]. This also offers the opportunity to study heterogeneity within the tumor.

There are a number of P-glycoprotein antibodies available at the moment for immunohistochemistry [27,28]. There is, however, a considerable variability in reactivity with P-glycoprotein between these antibodies. Therefore, a panel of antibodies may be necessary before it is possible to draw firm conclusions for the clinic with immunohistochemistry. Prospective studies are necessary to prove that high P-glycoprotein expression correlates with no response on natural products in the clinic. One of the possibilities of the above-mentioned techniques is to define and select patients, e.g., those with P-glycoprotein-positive tumors for treatment with compounds known to reverse MDR. These techniques, although they detect, e.g., P-glycoprotein expression, do not, however, give information about the function of the proteins or enzymes studied.

It is therefore relevant to study whether a particular phenomenon leading to resistance takes place in tumor cells of the patient. In vitro studies with tumor cells obtained from patients can determine whether the drug accumulation is disturbed and show whether reversal of the drug resistance with modulators is effective. It is clear that these types of studies are most easily performed in hematological malignancies, such as multiple myeloma and acute leukemia, or in pleural effusions and ascites of patients with solid tumors, sometimes containing a large number of single tumor cells.

Nooter et al. studied the effect of cyclosporin A on intracellular anthracycline accumulation with flow cytometry for the quantitation of cellular anthracycline [29]. This study was performed in bone marrow, peripheral blood, pleural fluid, and ascites of patients with leukemias and solid tumors. Tumor cells of a few patients showed defective drug accumulation. In several instances, cyclosporin A raised the intracellular anthracycline level. Another study reported the effect of verapamil on daunorubicin accumulation in blast cells with flow cytometry [30]. The increase in daunorubicin accumulation was $19.5 \pm 23.1\%$ in the 14 non-responders and $6.4 \pm 6.3\%$ in the 16 responding AML patients.

Dalton et al. demonstrated an increase of intracellular drug accumulation with radiolabelled doxorubicin and vincristine by verapamil in two P-glycoprotein-positive tumor specimens studied [31]. The Leukemia Intergroup studied *mdr1* gene expression with Northern blot analysis and daunomycin uptake in tumor cells of patients with ANLL [32]. They found for a standard risk group and a relapse group, a relation between this factor and complete remission percentage and response duration. There was, however, no relation between the results in the clinic and the levels of glutathione S-transferase or DNA polymerase B. Studies of daunomycin uptake showed that in some patients several agents (verapamil plus trifluoroperazine plus vincristine) were additive, while in others interference was detected [32]. Apart from the study of drug accumulation in whole cells, it may also be relevant, based on recent in vitro data, to study the distribution of anthracyclines over cell compartments [33–35]. In a MDR squamous lung carcinoma cell line, a shift of the anthracycline from the cytoplasm to the nucleus was found with laser scan and fluorescence microscopy after coincubation with verapamil [33,34].

Reversal of P-glycoprotein mediated multidrug resistance in the clinic

Until recently, treatment strategies to circumvent drug resistance consisted of the use of combination chemotherapy and high-dose chemotherapy with bone marrow reinfusion. In vitro studies with MDR cell lines show, in general, no change in sensitivity for antimetabolites and alkylating agents, although cross-resistance with the alkylating agent mitomycin C was described once [36]. Thus, in the case of MDR, treatment with drugs not known to participate in MDR may give better results. In MDR cells in vitro, an increased collateral sensitivity is found for compounds that could be used in the clinic, such as certain local anesthetics, glucocorticoids, and propranolol [37].

In the clinic many studies are performed in which for example drugs known not to participate in MDR were administered after MDR drugs. It remains unclear whether MDR really played a role in these studies. This is illustrated with a recent study. Patients with small-cell lung carcinoma first received etoposide, doxorubicin, and vincristine [38]. In the case of a complete or partial response, intensification with the alkylator ifosfamide was performed, but did not result in more complete responders. However, 43% of 14 patients unresponsive to the first treatment obtained a partial response but no complete response with ifosfamide. Recent data [21] indicate that MDR is uncommon in small-cell lung cancer, which may explain the disappointing results of an alkylator treatment after a treatment with drugs involved in MDR in this study.

174

Another approach is to add certain compounds known to reverse MDR in vitro in the laboratory to the chemotherapeutic drug treatment. A number of noncytotoxic agents have been studied and have been found to reverse MDR. This effect was shown in vitro by calcium-channel blockers, calmodulin inhibitors, isoprenoids [39], triparanol and triparanol analogs, and other agents, such as quinidine, amiodarone, and cyclosporin A. Zamora et al. studied the physical-chemical properties of compounds that modulated MDR in a human vinblastine-resistant cell line [40]. They found lipid solubility at physiological pH, cationic charge, and molar refractivity to be important properties of these compounds. In a second study, Pearce et al. described the essential features of the P-glycoprotein "pharmacophore" with a series of reserpine and yohimbine analogs [41]. They considered that the relative disposition of aromatic rings and the basic nitrogen atom was important for modulators of P-glycoprotein-associated MDR and suggested a ligand-receptor relationship for these agents. These two studies may help to synthesize new compounds with fewer side effects for MDR reversal in the clinic. A number of studies showed that some modulating agents, such as calcium-channel blockers and quinidine, bind at the same site as vinblastine, while for other agents this was not the case [42–44], suggesting that certain modulators can potentiate each other at the P-glycoprotein level.

The most extensive knowledge on reversing MDR in vitro and in vivo has been gathered on calcium-channel blockers. Calcium-channel blockers act at least partially by direct binding to the P-glycoprotein, resulting in increased accumulation of chemotherapeutic drugs. They have shown to be able to change subcellular distribution of chemotherapeutic drugs [33,34]. A number of clinical trials applying calcium-channel blockers given concurrently with chemotherapy regimens have been completed. In a phase I study of verapamil plus vinblastine, both drugs were administered as continuous infusion after a loading dose of verapamil. In the 17 patients treated, no responses were seen. The plasma concentrations of verapamil were lower (290 ng/ml during steady state) than the concentration required in vitro for increasing vincristine induced cytotoxicity [45]. In a study in children with ALL refractory to vincristine, the combination of this drug with diltiazem resulted in a cytolytic effect, but no complete response [46].

In patients with ovarian cancer, the addition of verapamil to doxorubicin did not produce a response. As in other studies, the verapamil plasma concentrations achieved without unacceptable cardiac toxicity were lower than the verapamil concentrations required in vitro (3000 ng/ml) for reversal of doxorubicin toxicity in ovarian cancer cell lines established from drug-resistant patients [47–49]. These cell lines also failed to demonstrate a decrease in drug accumulation [51]. The expression of P-glycoprotein in the tumor specimens of these patients was not measured.

Durie et al. showed that a low concentration of 100 ng/ml verapamil is effective in reversing resistance for doxorubicin and vincristine in a resistant myeloma cell line [51]. They reported a patient with multiple myeloma resistant to combination chemotherapy consisting of vincristine, doxorubicin, and dexamethason, who responded after the addition of oral verapamil. Interestingly, the verapamil (plus metabolite) trough level was low, 74 ng/ml (0.15 µM), 14 hr after oral administration of verapamil [51]. In a more extensive study, Dalton et al. reported eight patients — six with myeloma, one with plasma-cell leukemia, and one with diffuse large-cell lymphoma — with progressive disease on the same combination chemotherapy. These patients received thereafter the identical chemotherapy combination and a continuous infusion of verapamil. Of the six patients with P-glycoprotein-positive tumors, three showed a response, two patients with multiple myeloma and one with diffuse large-cell lymphoma. The two patients with P-glycoprotein-negative tumors showed no response. All three responding patients had rather low verapamil serum levels (215, 397, and 1342 ng/ml, respectively) [31].

There may be a number of reasons for responses encountered after the addition of verapamil in this study: 1) The responders had P-glycoprotein-positive tumors. 2) B-cell neoplasms may be more sensitive to MDR reversal with low serum levels of verapamil. 3) The combination of drugs used in this treatment regimen may have influenced the results. Vincristine, as well as verapamil, can increase doxorubicin accumulation in tumor cells; and dexamethason, for which MDR cells may exhibit collateral sensitivity, might also have added to the effect. Fine et al. found no increase of bone marrow toxicity, as measured with myeloid and macrophage colony formation of cytotoxic drugs, if the bone marrow was coincubated with verapamil or nitrendipine [52].

Also, in most clinical studies with calcium-channel blockers, the clinical toxicity of the chemotherapeutic drugs was not increased. However, cardiac toxicity of the calcium-channel blocker was a major problem. This had to be very carefully monitored and was the dose-limiting toxicity. Due to the cardiac toxicity, it is difficult to achieve serum verapamil concentrations comparable to the concentrations necessary in vitro to reverse multidrug resistance. An advantage of the calcium-channel blocker bepridil is the fact that concentrations of 3–7 µM can be achieved without toxicity in the clinic. Bepridil, compared with verapamil, nifedipine, and diltiazem, has a larger volume of distribution and a longer half-life [53]. In addition, Schuurhuis et al. showed that bepridil is equally effective as verapamil in reversing resistance at clinically achievable plasma levels [54].

Following these findings, Van Kalken et al. performed a pilot study with bepridil in 14 patients with tumors resistant to doxorubicin-containing combinations [55]. The doxorubicin dose administered was kept unchanged. The aim was 1) to achieve a steady-state serum concentration equal to the effective concentration of in vitro experiments and 2) to acquire information of the drug at steady-state concentration. In most patients a plateau level of 3–7 µM was reached after 24 hr, with patients receiving a bolus injection and 36 hr infusion of bepridil. Of interest, in one patient with unexplained high serum levels of bepridil, the concentration in a removed subcutaneous metastasis appeared to be sevenfold higher than the serum concentration at the time of doxorubicin administration (24 hr after starting bepridil). This observation indicates that the high plasma protein binding of bepridil did not preclude the calcium-channel blocker from accumulating in tumor tissue. As no cardiac toxicity and no reversal of resistance was observed, a follow-up study is being conducted in which doses of bepridil are being escalated and accompanied by pharmacological investigations. These studies illustrate the complexity of the pharmacology that should accomplish clinical studies with reverting agents.

A high percentage of the calcium-channel blockers in the plasma is protein bound (diltiazem 78%, verapamil 90%, nifedipine 98%, bepridil 99%). This high protein binding could change plasma pharmacokinetics of the chemotherapeutic drug. In a study with mice, however, no change of doxorubicin pharmacokinetics and metabolism was found with combined treatment with verapamil in the plasma, heart, and spleen [56].

Calmodulin is a calcium-binding protein [57]; its antagonists can also reverse MDR by inhibiting the active efflux of the chemotherapeutic drugs. There are a wide variety of different classes of agents known to exhibit anticalmodulin activity, e.g., antidepressants, antidiarrheals, antiestrogens, antihistamines, antimalarials, antipsychotics, calcium-channel blockers, and local anesthetics. Miller et al. performed a phase I/II trial with the calmodulin-inhibitor trifluoperazine and doxorubicin in patients with de novo or acquired doxorubicin resistance [58]. The maximum tolerated dose of oral trifluoperazine was 60 mg/day on days 1–6. Responses did not occur in the 15 patients with de novo resistance, but they were seen in 7 out of 21 patients with acquired doxorubicin resistance. In this study, two variables may have influenced the results. The dose of doxorubicin administered in patients with acquired resistance was slightly higher than the initial dose, and the doxorubicin was now administered as a 96 hr continuous infusion. Whether the tumors expressed P-glycoprotein is not known. Plasma levels of trifluoperazine varied between 4.16 and 129.83 ng/ml. Again, these plasma levels are far below those needed in tissue culture to reverse MDR.

The cardiac agents quinidine and amiodarone are also considered to reverse MDR. As opposed to the calcium-channel blockers and calmodulin inhibitors mentioned above, it should be possible for these two drugs to achieve plasma concentrations in patients that are nearly equal to concentrations needed in vitro for MDR reversal [59–61]. The ability to increase the sensitivity for doxorubicin with quinidine was studied in tumor samples from patients with renal-cell carcinoma with a [³H] thymidine assay. The enhancing effect of quinidine (7.5 µg/ml) was only significant in the tumor samples with high *mdr1* RNA levels. Quinidine plasma levels of 2–5 µg/ml are considered therapeutic and safe concentrations [62]. Amiodarone reversed MDR in rat colon cancer cells in vitro and in vivo [63].

Chauffert et al. showed that amiodarone and its metabolite desethylamiodarone are equally efficient in vitro, and at equimolar concentrations amiodarone was more efficient than verapamil [60]. In patients, after oral administration of 400 mg amiodarone daily, serum levels of amiodarone plus its metabolite were above $3 \mu M$. After an intravenous loading dose of 450 mg amiodarone over 3 hr, the serum level was above $5.5 \mu M$ [60]. These concentrations are not likely to be associated with acute cardiac toxicity, but do reverse MDR in vitro. With long-term use, however, this drug can have its own toxicity [64]. Serum concentrations of up to $3.8 \mu M$ were found to not produce toxicity in a number of studies. The (acute elimination) half-life of distribution of amiodarone is 3.2–20.7 hr, and the terminal half-life of distribution is 13.7–52.6 days. Amiodarone has a large volume of distribution and it is highly bound to body tissues. Studies in rats and postmortem studies in humans revealed that fat, lung, liver, heart, pancreas, and kidney contain especially high concentrations. Fojo et al. have begun a study with quinidine and amiodarone for MDR reversal. Preliminary reports are that the objective response rate is low, but toxicity was not enhanced [65,66].

The addition of triparanol or triparanol analogs, such as tamoxifen, to a chemotherapeutic regimen may be attractive because of a different toxicity spectrum of tamoxifen compared to the cardiac agents. In a preliminary report of Cantwell et al., the effect of high-dose tamoxifen (120 mg daily) and oral etoposide (300 mg daily), both administered for 3 days and repeated at 21-day intervals, was described [67]. Of 46 evaluable patients, two patients achieved a complete remission and four a partial remission. DeGregorio et al. studied the effect of a new triphenylethylene, toremifene, on the growth of doxorubicin-exposed cells of a doxorubicin-resistant human breast cell line [68]. Toremifene and its metabolites sensitized the multidrug-resistant (MCF7) cells. Ultrafiltrate plasma of patients treated with toremifene was also added in an in vitro microtiter assay. At clinically achievable plasma concentrations, a potentiation of doxorubicin cytotoxicity was found in the resistant MCF7 cells. Tamoxifen and toremifene are active as single agents in estrogen receptor-positive breast cancer. The fact that high-dose toremifene can be administered and results in high plasma levels of this drug makes it attractive to combine toremifene with doxorubicin for MDR reversal.

There are a number of reasons why MDR modulators do not yet look very effective. 1) There may be much heterogeneity within a tumor as far as P-glycoprotein mediated MDR is concerned. 2) Other resistance mechanisms may play a role. 3) Serum levels of the modulator may be inadequate. 4) Little knowledge is available about the tumor tissue level of the modulator that can be achieved. This last aspect may be much more important. 5) Little is known about the pharmacokinetics of the interaction between the chemotherapeutic drug and the modulator. The fact that various modulators of MDR can act differently makes it interesting to consider, if clinically feasible, combinations of modulators in the future.

Monoclonal antibodies directed against 170 kDa P-glycoprotein were shown to reverse MDR resistance [69,70]. In an MDR human ovarian carcinoma cell line exposed to MRK-16, a monoclonal antibody that recognizes a cell-surface exposed epitope of P-glycoprotein resulted in an increase in vincristine but not daunorubicin accumulation. However, in the presence of verapamil (8 μM), MRK-16 increased not only vincristine but also daunorubicin accumulation. For clinical use, it is interesting to link a P-glycoprotein antibody with a radioactive or toxic compound. FitzGerald et al. showed in vitro that conjugates of the Pseudomonas toxin with P-glycoprotein antibody MRK-16 were toxic to MDR human KB cells [71]. The clinical use of these monoclonal antibodies will be hampered by the fact that many normal tissues do express the 170 kDa P-glycoprotein.

Reversal of other resistance mechanisms coexisting with P-glycoprotein mediated MDR

Glutathione plays a role in the detoxification of quinone-containing agents, such as doxorubicin. Apart from direct detoxification, it may also help to remove reactive oxygen species with the glutathione oxidation-reduction cycle. Glutathione depletion can result in a less efficient activity of the detoxifying enzymes GST and glutathione peroxidase, as they both need glutathione as substrate for their activity. Buthionine sulfoximine (BSO) is an agent that interacts with the enzyme τ-glutamyl cysteine synthetase, which is necessary for glutathione synthesis, resulting in decreased intracellular glutathione levels. In vitro BSO reversed, at least partially, MDR to doxorubicin in a variety of tumor cell lines [72,73]. Kramer et al. showed that BSO and verapamil both partially reversed MDR to doxorubicin. Although the combination of both potentiated this effect, this is no proof that the two drugs were affecting different mechanisms [74]. So far, BSO has only been studied in animals. Results from studies with this agent in humans are not yet available. GST mRNA expression was found to be variably expressed in both normal and malignant tissues. But comparison of paired specimens from the same patient indicated that GST expression was increased in many tumors relative to matched normal tissue [75]. However, the role of GST in doxorubicin resistance is not yet clear. The question of whether the use of effective modulating drugs in vitro, such as ethacrynic acid — an inhibitor of GST — is useful in the clinic still remains to be answered [76].

Recently, much more attention has been paid to a possible role of topoisomerase II in MDR, as well as in the so-called atypical drug resistance. Topoisomerase II is important for the handling of DNA during vital cellular processes. The DNA-topoisomerase II complex, an intermediate in the normal enzyme pathway, is stabilized by chemotherapeutic drugs and forms a cytotoxic "cleavable complex." Among the chemotherapeutic drugs involved are drugs also participating in MDR, namely, the anthracyclines and epipodophyllotoxins. Development of drug resistance is possible by downregulation of topoisomerase II or production of resistant mutants. Clinically, a substantial increase of topoisomerase II in tumor cells with a low topoisomerase II might result in an increased tumor cytotoxicity. In vitro effects are reported of estrogens, tumor necrosis factor, protein kinase C stimulators, and growth factors [77–81]. Theoretically one could speculate that clinically long-term exposure to chemotherapeutic drugs that exhibit at least partially their activity via the "cleavable complex" could also result in a higher antitumor activity of the drug. Even in the case of low topoisomerase II levels, many cleavable complexes can then be formed. There are not yet much clinical data available to underscore the importance of topoisomerase II.

Slevin et al. found that, despite identical plasma AUC of etoposide after a 24 hr and a 5-day infusion, the 5-day infusion was more effective in small-cell lung cancer [82]. In a phase I study in a group of patients who had all received previous chemotherapy, etoposide was administered orally for 21 days. The maximum tolerated dose was $50\,mg/m^2/day$. Five out of 16 evaluable patients had a partial response [83]. Although not conclusive for the role of topoisomerase II, these two studies show encouraging results for further studies with long-term low-dose etoposide exposure.

There are a number of agents that are considered to reverse drug resistance by alteration of the cell membrane that could also be useful. Docosahexaenoic acid, a fish oil, raised intracellular doxorubicin and increased doxorubicin cytotoxicity in a doxorubicin-resistant small-cell lung carcinoma cell line, while the lipid composition of the tumor cell membrane was changed [84]. In a phase I/II study, the effect of amphotericin B was evaluated [85]. When the patients became clinically drug resistant, they received the same regimen together with amphotericin B. In the 51 evaluable patients, the overall response rate was 12% (one complete response and five partial responses).

Clinically there is much experience with dipyridamole as an antithrombotic drug and a vasodilator [86,87]. Howell et al. showed potentiation of cytotoxicity of important drugs involved in MDR, namely, etoposide, doxorubicin, and vinblastine, in a human ovarian carcinoma cell line by dipyridamole [88]. The precise mechanism for this is not yet clear. Again, with this drug it is impossible in the clinic to reach the plasma concentrations necessary for drug resistance reversal in vitro [89]. Addition of this drug to intraperitoneal (ip) treatment may, however, be useful. When dipyridamole was administered ip, the ip concentrations were high enough [90].

Conclusion

Recently, much knowledge has been gathered on the existence of P-glycoprotein-positive tumor cells in various tumor types. Studies on combinations of chemotherapeutic drugs involved in MDR with modulators of

MDR have not, for a variety of reasons, been very successful until now. Refinement of techniques will make it possible, in the future, to study the cellular localization and quantitation of tumor cell expression of *mdr1* and other gene products related to resistance in individual cells in tumor specimens. This will offer the opportunity to study heterogeneity within tumors. In vitro functional assays, such as anthracycline accumulation with and without modulation, on human tumor samples may also help to predict whether the resistance mechanism is functionally present. Prospective studies with modulators in patients with tumors known to be P-glycoprotein positive are needed. In terms of clinical studies, additional attention will have to be paid to the coexistence of other resistance mechanisms. Each resistance mechanism may offer separate opportunities for modulation of drug resistance. In order to further unravel the drug resistance problem in the clinic, a close collaboration between laboratory and clinical workers is crucial.

References

1. Deffie, A.M., Batra, J.K., and Goldenberg, G.J. Direct correlation between DNA topoisomerase II activity and cytotoxicity in adriamycin-sensitive and -resistant P388 leukemia cell lines. Cancer Res. 49:58–62, 1989.
2. Deffie, A.M., Alam, T., Seneviratne, C., Beenken, S.W., Batra, J.K., Shea, T.C., Henner, W.D., and Goldenberg, G.J. Multifactorial resistance to adriamycin: relationship of DNA repair, glutathione transferase activity, drug efflux and P-glycoprotein in cloned cell lines of adriamycin-sensitive and -resistant P388 leukemia. Cancer Res. 48:3595–3602, 1988.
3. Sinha, B.K., Haim, N., Dusre, L., Kerrigan, D., and Pommier, Y. DNA strand breaks produced by etoposide (VP-16,213) in sensitive and resistant human breast tumor cells: implications for the mechanism of action. Cancer Res. 48:5096–5100, 1988.
4. Batist, G., Tulpule, A., Sinha, B.K., Katki, A.G., Myers, C.E., and Cowan, K.H. Overexpression of a novel anionic glutathione transferase in multidrug-resistant human breast cancer cells. J. Biol. Chem. 261:15544–15549, 1986.
5. Ido, M., Sato, K., Sakurai, M., Inagaki, M., Saitoh, M., Watanabe, M., and Hidaka, H. Decreased phorbol ester receptor and protein kinase C in P388 murine leukemic cells resistant to etoposide. Cancer Res. 47:3460–3463, 1987.
6. Fine, R.L., Platel, J., and Chabner, B.A. Phorbol esters induce multidrug resistance in human breast cancer cells. Proc. Natl. Acad. Sci. USA 85:582–586, 1988.
7. De Vries, E.G.E., Meijer, C., Timmer-Bosscha, H., Berendsen, H.H., de Ley, L., Scheper, R.J., and Mulder, N.H. Resistance mechanisms in three human small cell lung cancer cell lines established from one patient during clinical follow-up. Cancer Res. 49:4175–4178, 1989.
8. Shen, D.W., Fojo, A., Chin, J.E., Roninson, I.B., Richert, N., Pastan, I., and Gottesman, M.M. Human multidrug-resistant cell lines: increased mdr1 expression can precede gene amplification. Science 232:643–645, 1986.
9. Bradley, G., Naik, M., and Ling, V. P-glycoprotein expression in multidrug-resistant human ovarian carcinoma cell lines. Cancer Res. 49:2790–2796, 1989.
10. Fojo, A.T., Ueda, K., Slamon, D.J., Poplack, D.G., Gottesman, M.M., and Pastan, I. Expression of a multidrug-resistance gene in human tumors and tissues. Proc. Natl. Acad. Sci. USA 84:265–269, 1987.

11. Thiebaut, F., Tsuruo, T., Hamada, H., Gottesman, M.M., Pastan, I., and Willingham, M.C. Cellular localization of the multidrug-resistance gene product P-glycoprotein in normal human tissues. Proc. Natl. Acad. Sci. USA 84:7735–7738, 1987.

12. Van der Valk, P., van Kalken, C.K., Ketelaars, H., Broxterman, H.J., Scheffer, G.L., Kuiper, C.M., Tsuruo, T., Lankelma, J., Meyer, C.J.L.M., Pinedo, H.M., and Scheper, R.J. Distribution of multidrug resistance-associated P-glycoprotein in normal and neoplastic human tissue. Ann. Oncol. 1:56–64, 1990.

13. Goldstein, L.J., Galski, H., Fojo, A., Willingham, M., Lai, S.-L., Gadzdar, A., Pirker, R., Green, A., Crist, W., Brodeur, G.M., Lieber, M., Cossman, J., Gottesman, M.M., and Pastan, I. Expression of a multidrug resistant gene in human cancers. J. Natl. Cancer Inst. 81:116–124,1989.

14. Bell, D.R., Gerlach, J.H., Kartner, N., Buick, R.N., and Ling, V. Detection of P-glycoprotein in ovarian cancer; a molecular marker associated with drug resistance. J. Clin. Oncol. 3:311–315, 1985.

15. Holmes, J., Jacobs, A., Carter, G., Janouski-Wieczorek, A., and Padua, R.A. Multidrug resistance in haematopoietic cell lines, myelodysplastic syndromes and acute myeloblastic leukaemia. Br. J. Haematol. 72:40–44, 1989.

16. Epstein, J., Xiao, H., and Oba, B.K. P-glycoprotein expression in plasma-cell myeloma is associated with resistance to VAD. Blood 74:913–917, 1989.

17. Bourhus, J., Goldstein, L.J., Riou, G., Pastan, I., Gottesman, M.M., and Bénard, J. Expression of a human multidrug resistance gene in ovarian carcinoma. Cancer Res. 49:5062–5096, 1989.

18. Rothenberg, M., Mickley, L., Cole, D.E., Balis, F.M., Tsuruo, T., Poplack, D.G., and Fojo, A.T. Expression of the mdr-1/P-170 gene in patients with acute lymphoblastic leukemia. Blood 74:1388–1395, 1989.

19. Gerlach, J.H., Bell, D.R., Karakousis, C., Slocum, A.K., Kartner, N., Rustum, Y.M., Ling, V., and Baker, R.M. P-glycoprotein in human sarcoma, evidence for multidrug resistance. J. Clin. Oncol. 5:1452–1460, 1987.

20. Ma, D.D.F., Davey, R.A., Harman, D.H., Isbister, J.P., Scurr, R.D., Mackertich, S.M., Dowden, G., and Bell, D.R. Detection of a multidrug resistant phenotype in acute non-lymphoblastic leukaemia. Lancet 1:135–137, 1987.

21. Lai, S.-L., Goldstein, L.J., Gottesman, M.M., Pastan, I., Tsai, C., Johnson, B.E., Mulshine, J.L., Ihde, D.C., Kayser, K., and Gazdar, A.F. MDR1 gene expression in lung cancer. J. Natl. Cancer Inst. 81:1144–1150, 1989.

22. Merkel, D.E., Fuquo, S.A.W., Tandon, A.K., Hill, S.M., Buzdar, A.U., and McGuire, W.L. Electrophoretic analysis of 248 clinical breast cancer specimens for P-glycoprotein overexpression or gene amplification. J. Clin. Oncol. 7:1129–1136, 1989.

23. Salman, S.E., Grogan, T.M., Miller, T., Scheper, R., and Dalton, W.S. Prediction of doxorubicin resistance in vitro in myeloma, lymphoma, and breast cancer by P-glycoprotein staining. J. Natl. Cancer Inst. 81:696–701, 1989.

24. Kacinski, B.M., Yee, L.D., and Carter, D. Quantitation of tumor cell expression of the P-glycoprotein (mdr1) gene in human breast carcinoma clinical specimens. Cancer Bull. 41:44–48, 1989.

25. Shen, D.-W., Pastan, I., and Gottesman, M.M. In situ hybridization analysis of acquisition and loss of the human multidrug resistance gene. Cancer Res. 48:4334–4339, 1988.

26. Dalton, W.S., Grogan, T.M., Rybski, J.A., Scheper, R.J., Richter, L., Kailey, J., Broxterman, H.J., Pinedo, H.M., and Salmon, S.E. Immunohistochemical detection and quantitation of P-glycoprotein in multidrug resistant human myeloma cells: association with level of drug resistance and drug accumulation. Blood 73:747–752, 1989.

27. Wooten, P., Cuddy, D., Felsted, P., Pan, S., and Ross, D. Comparison of anti-P-glycoprotein monoclonal antibodies MRK16, 265/F4 and C219 in the detection of multidrug resistant cells. Proc. Am. Assoc. Cancer Res. 30:2105, 1989.

28. Scheper, R.J., Bulte, J.W.M., Brakkee, J.G.P., Quak, J.J., van der Schoot, E., Balm, A.J.M., Meyer, C.J.L.M., Broxterman, H.J., Kuiper, C.M., Lankelma, J., and Pinedo,

H.M. Monoclonal antibody JSB-1 detects a highly conserved epitope on the P-glycoprotein associated with multi-drug-resistance. Int. J. Cancer 42:389–394, 1988.

29. Nooter, K., Herweyer, H., Sonneveld, P., Verwey, J., Hagenbeek, A., and Stoter, G. Detection of multidrug resistance in refractory cancer patients (obstr.). Proc. Am. Assoc. Cancer Res. 30:2092, 1989.

30. Marayana, Y., Murohashi, I., Nara, N., and Aoki, N. Effects of verapamil on the cellular accumulation of daunorubicin in blast cells and on the chemosensitivity of leukaemic blast progenitors in acute myelogenous leukaemia. Br. J. Haematol. 72:357–362, 1989.

31. Dalton, W.S., Grogan, T.M., Meltzer, P.S., Scheper, R.J., Durie, B.G.M., Taylor, C.W., Miller, T.P., and Salmon, S.E. Drug-resistance in multiple myeloma and non-Hodgkin's lymphoma: detection of P-glycoprotein and potential circumvention by addition of verapamil to chemotherapy. J. Clin. Oncol. 7:415–424, 1989.

32. Preisler, H.D., Gottesman, M., Raza, A., Pastan, I., and Day, R. The clinical significance of expression of the multidrug resistance (MDR) gene in acute nonlymphocytic leukemia (ANLL). Proc. ASCO 8:782, 1989.

33. Keizer, H.G., Schuurhuis, G.J., Broxterman, H.J., Lankelma, J., Schoonen, W.G.E.J., van Rijn, J., Pinedo, H.M., and Joenje, H. Correlation of multidrug resistance with decreased drug accumulation, altered subcellular drug distribution and increased P-glycoprotein expression in cultured SW-1573 human lung tumor cells. Cancer Res. 49: 2988–2993, 1989.

34. Schuurhuis, G.J., Broxterman, H.J., Cervantes, A., Van Heyningen, T.H., De Lange J.H., Baak, J.D., and Pinedo, H.M. Quantitative determination of factors contributing to doxorubicin resistance in multidrug-resistant cells. J. Natl. Cancer Inst. 81:1887–1892, 1989.

35. Hindenburg, A.A., Gervasoni, J.E., Krishna, S., Stewart, V.J., Rosado, M., Lutzky, J., Bhalla, K., Baker, M.A., and Taub, R.N. Intracellular distribution and pharmacokinetics of daunorubicin in antracylcine-sensitive and -resistant HL-60 cells. Cancer Res. 49: 4607–4614, 1989.

36. Dorr, R.T., Liddil, J.D., Trent, J.M., and Dalton, W.S. Mitomycin C resistant L1210 leukemia cells: association with pleiotropic drug resistance. Biochem. Pharmacol. 36: 3115–3120, 1987.

37. Beck-Hansen, N.T., Till, J.E., and Ling, V. Pleiotropic phenotype of colchicine-resistant CHO cells: cross-resistance and collateral sensitivity. J. Cell Physiol. 88:23–32, 1976.

38. Cantwell, B.M.J., Bozzino, J.M., Corris, P., and Harris, A.L. The multidrug resistant phenotype in clinical practice; evaluation of cross resistance to ifosfamide and mesna after VP 16–213, doxorubicin and vincristine (VPAV) for small cell lung cancer. Eur. J. Cancer Clin. Oncol. 24:123–129, 1988.

39. Nakagawa, M., Akiyama, S., Yamaguchi, T., Shiraishi, N., Ogata, J., and Kuwano, M. Reversal of multidrug resistance by synthetic isoprenoids in the KB human cancer cell line. Cancer Res. 46:4453–4457, 1986.

40. Zamora, J.M., Pearce, H.L., and Beck, W.T. Physical-chemical properties shared by compounds that modulate multidrug resistance in human leukemic cells. Mol. Pharmacol. 33:454–462, 1988.

41. Pearce, H.L., Safa, A.R., Bach, N.J., Winter, M.A., Cirtain, M.C., and Beck, W.T. Essential features of the P-glycoprotein pharmacophore as defined by a series of reserpine analogs that modulate multidrug resistance. Proc. Natl. Acad. Sci. 86:5128–5132, 1989.

42. Akiyama, S.-I., Cornwell, M.M., Kuwano, M., Pastan, I., and Gottesman, M.M. Most drugs that reverse multidrug resistance also inhibit photoaffinity labeling of P-glycoprotein by a vinblastine analog. Mol. Pharmacol. 34:180–185, 1988.

43. Beek, W.T., Cirtain, M.C., Glover, C.J., et al. Effects of indole alkaloids on multidrug resistance and labeling of P-glycoprotein by a photoaffinity analog of vinblastine. Biochem. Biophys. Res. Commun. 153:959–966, 1988.

44. Cornwell, M.M., Pastan, I., and Gottesman, M.M. Certain calcium channel blockers bind specifically to multidrug resistant human KB carcinoma membrane vesicles and inhibit drug

binding to P-glycoprotein. J. Biol. Chem. 262:2166–2170, 1987.

45. Benson, A.B., Trump, D.L., Koeller, J.M., Egorin, M.I., Olman, E.A., Witte, R.S., Davis, T.E., and Tormey, D.C. Phase 1 study of vinblastine and verapamil given by concurrent IV infusion. Cancer Treat. Rep. 69:795–799, 1985.
46. Bessho, F., Kinumaki, H., Kobayashi, M., Habu, H., Nakamura, K., Yohata, S., Tsuruo, T., and Kobayashi, N. Treatment of children with refractory acute lymphocytic leukemia with vincristine and diltiazem. Med. Ped. Oncol. 13:199–202, 1985.
47. Rogan, A.M., Hamilton, T.C., Young, R.C., Klecker, R.W., and Ozols, R.F. Reversal of adriamycin resistance by verapamil in human ovarian cancer. Science 224:994–996, 1984.
48. Ozols, R.F., Cunnion, R.E., Klecker, R.W., Hamilton, T.C., Ostchega, Y., Parrillo, J.E., and Young, R.C. Verapamil and adriamycin in the treatment of drug-resistant ovarian cancer patients. J. Clin. Oncol. 5:641–647, 1987.
49. Louie, K.G., Hamilton, T.C., and Winker, M.A. Adriamycin accumulation and metabolism in adriamycin-sensitive and resistant human ovarian cancer cell lines. Biochem. Pharmacol. 35:467–472, 1986.
50. Fojo, A., Hamilton, T.C., Young, R.C., and Ozols, R.F. Multidrug resistance in ovarian cancer. Cancer 60:2075–2080, 1987.
51. Durie, B.G.M. and Dalton, W.S. Reversal of drug-resistance in multiple myeloma with verapamil. Br. J. Haematol. 68:203–206, 1988.
52. Fine, R.L., Koizumi, S., Curt, G.A., and Chabner, B.A. Effect of calcium channel blockers on human CFU-GM with cytotoxic drugs. J. Clin. Oncol. 5:489–495, 1987.
53. Benet, L.Z. Pharmacokinetics and metabolism of bepridil. Am. J. Cardiol. 55:8C–13C, 1985.
54. Schuurhuis, G.J., Broxterman, H.J., van der Hoeven, J.J.M., Pinedo, H.M., and Lankelma, J. Potentiation of doxorubicin cytotoxicity by the calcium antagonist bepridil in antracycline-resistant and -sensitive cell lines. Cancer Chemother. Pharmacol. 20:285–290, 1987.
55. Van der Hoeven, J.J.M., van Kalken, C.K., Maessen, P., van der Vijgh, W.J.F., and Pinedo, H.M. Combination of doxorubicin (Dox) and the calcium channel blocker bepridil (Bp) in patients with Dox resistant tumors,. In: 5th European Conference on Clinical Oncology (abstr. no O-0428) 1989.
56. Formelli, F., Cleris, L., and Carsana, R. Effect of verapamil on doxorubicin activity and pharmacokinetics in mice bearing resistant and sensitive solid tumors. Cancer Chemother. Pharmacol. 21:329–336, 1988.
57. Hait, W.N., and Lazo, J.S. Calmodulin: a potential target for cancer chemotherapeutic agents. J. Clin. Oncol. 4:994–1012, 1986.
58. Miller R.L., Bukowski, R.M., Budd, T., Purvis, J., Weick, J.K., Shepard, K., Midha, K.K., and Ganapathi, R. Clinical modulation of doxorubicin resistance by the cadmodulin-inhibitor, trifluoperazine. A phase I/II trial. J. Clin. Oncol. 6:880–888, 1988.
59. Fojo, A.T., Shen, D.-W., Mickley, L.A., Pastan, I., and Gottesman, M.M. Intrinsic drug resistance in human kidney cancer is associated with expression of a human multidrug-resistance gene. J. Clin. Oncol. 5:1922–1927, 1987.
60. Chauffert, B., Rey, D., Coudert, B., Duras, M., and Martin, F. Amiodarone is more efficient than verapamil in reversing resistance to anthracyclines in tumour cells. Br. J. Cancer 56:119–122, 1987.
61. Kanamaru, H., Kakehi, Y., Yoshida, O., Nakanishi, S., Pastan, I., and Gottesman, M.M. MDR1 RNA levels in human renal cell carcinomas: correlation with grade and prediction of reversal of doxorubicin resistance by quinidine in tumor explants. J. Natl. Cancer Inst. 81:844–849, 1989.
62. Benet, L.Z. and Williams, R.L. Design and optimization of dosage regimens: pharmacokinetic data. In: The Pharmacological Basis of Therapeutics, Goodman Gilman, A., Rall, T.W., Nies, A.S., Taylor, P. (eds.). Pergamon Press, New York, p. 1705, 1990.
63. Chauffert, B., Martin, M., Hamman, A., Michel, M.F., and Martin, F. Amiodarone-induced enhancement of doxorubicin and 4'-deoxydoxorubicin cytotoxicity to rat colon

cancer cells in vitro and in vivo. Cancer Res. 46:825–830, 1986.

64. Singh, B.N., Venkatesh, N., Nademanee, K., Josephson, M.A., and Kannan, R. The historical development, cellular electrophysiology and pharmacology of amiodarone. Progress Cardiovasc. Dis. 31:249–281, 1989.

65. Fojo, T., McAtee, N., Allegra, C., Bates, S., Mickley, L., Keiser, H., Linehan, M., Steinberg, S., Tucker, E., Goldstein, L., Gottesman, M.M., and Pastan, I. Use of quinidine and amiodarone to modulate multidrug resistance mediated by mdr1 gene. Proc. ASCO 8:262. 1989.

66. Rothenberg, M. and Ling V. Multidrug resistance: molecular biology and clinical relevance. J. Natl. Cancer Inst. 81:907–910, 1989.

67. Cantwell, B., Carmichael, J., Millward, M., Chatterjee, M., and Harris, A.L. Intermittent high dose tamoxifen with oral etoposide (epo): phase I and II clinical studies. Proc. ASCO 8:252. 1989.

68. DeGregorio, M.W., Ford, J.M., Benz, C.C., and Wiebe, V.J. Toremifene: pharmacologic and pharmacokinetic basis of reversing multidrug resistance. J. Clin. Oncol. 7:1359–1364, 1989.

69. Hamada, H. and Tsuruo T. Functional role for the 170- to 180-kDa glycoprotein specific to drug-resistant tumor cells as revealed by monoclonal antibodies. Proc. Natl. Acad. Sci. USA 83:7785–7789, 1986.

70. Broxterman, H.J., Kuiper, C.M., Schuurhuis, G.J., Tsuruo, T., Pinedo, H.M., and Lankelma, J. Increase of daunorubicin and vincristine accumulation in multidrug resistant human ovarian carcinoma cells by a monoclonal antibody reacting with P-glycoprotein. Biochem. Pharmacol. 37:2389–2393, 1988.

71. FitzGerald, D.J., Willingham, M.C., Cardarelli, C.O., Hamada, H., Tsuruo, T., Gottesman, M.M., and Pastan, I. A monoclonal antibody Pseudomonas toxin conjugate that specifically kills multidrug-resistant cells. Proc. Natl. Acad. Sci. USA 84:4288–4292, 1987.

72. Hamilton, T.C., Winker, M.A., Konie, K.G., Batist, G., Behrens, B.C., Tsuruo, T., Grotzinger, K.R., McKoy, W.M., Young, R.G., and Ozols, R.F. Augmentation of adriamycin, melphalan and cisplatin cytotoxicity in drug-resistant and sensitive human ovarian carcinoma cell lines by buthionine sulfoximine mediated glutathione depletion. Biochem. Pharmacol. 34:2583–2586, 1985.

73. Dusre, L., Mimnaugh, E.G., Myer, S.C.E., and Sinha, B.K. Potentation of doxorubicin cytotoxicity by buthionine sulfoximine in multidrug-resistant human breast tumor cells. Cancer Res. 49:511–515, 1989.

74. Kramer, R.A., Zakher, J., and Kim, G. Role of the glutathione redox cycle in acquired and de novo multidrug resistance. Science 241:694–697, 1988.

75. Moscow, J.A., Fairchild, C.R., Madden, M.J., Ramson, D.T., Wieand, H.S., O'Brien, E.E., Poplack, D.G., Cossman, J., Myers, C.E., and Cowan, K.H. Expression of anionic glutathione-S-transferase and P-glycoprotein genes in human tissues and tumors. Cancer Res. 49:1422–1428, 1989.

76. Nagourney, R.A., Messenger, J.C., Kern, D.H., and Weisenthal, L.M. In vitro enhancement of doxorubicin (Dox) and nitrogen mustard (NM) cytotoxicity in drug resistant human neoplasms by ethacrynic acid (EA). Proc. Am. Assoc. Cancer Res. 30:2283, 1989.

77. Epstein, R.J. and Smith, P.J. Estrogen-induced potentiation of DNA damage and cytotoxicity in human breast cancer cells treated with topoisomerase II-interactive antitumor drugs. Cancer Res. 48:297–303, 1988.

78. Alexander, R.B., Nelson, W.G., and Coffey, D.S. Synergistic enhancement by tumor necrosis factor of in vitro cytotoxicity from chemotherapeutic drugs targeted at DNA topoisomerase II. Cancer Res. 47:2403–2406, 1987.

79. Zwelling, L.A., Chan, D., Hinds, M., Mayes, J., Silberman, L.E., and Blick, M. Effect of phorbol ester treatment on drug-induced topoisomerase II-mediated DNA cleavage in human leukemia cells. Cancer Res. 48:6625–6633, 1988.

80. Sahyoun, N., Wolf, M., Besterman, J., Hsieh, T.-S., Sander, M., LeVine, III H., Chang,

K.-J., and Cuatrecasas, P. Protein kinase C phosphorylates topoisomerase II: topoisomerase activation and its possible role in phorbol ester-induced differentiation of HL-60 cells. Proc. Natl. Acad. Sci. 83:1603–1607, 1986.

81. Miskimins, R., Miskimins, W.K., Bernstein, H., and Shimizu, N. Epidermal growth factor-induced topoisomerase(s). Intracellular translocation and relation to DNA synthesis. Exp. Cell Res. 146:53–62, 1983.

82. Slevin, M.L., Clark, P.I., Joel, S.P., Malik, S., Osborne, R.J., Gregory, W.M., Lowe, D.G., Reznek, R.H., and Wringley, P.F.M. A randomized trial to evaluate the effect of schedule on the activity of etoposide in small-cell lung cancer. J. Clin. Oncol. 7: 1333–1340, 1989.

83. Hainsworth, J.D., Johnson, D.H., Frazier, S.R., and Greco, F.A. Chronic daily administration of oral etoposide. A phase I trial. J. Clin. Oncol. 7:396–401, 1989.

84. Zijlstra, J.G., de Vries, E.G.E., Muskiet, F.A.J., Martini, I.A., Timmer-Bosscha, H., and Mulder, N.H. Influence of docosahexaenoic acid in vitro on intracellular adriamycin concentration in lymphocytes and human adriamycin-sensitive and -resistant small-cell lung cancer cell lines, and on cytotoxicity in the tumor cell lines. Int. J. Cancer 40: 850–856, 1987.

85. Presant, C.A., Multhauf, P., and Metter, G. Reversal of cancer chemotherapeutic resistance by amphotericin B: a broad based phase I-II pilot study. Eur. J. Cancer Clin. Oncol. 23:683–687, 1987.

86. Willson, J.K.V., Fisher, P.H., Tutsch, K., Alberti, D., Simon, K., Hamilton, R.D., Bruggink, J., Koeller, J.M., Tormey, D.C., Earhart, R.H., Ranhosky, A., and Trump, D.L. Phase 1 clinical trial of a combination of dipyridamole and acivicin based upon inhibition of nucleoside salvage. Cancer Res. 48:5585–5590, 1988.

87. FitzGerald, G.A. Drug therapy: Dipyridamole. N. Engl. J. Med. 20:1247–1257, 1987.

88. Howell, S.B., Hom, D., Sanga, R., Vick, J.S., and Abramson, I.A. Comparison of the synergistic potentiation of etoposide, doxorubicin and vinblastine cytotoxicity by dipyridamole. Cancer Res. 49:3178–3183, 1989.

89. Willson, J.K.V., Fisher, P.H., Remick, S.C., Tutsch, K.D., Grem, J.L., Nieting, L., Alberti, D., Bruggink, J., and Trump, D.L. Methotrexate and dipyridamole combination chemotherapy based upon inhibition of nucleoside salvage in humans. Cancer Res. 49: 1866–1870, 1989.

90. Chan, T.C.K., Coppoc, G.L., Zimm, S., Cleary, S., and Howell, S.B. Pharmacokinetics of intraperitoneally administered dipyridamole in cancer patients. Cancer Res. 48:215–218, 1988.

186

9. The role of P-glycoprotein in drug-resistant hematologic malignancies

William S. Dalton, Thomas M. Grogan, and Thomas P. Miller

Introduction

In the past two decades, remarkable accomplishments have been made in the treatment of hematologic tumors, resulting in many patients being cured. The role of chemotherapy in the treatment of acute leukemia in children constitutes one of the true success stories of modern clinical oncology. Modern chemotherapeutic regimens are capable of producing remissions in approximately 90–100% of children, and ultimately over half of these patients are cured of their disease [1]. In adults, remissions are also common in both acute lymphocytic and nonlymphocytic leukemias; however, long-term remissions and possible cures are achieved in only approximately 30% of the patients [2]. Treatment of relapsed leukemia is less rewarding, and ultimately patients become refractory to all drugs. The drug resistance that eventually develops in patients with recurrent acute leukemia is an acquired resistance. In other words, drugs that were initially effective in reducing tumor burden become ineffective by selecting for drug-resistant cells over time.

Like the leukemias, malignant lymphomas also commonly manifest acquired drug resistance. Both Hodgkin's disease and the non-Hodgkin's lymphomas routinely respond to a wide variety of chemotherapeutic agents at the time of initial diagnosis. However, among lymphoma patients, especially those with higher tumor burden, relapses are frequent. Subsequent responses to additional combination chemotherapy are less frequent and less durable. Eventually, resistant disease develops to the chemotherapy drugs used as initial treatment and to all available alternative regimens. Cures following a relapse of initial chemotherapy in patients with malignant lymphomas are uncommon events [3–5].

For purposes of illustration, consider the clinical course of patients with diffuse large-cell lymphoma, the most common subtype of potentially curable non-Hodgkin's lymphomas [6]. The clinical course and response to treatment of patients with diffuse large-cell lymphoma is directly related to stage at the time of initial diagnosis. In general, the stage of disease correlates with tumor burden, even though the Ann Arbor system used for nomenclature is based on an anatomical pattern of spread [7]. Patients with very

Robert F. Ozols (ed.), MOLECULAR AND CLINICAL ADVANCES IN ANTICANCER DRUG RESISTANCE. Copyright © 1991.
Kluwer Academic Publishers, Boston. All rights reserved. ISBN 0-7923-1212-0

localized disease, stage I, have consistently been shown to have complete remissions in the range of 90–97% [8]. Long-term follow up of these patients demonstrates few relapses and an overall survival of approximately 90%. Stage II disease, generally representing a higher tumor burden at the time of diagnosis, is associated with a correspondingly lower remission rate of approximately 75% and long-term survival of approximately 80%. Patients with far advanced disease and high tumor burdens, stage III and IV disease, have complete remission rates that vary by investigator, but range from approximately 60% to 85% [9–12]. Some recent unconfirmed series demonstrate that overall survival may be in the range of 60% [10,11], but studies performed in multiinstitutional cooperative group trials with very long-term follow up demonstrate that approximately 30% of patients are cured [13]. In any case, a high proportion of patients with high tumor burdens at the time of initial diagnosis eventually relapse and die of drug-resistant disease. The observation that increased tumor burden is associated with reduced response rates and increased relapse rates is compatible with the Goldie-Coldman model, suggesting that spontaneous mutations occur that confer drug resistance and that new clones eventually dominate as drug-resistant cells are selected by continued treatment [14]; that is, with higher tumor burdens, the probability of a spontaneous mutation associated with acquired drug resistance is increased. Furthermore, the observation that initial chemotherapy results in a high proportion of remissions is compatible with the suggestion that the majority of a tumor at the time of diagnosis contains drug-sensitive cells and that chemotherapy becomes a selective factor, leaving behind a smaller population of drug-resistant cells, which eventually expand to appear as recurrent and drug-resistant lymphoma.

Multiple myeloma, a tumor associated with the proliferation of immunoglobulin-secreting cells that are derived from the B-cell series of immunocytes, is another hematologic tumor that has recently been studied for the problem of acquired drug resistance [15,16]. Systemic chemotherapy induces a response in the majority of patients; however, 15–20% of patients manifest an intrinsic resistance to even aggressive chemotherapy at the time of initial presentation and develop progressive myeloma. Prior to the development of effective chemotherapy, the median survival was less than a year. With the advent of effective chemotherapy, median survival is now in the range of 3–4 years, and a few patients may live as long as 5–10 years and occasionally longer. Unfortunately, all patients eventually relapse and become refractory to chemotherapy, despite an initial response.

Alkylating agents, especially melphalan, are the primary drugs used in the treatment of multiple myeloma. In the past decade, the natural products vincristine and doxorubicin have been found to be effective chemotherapeutic drugs in patients with myeloma refractory to alkylating agents. Recently, Barlogie et al. reported the effectiveness of continuous infusion vincristine plus doxorubicin with oral dexamethasone (VAD) in patients with myeloma in relapse [17]. This regimen is particularly useful in patients who initially respond but then subsequently relapse; however, ultimately this treatment also fails. Like the leukemias and malignant lymphomas mentioned above, multiple myeloma appears to be a suitable clinical model for studying the development of acquired drug resistance.

The *Vinca* alkaloids, vincristine and vinblastine, and the anthracyclines, daunorubicin and doxorubicin, are major chemotherapeutic drugs used in the treatment of leukemias, lymphomas, and multiple myeloma. One type of resistance that develops following repeated exposure to natural chemotherapeutic agents, such as vincristine and doxorubicin, is termed *multiple-drug resistance* (MDR) [18,19]. In MDR, malignant cells not only become resistant to one drug, but develop resistance to many drugs that share little structural similarity or mechanism of action. Thus, tumors that exhibit this multidrug resistant phenotype are likely to become resistant to even combination chemotherapy.

The most important finding in the understanding of the multidrug resistant phenotype has been the discovery of an integral membrane protein termed the *P-glycoprotein* (P-gly) [18–20]. The multidrug resistant gene (*mdr1*) has been isolated and found to be responsible for the expression of P-glycoprotein. (P-gly). The mechanism of resistance associated with P-gly is energy dependent and decreases drug accumulation in tumor cells by enhancing drug efflux. Thus, overexpression of P-gly results in a reduced net intracellular concentration of drugs in resistant cells.

P-glycoprotein has recently been detected in both solid tumor cells as well as hematologic tumor cells, including leukemias, malignant lymphomas, and multiple myeloma [21–24]. A number of analytical, methods have been used for P-glycoprotein detection in these tumor samples, including immunoblotting, immunocytochemistry, and RNA analysis. Studies are currently being conducted to examine the functional role of P-glycoprotein expression and response to chemotherapy in these hematologic tumors.

If P-glycoprotein overexpression is responsible for the development of multidrug resistance in these hematologic tumors, it may be possible to circumvent this resistance by inactivating this protein or by using drugs to which MDR cells are not cross-resistant or even collaterally sensitive. The use of prednisone or dexamethasone as single agents in patients with drug-resistant multiple myeloma represents an example of using collaterally sensitive drugs in patients with drug-resistant myeloma [25]. It is also possible that biological response modifiers, such as interferon or tumor necrosis factor, may be effective in multidrug resistant disease [26].

A great deal of attention has been focused on the discovery that calcium-channel blocking agents, such as verapamil, are capable of circumventing multidrug resistance [27–30]. A variety of other compounds have been found to have similar chemosensitizing capabilities, including calmodulin inhibitors [31,32], such as trifluoperazine, lysosomotropic agents [33], and some cyclosporins [34,35]. The mechanism of these agents in overcoming drug resistance appears to be related to the blocking of enhanced drug efflux

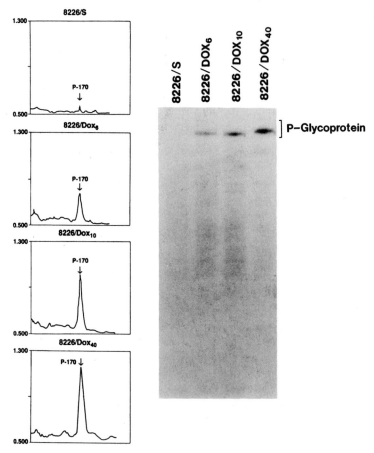

Figure 1. Western blot analysis of P-glycoprotein in human myeloma cell lines with increasing levels of multidrug resistance. Densitometry tracings with P-glycoprotein (p 170) of each cell line are noted on the left-hand side of the figure.

from cells, leading to increased intracellular drug accumulation. Clinical studies are currently being performed to investigate the efficacy and feasibility of using these types of chemosensitizers in patients with hematologic tumors.

Methods of detection of P-glycoprotein in clinical samples

A number of methods have been used to detect the presence of P-glycoprotein in clinical samples, including immunoblotting, immunocyto-chemistry, and detection of P-glycoprotein RNA [22,36,37,38]. While all these methods have demonstrated the ability to detect P-glycoprotein in clinical samples, there are certain clinical exigencies that influence the utility of various methods: 1) sample size (small number of tumor cells), 2) time delay in analysis of specimen (which might allow for degradation of RNA), and 3) admixture of tumor cells and stromal elements. While methods, such as Northern blotting to detect RNA or western blotting to detect P-glycoprotein, in tumor samples have been demonstrated to be specific for the P-glycoprotein, these methods sacrifice the sensitivity and resolution needed for the examination of heterogenous tissues, where the multidrug-resistant cell populations may exist in small numbers. Methods such as immunocytochemistry and RNA in situ hybridization, which examine P-glycoprotein in single cells, are likely to be superior for tumor specimens that are heterogeneous for drug-resistant cells.

Western blot analysis of cell membrane preparations using monoclonal antibodies specifically developed for P-glycoprotein have demonstrated in-creased concentrations of P-glycoprotein in multidrug-resistant cultured cell lines and human tumor specimens [18,39,40]. This method relies on the homogenization and extraction of cell membranes from whole tumor tissue and often requires $10^7 - 10^8$ cells in order to detect P-glycoprotein. Figure 1 shows the western blot analysis of P-glycoprotein in human myeloma cell lines that were selected for drug resistance. Analysis of cell lines with gradually increasing levels of multidrug resistance (8226/S, 8226/Dox$_6$, 8226/Dox$_{10}$, and 8226/Dox$_{40}$, where cells are exposed to 6, 10, and 40 times the amount of doxorubicin, respectively) demonstrated a close association be-tween the level of resistance to doxorubicin and the amount of P-glycoprotein in these tumor cell lines [36]. Western blot analyses are limited by the fact that one value is obtained for an entire population of cells, because the entire tumor must be homogenized and analyzed as one specimen. The western blot analysis, therefore, gives no indication of the degree of hetero-geneity among tumor cells in their expression of P-glycoprotein and would almost certainly fail to detect a small number of drug-resistant cells in a tumor population [37,41]. In contrast, immunocytochemical assays work at the level of the single cell, allowing for a high degree of sensitivity of detection of drug-resistant cells in the entire cell population. In addition, immunocytochemistry allows for direct visualization of the cell being analyzed; separating tumor cells from normal cells may be important in that certain normal tissues may express P-glycoprotein. Figure 2 shows the immuno-cytochemical detection of P-glycoprotein in a patient sample compared to the drug-resistant myeloma cell line, 8226/Dox$_6$. The intensity of staining increases with increasing doxorubicin resistance. The staining is particularly intense in the plasma membrane, with occasional staining of the Golgi apparatus in the cytoplasm. There are a number of monoclonal antibodies that have been developed for P-glycoprotein that may be used in an immuno-cytochemical assay. We have optimized the conditions for three different antibodies (C219, JSB1, and MRK16) in myeloma and found that the fixation conditions are different for each antibody [41]. Thus, in developing immunocytochemistry assays the fixation conditions for each antibody must

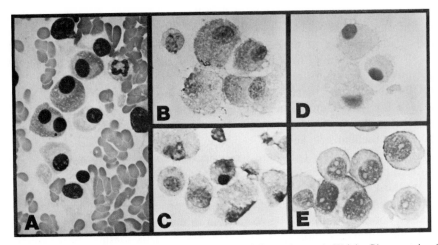

Figure 2. Immunocytochemistry of a patient with multiple myeloma. *A*: Wright-Giemsa stain of a patient's myeloma cells. *B*: Staining for P-glycoprotein, noted by brown discoloration. *C*: The same patient's cells, with staining prominently noted in the cell membrane as well as the golgi apparatus. *D*: Negative control using an irrelevant antibody. *E*: Immunocytochemistry staining for 8226/Dox$_6$ as a positive control.

be considered for a given type of tumor to be analyzed. A method for immunocytochemical detection of P-glycoprotein in hematologic tumors may not be necessarily suitable for solid tumors, and appropriate controls need to be performed to determine specificity, as well as sensitivity.

Having developed a sensitive immunocytochemical assay for the detection of P-glycoprotein in myeloma cells, we have also developed a method to quantitate the amount of P-glycoprotein on single cells [36,41]. In this system, the average optical density of individual cells stained is measured with a computer-assisted image analysis program (CAS100, Becton Dickinson, Mountain View, Cal). The system includes a light microscope from which the images are collected by a charge-coupled device video camera. Using this instrument, each cell's optical density is compared and relates to the degree of staining intensity. As shown in Figure 3, the mean optical density for approximately 50 cells of a patient specimen with multiple myeloma is compared to standard drug-resistant cell lines 8226/Dox$_6$ and 8226/Dox$_{40}$. This particular patient's cells appeared to have slightly more P-glycoprotein than the Dox$_6$ cell line, which is approximately 10-fold resistant compared to its sensitive parent cell line. This method allows the quantitation of P-glycoprotein on individual cells by measuring the average optical density of each cell stained immocytochemically and compares the values obtained to cell lines expressing known amounts of P-glycoprotein (positive standards) and those without P-glycoprotein (negative control). Thus, this method would both determine the percent of positive cells that express P-glycoprotein in a tumor specimen and quantitate the amount of P-

192

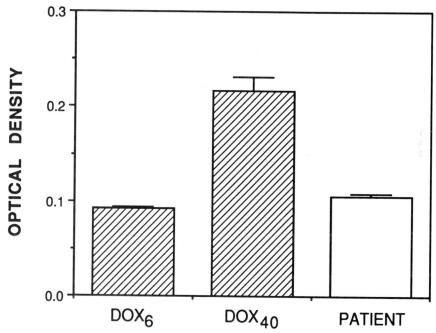

Figure 3. The mean optical density for two standard cell lines, 8226/Dox$_6$ and 8226/Dox$_{40}$, in comparison with a patient's myeloma cells. (Reprinted with permission, see reference 36).

glycoprotein on individual cells that may be of value in determining the significance of P-glycoprotein in clinical drug resistance.

Measuring levels of P-glycoprotein RNA has also been used as a means of detecting and quantitating P-glycoprotein in human tumors. Goldstein et al. [22] used an RNA slot blot analysis as well as RNase protection assay to detect P-glycoprotein RNA in over 400 human cancers. These investigators developed a quantitative method by comparing unknown tumor samples to known multidrug-resistant cell lines that expressed a standard amount of RNA. Using this method, the authors were able to categorize tumors as being low or high expressors of P-glycoprotein. More recently, this same group of investigators has developed an RNA in situ hybridization technique to detect messenger RNA at the level of the single cell [38]. Therefore, like the immunocytochemical assay, the in situ hybridization method of analysis of tumor specimens should allow for the detection of multidrug resistant tumor cells in heterogeneous cell populations.

Occurrence of P-glycoprotein in hematologic tumors

With the development of more sensitive techniques for the detection of P-glycoprotein, the incidence of P-glycoprotein expression in hematologic tumors is now being reported. Using the monoclonal antibody C-219, Ma et al. [42] reported an immunocytochemical technique for detecting P-glycoprotein in individual cells of two patients with acute nonlymphocytic leukemia. They demonstrated that as the disease progressed in these two patients, the percentage of cells that were P-glycoprotein positive increased. Thus, at least in these two patients, the emergence of clinical drug resistance was associated with increased expression of P-glycoprotein in these leukemic cells.

Table 1 lists six hematologic tumors that have been found to express P-glycoprotein when tumor specimens were analyzed from patients with these various diseases. When possible, the tumors were classified as untreated or treated, depending on whether the patients had received chemotherapy prior to the time of biopsy and analysis for P-glycoprotein. Goldstein et al. [22] analyzed the RNA of nine patients with chronic myelogenous leukemia. Three patients were in the chronic phase of their CML and six patients were in the blastic phase. All three patients who were in the chronic phase of their disease showed no P-glycoprotein expression on their leukemic cells. In contrast, five out of six patients in the blastic phase of their disease showed an overexpression of P-glycoprotein on their leukemic cells. Similarly, two different studies using either immunocytochemistry or RNA analysis found that 50% of patients in the blastic phase of their chronic myelogenous leukemia expressed P-glycoprotein on their cells [43,44]. These preliminary results indicate that, even at the time of diagnosis prior to treatment of the blastic phase, a high percentage of patients with CML will express P-glycoprotein on their cells. This may explain, in part, the poor results of teatment for blastic phase of chronic myelogenous leukemia. Although results are preliminary, it is also interesting that only cells from patients in blast crisis express P-glycoprotein, as opposed to cells in the chronic phase of the disease. It is possible that by further studying patients

Table 1. P-glycoprotein expression in hematologic tumors

Disease	Untreated (%)	Treated (%)	Reference
1. Chronic myelogenous leukemia			
Chronic phase	0/3 (0)		22
Blastic phase	3/3 (100)	2/3 (66)	22
	3/6 (50)		43
	2/4 (50)		44
2. Acute lymphocytic leukemia	1/9 (11)	3/19 (16)	45
	2/15 (13)	1/1 (100)	22
3. Acute non-lymphocytic leukemia	3/24 (13)	4/5 (80)	22
	2/8 (25)	5/8 (62)	46
4. Myelodysplastic syndrome	7/19 (37)		46
5. Myeloma	2/51 (4)	5/7 (71)	23,41
		8/14 (57)	47
6. Non-Hodgkin's lymphoma	1/39 (3)	6/8 (75)	48
	4/11 (36)	4/11 (36)	49

194

with chronic myelogenous leukemia, information may be obtained as to whether P-glycoprotein is expressed in only the mature well-differentiated cells versus more immature, progenitor cells with a pluripotential capacity. Analyzing early B-cells for immunoglobulin gene rearrangement in patients with myeloma, for example, may reveal at what stage of development these cells are able to express P-glycoprotein.

Patients with acute lymphocytic leukemia, both childhood and adult, appear to have low level of expression of P-glycoprotein, with approximately 10–15% of patients expressing the drug-resistant molecule on their cells. In a study of 28 patients with acute lymphoblastic leukemia, Rothenberg et al. [45] found that four patients (three after multiple relapses, one at presentation) overexpressed P-glycoprotein. In contrast to patients with acute lymphocytic leukemia, patients with acute nonlymphocytic leukemia appear to have a high overexpression of P-glycoprotein if they have been previously treated. Goldstein et al. [22] found that 3 of 24 patients or 13% expressed P-glycoprotein in their leukemic cells at time of diagnosis; however, 4 of 5 patients expressed P-glycoprotein on their leukemic cells if they had received prior chemotherapy. Similarly, Holmes and coworkers [46] found that 62% of patients who had received prior chemotherapy expressed elevated levels of P-glycoprotein compared to 25% of patients who were newly diagnosed. These same investigators also found elevated P-glycoprotein RNA expression in 4 out of 5 patients with the diagnosis of secondary acute leukemia. Therefore, in the case of acute nonlymphocytic leukemia, P-glycoprotein overexpression is associated with the emergence of clinical drug resistance. Patients with myelodysplastic syndromes (pre- leukemia) are also known to have drug-resistant disease, with essentially no patients being cured by chemotherapy. Holmes et al. [46] found that 37% of patients with myelodysplastic syndrome had P-glycoprotein expression on their leukemic cells.

Patients with newly diagnosed multiple myeloma versus those who have been previously treated with *Vinca* alkyloids or doxorubicin have also been analyzed for the overexpression of P-glycoprotein [23,24,47]. Using immunocytochemical techniques with RNA analysis as a means of confirmation in some patients, we have found a low incidence of P-glycoprotein expression (4%) in newly diagnosed myeloma patients. In contrast, in patients who have received extensive prior chemotherapy including continuous infusion vincristine and adriamycin, there appears to be a high percentage of patients whose cells express the drug-resistant protein [23,36]. We recently reported that 5 out of 7 patients who had progressed on continuous infusion vincristine and adriamycin (VAD) had elevated levels of P-glycoprotein [23]. Similarly, Epstein and colleagues [47], using the C219 monoclonal antibody and flow cytometry to analyze myeloma cells, found that the majority of patients who failed VAD treatment had P-glycoprotein positive myeloma cells.

In order to determine if the P-glycoprotein was expressed in patients with non-Hodgkin's lymphomas, we tested tumor biopsies for the presence of P-glycoprotein in 39 consecutive untreated patients using an immunohisto-chemical [48]. The presence of P-glycoprotein was found in 1 of 39 patients who were newly diagnosed and untreated at the time of biopsy. On the other hand, among 8 biopsies from previously treated and clinically drug refractory patients, 6 of the patients (75%) expressed detectable levels of P-glycoprotein on their tumor cells. We, therefore, concluded that P-glycoprotein was infrequently expressed among untreated non-Hodgkin's lymphoma patients and was relatively common in selected drug refractory patients. Those patients had received multiple drug combinations, including *Vinca* alkaloids and doxorubicin, appeared more likely to overexpress P-glycoprotein on their tumor cells.

In a similar study by Moscow et al. [49], P-glycoprotein positive cells were found in a series of 23 non-Hodgkin's lymphomas. Information was available on 22 of the 23 patients regarding prior treatment with chemo-therapy. In this series, 4 of 11 patients in the previously treated group and 4 of 11 patients in the untreated group, were positive for P-glycoprotein. Thus, in this study there was no apparent relationship between P-glycoprotein levels and exposure to prior chemotherapy, as was seen in the study by Miller et al. [48]. This apparent discrepancy actually demonstrates the importance of defining "prior treatment" in patients biopsied for detection of P-glycoprotein. Prior treatment of indolent lymphomas with chlorambucil cannot be expected to select for the same type or degree of drug resistance as prior treatment with combined chemotherapy containing vincristine and doxorubicin for patients with intermediate or high-grade lymphoma.

Reversal of P-glycoprotein function

Attempts to overcome drug resistance attributable to P-glycoprotein might include the following possibilities: 1) the use of non-cross-resistant regimens, as proposed by the Goldie-Coldman hypothesis; 2) high-dose chemotherapy, as would be used in autologous bone marrow transplants in lymphoma; 3) targeting P-glycoprotein positive cells with monoclonal antibodies or monoclonal antibody conjugates; and 4) the use of chemosensitizing agents or agents that are able to inhibit the function of P-glycoprotein. The use of non-cross-resistant therapeutic regimens is perhaps best illustrated in the new regimens for Hodgkin's disease and non-Hodgkin's lymphoma. In these regimens, the largest possible number of active agents are combined at the highest dose possible assuming that mutations conferring resistance to some drugs will not convey cross-resistance to others, as described in the Goldie-Coldman hypothesis. Recent studies have indicated that these newer regi-mens produce improved remission rates and may improve long-term survival, but confirmatory studies are needed with long-term follow-up [50,51].

High-dose chemotherapy or radiation therapy with bone marrow trans-plantation, as used for chronic myelogenous leukemia and malignant

196

lymphomas, represents another approach in overcoming drug resistance [52–54]. This form of therapy is currently the only possibility of cure for chronic myelogenous leukemia [52]. The assumption is that, despite resistance to standard doses of drugs, a dose response phenomenon does exist for these drug resistant tumors and that high doses of drugs or radiation therapy are able to overcome drug resistance. If it is assumed that P-glycoprotein functions by decreasing the intracellular drug accumulation, then perhaps the use of high doses of chemotherapy can overcome this phenomenon. No studies to date have tested this possibility in the clinic.

Another approach in overcoming P-glycoprotein-induced drug resistance would be specifically targeting cells using monoclonal antibody therapy. Tsuruo and colleagues [55] investigated the effectiveness of a monoclonal antibody developed against an external epitope of P-glycoprotein in treating multidrug-resistant human ovarian cancer xenografts in athymic nude mice. These monoclonal antibodies were able to either inhibit tumor formation in athymic mice or actually reduce tumor volume in mice who were treated after tumor development [55]. A second approach would be to conjugate monoclonal antibodies with a toxin, such as pseudomonas toxin, thereby enhancing the cytotoxicity of the monoclonal antibody [56]. Using monoclonal antibodies against P-glycoprotein to purge multidrug-resistant cells from bone marrow prior to the use of autologous bone marrow transplantation has also been theorized. Tong et al. [57] recently demonstrated in vitro that the use of monoclonal antibodies against myeloma cells and multidrug-resistant myeloma cells were effective in eradicating tumor cells, but spared normal progenitor cells that would allow marrow engraftment.

The area that was received the most attention, both in the laboratory and more recently in the clinic, is the use of chemosensitizers to reverse P-glycoprotein function. This work is primarily based on the observation by Tsuruo et al. who observed that the calcium antagonist, verapamil, and other compounds were able to overcome resistance to vincristine and adriamycin [27,31]. The chemosensitizers that reverse multidrug resistance seem to share the property of binding P-glycoprotein, thereby inhibiting its function [58,59]. Although calcium-channel blockers as a class of reagents are very effective in binding P-glycoprotein and inhibiting P-glycoprotein function, calcium ion involvement appears to have little to do with this activity [60]. A second possibility involves the phosphorylation of P-glycoprotein; agents such as verapamil and trifluoperazine are able to hyperphosphorylate P-glycoprotein, which may effectively inactivate it [61].

Studies of structure activity relationships of chemosensitizers performed by Beck and colleagues have demonstrated that modulators of P-glycoprotein are generally lipid soluble at physiological pH and possess a basic nitrogen atom and two planar aromatic rings [62,63]. Changes in the structure of P-glycoprotein by spontaneous mutations of the *mdr1* gene might also affect binding of chemomodifying agents, making one class of chemosensitizers more effective than others [64].

197

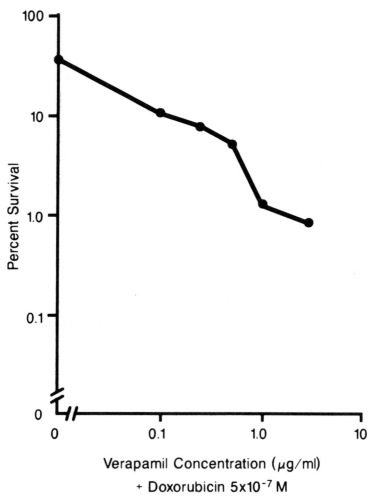

Figure 4. Cell survival of 8226/Dox$_{40}$ when cells are exposed to a constant dose of doxorubicin (5×10^{-7} M) plus varying doses of verapamil.

Using multidrug-resistant human myeloma cells, we have examined the efficacy of verapamil and other chemosensitizers in reversing resistance to vincristine and adriamycin [29,65,66]. We observed that verapamil was very effective in reversing resistance for both vincristine and adriamycin, even at a dose as low as 0.1 µg/ml. The in vitro cytotoxicity studies showed that verapamil was most effective when used by continuous exposure and that the ability of verapamil to reverse doxorubicin resistance was related to the dose of verapamil (Figure 4). A clear dose-response effect for verapamil in increasing net intracellular doxorubicin in the resistant cells was also observed (Figure 5). This increase in net accumulation of doxorubicin seen with verapamil in these myeloma cell lines is due to the blocking of enhanced drug efflux [29].

Table 2 lists the effectiveness of various chemosensitizers on the multidrug-resistant human myeloma cell line. Compounds are compared by their ability to reduce the concentration of doxorubicin requried to kill 50% of the colonies (ID50). The dose modifying factor (DMF) is defined by divid-

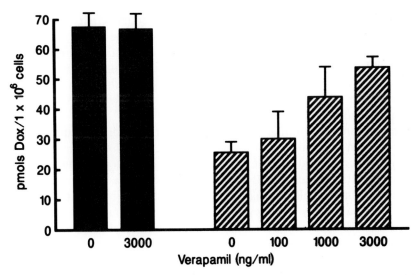

Figure 5. Dose response effect of verapamil on the intracellular accumulation of doxorubicin in 8226/Dox$_{40}$ cells (hatched bars) and sensitive, 8226/S cells (solid bars).

Table 2. Drug resistance in hematologic Tumors: Effectiveness of various chemosensitizers on a P-glycoprotein-positive human myeloma cell line

| Modifier | 6 μM | | 1 μM | |
	ID$_{50}$ Dox	DMF[a]	ID$_{50}$ Dox	DMF
Dox alone	3.0×10^{-6}		3.0×10^{-6}	
± Verapamil	1.5×10^{-7}	20	9.9×10^{-7}	3.0
R-verapamil	1.2×10^{-7}	25		
S-verapamil	1.5×10^{-7}	20		
± Gallopamil	2.2×10^{-7}	13	9.6×10^{-7}	3.0
R-gallopamil	1.4×10^{-7}	21		
S-gallopamil	5.6×10^{-7}	5		
Quinine	8.0×10^{-7}	4		
Quinidine	5.3×10^{-7}	6		
Trifluoperazine			2.6×10^{-6}	1.2
Diltiazem	4.5×10^{-7}	7		
Tween 80	1.9×10^{-7}	16		

[a] DMF = dose modifying factor defined by dividing the ID$_{50}$ Dox alone by ID$_{50}$ Dox + modifier.

ing the ID_{50} of doxorubicin alone by the ID_{50} of doxorubicin plus the modifier at a dose of 1 or 6 μm. When possible, optical isomers were studied to determine if a structural activity relationship existed for a specific compound. Both the R and S isomers of verapamil were equally effective with a DMF of approximately 20. Keilhauer and colleagues also demonstrated equal efficacy of the R and S isomers of verapamil, but reported that the S isomer was 10 times as cardiotoxic compared to the R isomer [67]. In contrast, the R-isomer of gallopamil appeared to be more active than the S-isomer with the racemic mixture being intermediate in activity. The optical isomers, quinine and quinidine, appeared to have equal activity with a DMF of approximately 5. Quinine is less toxic than quinidine, however, and the therapeutic index for quinine would likely be greater in the clinical setting. It is possible that by taking advantage of differences in toxicity for optical isomers, such as with quinine and quinidine, and possibly with R- kand S-verapamil, that the therapeutic index might be increased by using the less toxic optical isomer.

Given that reduced intracellular chemotherapeutic drug accumulation is the mechanism associated with P-glycoprotein expression on drug-resistant cells, a number of studies have now investigated cytotoxic drug accumulation in clinical specimens [23,45,68,69]. Drug uptake in cells was measured using either radiolabelled drug or by flow cytometry measuring cellular fluorescence caused by anthracyclines. The latter technique of fluorimetric analysis tended to demonstrate heterogeneity of daunorubicin accumulation in tumor cells, with drug-resistant cells presumably taking up less drug [45,68,69]. In a study of patients with acute nonlymphocytic leukemia, patients achieving complete remission showed a tendency of higher daunorubicin accumulation in leukemic blast cells than did partial responders [69].

The effects of chemosensitizers, such as verapamil, on cytotoxic drug accumulation has also been investigated in tumor cells from patients with drug-resistant disease [23,45,70,71]. In these studies of patients with multiple myeloma, chronic lymphocytic leukemia, chronic myelogenous leukemia, acute lymphocytic, and nonlymphocytic leukemia, verapamil appeared to increase the accumulation of either vincristine or daunorubicin. In two separate studies of patients with myeloma and acute lymphocytic leukemia, verapamil increased drug accumulation in cells shown to express P-glycoprotein. Thus, this in vitro analysis of human tumor cells obtained from patients with drug-resistant, P-gly-positive disease demonstrated that drug accumulation can be increased by the addition of verapamil. What remains to be demonstrated, however, is an increase in cellular drug accumulation when verapamil is given in vivo in the clinical situation.

With the evidence that P-glycoprotein overexpression occurs in patients with drug-resistant myeloma and non-Hodgkin's lymphoma, we have conducted a pilot study to determine if verapamil is capable of overcoming drug resistance [23]. Five of 7 patients with drug-resistant multiple myeloma overexpressed P-glycoprotein on their tumor cells, as determined by immunohistochemical staining and RNA analysis. All patients had developed progressive disease while receiving a regimen containing vincristine and doxorubicin (VAD). At the time of progressive disease, continuous infusion verapamil was added to the VAD regimen. Two of the seven patients who were refractory to vincristine and doxorubicin alone responded when verapamil was added to VAD. Both patients who responded had P-glycoprotein-positive tumors. Verapamil increased the intracellular accumulation of doxorubicin and vincristine in vitro for both patients whose tumors overexpressed P-glycoprotein. To date, 22 patients have been treated, with five patients showing a partial response. Durations of response have been short, however, with the median duration of response being less than 6 months.

Two other studies have reported preliminary clinical observations in patients with drug-resistant multiple myeloma [72,73]. In a preliminary report by Gore et al. seven patients who were resistant to 4 day continuous infusion vincristine and adriamycin were administered a low dose of verapamil by continuous infusion. Four out of 7 patients had a further reduction in paraprotein levels of greater than 25%. Two of the responders had a greater than 50% response with the addition of verapamil to the chemotherapeutic regimen. A second pilot study reported by Trumper et al. [73] studied 10 patients who had developed drug-resistant multiple myeloma. Only 1 of 10 patients responded when verapamil was added to the VAD regimen. Based on the results of these pilot studies, prospective, randomized, controlled studies are now indicated. A study of VAD versus VAD plus verapamil in multiple myeloma is now being conducted in the Southwest Oncology Group.

We have recently conducted a similar pilot study in patients with drug-refractory non-Hodgkin's lymphoma [48]. In order to achieve maximally tolerated doses of verapamil, the verapamil was administered as a continuous infusion for 5 days, beginning at a dose 0.2mg/kg/hr and increasing the dose by 0.05 mg/kg/hr each day as toxicity permitted. The chemotherapy consisted of $600 \, mg/m^2$ cyclophosphamide (C) on day 1, 0.4 mg/day vincristine (V), and $10 \, mg/m^2/day$ doxorubicin (A) as 24-h infusions on days 1–4, and 8 mg of dexamethasone (D) given by mouth on days 1–4 (C-VAD). Fourteen patients with recurrent and drug-refractory malignant lymphoma were treated with C-VAD and high-dose infusion verapamil. Among 11 evaluable patients, 10 (91%) responded to treatment with at least a partial response. Three patients (27%) had a complete remission. It was concluded that C-VAD plus high doses of verapamil resulted in a high response rate among heavily pretreated and drug-refractory patients. This initial success has led to further trials to gain experience with a larger number of patients in order to correlate response and survival with the presence or absence of P-glycoprotein.

The toxicity noted for patients with multiple myeloma and non-Hodgkin's lymphoma given continuous infusion verapamil with chemotherapy was clinically significant. All patients required hospitalization with continuous cardiac monitoring. Cardiovascular side effects were dose limiting, but no patient died from toxicity and hospitalizations were not prolonged. Hypotension was essentially a universal finding, with an average drop in mean blood pressure of 10 mmHg. An increase in PR interval was also frequent, occurring in most patients. A junctional rhythm with nodal escape occurred in approximately 14% of the patients. Patients were generally asymptomatic from these cardiovascular side effects. Non-cardiovascular side effects included constipation, weight gain, peripheral edema, and occasional headache. Myelosuppression was not significantly increased by the addition of verapamil to VAD. Other toxicities, such as peripheral neuropathy secondary to vincristine or nausea/vomitting secondary to doxorubicin, were not increased by verapamil.

Our findings are in agreement with those of Ozols et al. [74] in that the dose-limiting toxicity of verapamil combined with chemotherapeutic drugs is transient cardiotoxicity. Given that P-glycoprotein occurs in normal tissues, it is conceivable that toxicity in these organs might be increased when verapamil is added to chemotherapeutic agents. Recently, Horton et al. [75] studied the modulation of vincristine by verapamil and the associated toxicity in mice. These investigators showed that verapamil markedly increased the uptake and retention of vincristine in small intestine, liver, and kidney of mice [75]. Recently, Cordon-Cardo et al. [76] reported that endothelial cells of human capillary blood vessels at the blood-brain barrier expressed P-glycoprotein. It is conceivable, therefore, that verapamil might actually increase the concentration of certain chemotherapeutic agents in the brain and that neurotoxicity could be manifested. In the clinical studies performed to date, no untoward neurological side effects have been reported, with the exception of occasional patients complaining of headache while on continuous infusion vincristine, adriamycin, and verapamil [23].

Clearly, new chemosensitizers need to be developed that are, by themselves, less toxic and will not enhance the toxicity of the chemotherapeutic agents. It will be difficult to evaluate the clinical role of drug-resistance modulators on a large-scale basis until new chemosensitizers are developed.

Conclusions

The hematologic tumors multiple myeloma, chronic and acute leukemias, and the malignant lymphomas appear to be excellent clinical models for the study of acquired drug resistance. Preliminary data from human specimens indicates that P-glycoprotein does play a role in the acquisition of resistance to natural products, such as vincristine and adriamycin. Pilot studies have also shown that verapamil and other chemosensitizers, such as trifluoperazine [77], may reverse resistance in a subset of patients. These same preliminary studies also indicate that drug resistance in hematologic tumors is multifactorial, given that not all drug-resistant patients have positive

P-glycoprotein tumor cells and only a minority of patients appear to benefit from the use of chemosensitizers. These findings suggest that verapamil, at the doses administered, is either an incomplete modulator of P-glycoprotein or other mechanisms of tumor escape from therapy exist. These mechanisms may include the simultaneous or sequential development of other cell membrane proteins, which are not detectable by the current methods used and/or not reversible with verapamil [78–80]. Furthermore, tumors may escape control with treatment for a variety of reasons not associated with drug resistance. For example, we and others have previously shown that the absence of HLA-DR on biopsies from patients with diffuse large-cell lymphoma portends an extremely poor outcome [81]. It is possible that cell surface proteins responsible for cell-cell contact and identification are essential for the host response. Tumors that have lost the HLA-DR antigen may have a low number of tumor-infiltrating lymphocytes, resulting in a poor prognosis. The rate of cell proliferation in tumor growth may be another example of a mechanism for treatment failure and unrelated to drug resistance in patients with large-cell lymphoma or myeloma [23,82,83]. Thus, it may be possible for tumors to relapse and progress, in spite of treatment with effective chemotherapy, as measured by drug sensitivity or resistance. Most investigators have observed patients who have very dramatic responses to combination chemotherapy only to relapse before bone marrow recovery, thus limiting the frequency of effective treatment.

In summary, we believe that hematologic malignancies represent a clinical corollary for studies of clinical drug resistance related to the P-glycoprotein. We would recommend that randomized, prospective, controlled, clinical studies be performed using chemosensitizers. Several major factors must be considered when disigning these types of trials: 1) prior treatment of patients registered in these trials (conceivably treating patients with chemosensitizers early in the course of their disease could actually prevent or at least delay the expression of P-glycoprotein); 2) the type and dose of chemosensitizer used; 3) the presence or absence of P-glycoprotein on individual patient's tumor cells at the time of adding chemosensitizers to therapy; and 4) the method by which both chemotherapy and chemosensitizers are administered to patients. Continuous infusion of both chemotherapeutic drugs and chemosensitizers may be the best form of administration based on preclinical studies that have shown that the continuous presence of verapamil is necessary to inhibit drug efflux and that the effects are rapidly reversible [84,85].

References

1. Poplack, D.G., Kun L.E., Cassady J.R., et al. Leukemias and lymphomas of childhood. In: DeVita, V.T., Hellman, S., Rosenberg, S.A. (eds). Cancer Principles and Practice of Oncology, Philadelphia, J.B. Lippincott, p. 1671. 1989.
2. Wiernik P. Acute leukemias. In: Cancer Principles and Practice of Oncology DeVita, V.T., Hellman, S., and Rosenberg, S.A. (eds). J.B. Lippincott, Philadelphia, 1989.

3. Buzaid, A.C., Lippman S.M., and Miller, T.P. Salvage therapy of advanced Hodgkin's disease. Critical appraisal of curative potential. Am. J. Med. 83:523–532, 1987.
4. Cabanillas, F., Hagemeister, F.B., McLaughlin, P., et al. MIMI combination chemotherapy for refractory or recurrent lymphomas. J. Clin. Oncol. 5:407–412, 1987.
5. Velasquez W.S., Cabanillas, F., Salvador, P., et al. Effective salvage therapy for lymphoma with cisplatin in combination with high-dose Ara-C and dexamethasone (DHAP). Blood 71:117–122, 1988.
6. The Non-Hodgkin's Lymphoma Pathologic Classification Project Writing Committee. National Cancer Institute sponsored study of classifications of non-Hodgkin's lymphomas. Cancer 49:2112–2135, 1982.
7. Carbone, P.P., Kaplan, H.S., Musshoff, K., et al. Report of the committee on Hodgkin's disease staging classification. Cancer Res. 31:1860–1861, 1971.
8. Miller, T. Therapy of localized non-Hodgkin's lymphmas. In: Cancer: Principles and Practice of Oncology Updates 3(6), DeVita, D.V. Jr., Hellman, S. and Rosenbert, S.A. (eds). J.B. Lippincott, Philadelphia, 1989.
9. Jones, S.E., Grozea, P.N., Metz, E.N., et al. Improved complete remission rates and survival for patients with large cell lymphoma treated with chemoimmunotherapy. Cancer 51:1083–1090, 1983.
10. Klimo, K. and Connors, J.M. MACOP-B chemotherapy for the treatment of diffuse large-cell lymphoma. Ann. Intern. Med. 102:596–602, 1985.
11. Coleman, M., Gerstein, G., Topilow, A., et al. Advances in therapy for large cell lymphoma. Semin. Hematol 24:8, 1987.
12. Miller, T.P., Dana, B.W., and Weick, J.K. Southwest Oncology Group clinical trials for intermediate and high grade non-Hodgkin's lymphomas. Semin. Hematol. 25:17–22, 1988.
13. Coltman, C.A., Dahlbert, S., Jones, S.E., et al. CHOP is curative in thirty percent of patients with large cell lymphoma: a twelve year Southwest Oncology Group follow-up. Proc. Am. Soc. Clin. Oncol. 5:197, 1986.
14. Goldie, J.H. and Coldman A.J. The genetic origin of drug resistance in neoplasms: implications for systemic therapy. Cancer Res. 44:3643–●●●●, 1984.
15. Kyle, R.A. Diagnosis and management of multiple myeloma and related disorders. Prog. Hematol. 14:257–282, 1986.
16. Buzaid, A.C. and Durie, B.G.M. Management of refractory myeloma: a review. J. Clin. Oncol. 6:889–905, 1988.
17. Barlogie, B., Smith, L., and Alezanian, R. Effective treatment of advanced multiple myeloma refractory to alkylating agents. N. Engl. J. Med. 310:1353–1356, 1984.
18. Gerlach, J.H., Kartner, N., Bell, D.R., et al. Multidrug resistance. Cancer Surv. 5:24–26, 1986.
19. Pastan, I. and Gottesman, M. Multiple-drug resistance in human cancer. N. Engl. J. Med. 316:1388–1393, 1987.
20. Kartner, N., Evernden-Porelle, D., Bradley, G., et al. Detection of P-glycoprotein in multidrug-resistant cell lines by monoclonal antibodies. Nature 316:820–823, 1985.
21. Fojo, A.T., Ueda, K., Slamon, D.J., et al. Expression of a multidrug resistance gene in human tumors and tissues. Proc. Natl. Acad. Sci. USA 84:265–269, 1987.
22. Goldstein, L.J., Galski, H., Fojo, A., et al. Expression of a multidrug resistance gene in human cancers. J. Natl. Cancer Inst. 81:116–124, 1989.
23. Dalton, W.S., Grogan, T.M., Meltzer, P.S., et al. Drug-resistance in multiple myeloma and non-Hodgkin's lymphoma: detection of P-glycoprotein and potential circumvention by addition of verapamil to chemotherapy. J. Clin. Oncol. 7:415–424, 1989.
24. Salmon, S.E., Grogan, T.M., Miller, T., et al. Prediction of doxorubicin resistance in vitro in myeloma, lymphoma, and breast cancer by P-glycoprotein staining. J. Natl. Cancer Inst. 81, 1989.
25. Salmon, S.E., Shadduck, R.K., and Schilling, A. Intermittent high dose prednisone therapy for multiple myeloma. Cancer Chemother. Rep. 51:179–187, 1967.

26. Salmon, S.E., Soehnlen, B., Dalton, W.S., et al. Effects of tumor necrosis factor on sensitive and multidrug resistant human leukemia and myeloma cell lines. Blood 74:1723–1727, 1989.
27. Tsuruo, T., Iida, H., Tsukagoshi, S., et al. Overcoming of vincristine resistance in P388 leukemia *in vivo* and *in vitro* through enhanced cytotoxicity of vincristine and vinblastine by verapamil. Cancer Res. 41:1967–1972, 1981.
28. Tsuruo, T., Iida, H., Nojiri, M., et al. Circumvention of vincristine and adriamycin resistance in vitro by calcium influx blockers. Cancer Res. 43:2905–2910, 1983.
29. Bellamy, W.T., Dalton, W.S., Kailey, J.M., et al. Verapamil reversal of doxorubicin resistance in multidrug-resistant human myeloma cells and association with drug accumulation and DNA damage. Cancer Res. 48:6365–6370, 1988.
30. Beck, W.T., Cirtain, M.C., Look, A.T., et al. Reversal of *Vinca* alkaloid resistance but not multiple drug resistance in human leukemic cells by verapamil. Cancer Res. 46:778–784, 1986.
31. Tsuruo, T., Iida, H., Tsukagoshi, S., et al. Potentiation of vincristine and adriamycin effects in human hemopoietic tumor cell lines by calcium antagonists and calmodulin inhibitors. Cancer Res. 43:2267–2272, 1983.
32. Ganapathi, R. and Grabowski, D. Enhancement of sensitivity to adriamycin in resistant P388 leukemia by the calmodulin inhibitor trifluoperazine. Cancer Res. 43:3696–3699, 1983.
33. Shiraishi, N. Akiyama, S., Kobayashi, M., et al. Lysosomotropic agents reverse multiple drug resistance in human cancer cells. Cancer Lett. 30:251–259, 1986.
34. Slater, L.M., Sweet, P., Stupecky, M., et al. Cyclosporin A reverses vincristine and daunorubicin resistance in acute lymphatic leukemia in vitro. J. Clin. Invest. 77:1405–1408, 1986.
35. Twentyman, P.I. Modification of cytotoxic drug resistance by non-immune-suppressive cyclosporins. Br. J. Cancer 57:254–258, 1988.
36. Dalton, W.S., Grogan, T.M., Rybski, J.A., et al. Immunohistochemical detection and quantitation of P-glycoprotein in multiple drug-resistant human myeloma cells: association with level of drug resistance and drug accumulation. Blood 74:747–752, 1989.
37. Friedlander, M.L., Bell, D.R., Leary, J., et al. Comparison of western blot analysis and immunocytochemical detection of P-glycoprotein in multidrug resistant cells. J. Clin. Pathol. 42:719–722, 1989.
38. Chabner, B.A. and Fojo, A Multidrug resistance: P-glycoprotein and its allies — the elusive foes. J. Natl. Cancer Inst. 8:907–913, 1989.
39. Dalton, W.S., Durie, B.G.M., Alberts, D.S., et al. Characterization of a new drug-resistant human myeloma cell line that expresses P-glycoprotein. Cancer Res. 46:5125–5130, 1986.
40. Bell, D.R., Gerlach, J.H., Kartner, N., et al. Detection of P-glycoprotein in ovarian cancer: a molecular marker associated with multidrug resistance. J. Clin. Oncol. 3:311–315, 1985.
41. Grogan, T., Dalton, W., Rybski, J., et al. P-glycoprotein assessment in multiple myeloma: comparison of methods and antibodies leading to development of a clinically useful immunocytochemical assay. Lab Invest.
42. Ma, D.D.F., Davey, R.A., Harman, D.H., et al. Detection of a multidrug resistant phenotype in acute non-lymphoblastic leukaemia. Lancet 1:135–137, 1987.
43. Tsuruo, T., Sugimoto, Y., Hamada, H., et al. Detection of multidrug resistance markers, P-glycoprotein and mdr1 mRNA, in human leukemia cells. Jpn. J. Cancer Res. 78:1415–1419, 1987.
44. Carulli, G., Petrini, M., Marini, A., et al. P-glycoprotein in acute nonlymphoblastic leukemia and in the blastic crisis of myeloid leukemia. N. Engl. J. Med. 319:797–798, 1988.
45. Rothenberg, M.L., Mickley, L.A., Cole, D.E., et al. Expression of the *mdr1*/P-170 gene

in patients with acute lymphoblastic leukemia. Blood 74:1388–1395, 1989.

46. Holmes, J., Jacobs, A., Carter, G., et al. Multidrug resistance in haemopoietic cell lines, myelodysplastic syndromes and acute myeloblastic leukaemia. Br. J. Haematol. 72:40–44, 1989.

47. Epstein, J., Xiao, H., and Oba, B.K. P-glycoprotein expression in plasma-cell myeloma is associated with resistance to VAD. Blood 74:913–917, 1989.

48. Miller, T.P., Grogan, T.M., Spier, C.M., et al. High dose verapamil infusion added to chemotherapy reverses drug resistance in lymphoma patients in relapse. Proc. Am. Soc. Clin. Oncol. 8:252, 1989.

49. Moscow, J.A., Fairchild, C.R., Madden, M.J., et al. Expression of anionic glutathione-S-transferase and P-glycoprotein genes in human tissues and tumors. Cancer Res. 49:1422–1428, 1989.

50. Bonadonna, G., Valegusso, P., and Santoro, A. Alternating non-cross-resistant combination chemotherapy with ABVD or MOPP in stage IV Hodgkin's disease: report of eight year results. Ann. Intern. Med. 104:739–746, 1986.

51. Longo, D.L., DeVita, V., Diffy, P., et al. Randomized trial of ProMACE-MOPP (day 1, day 8) vs. ProMACE-CytaBOM in stage II-IV aggressive non-Hodgkin's lymphoma. Proc. Am. Soc. Clin. Oncol. 6:206, 1987.

52. Thomas, E.D. and Clift, R.A. Indications for marrow transplantation in chronic myelogenous leukemia. Blood 74:861–864, 1989.

53. Applebaum, F.R., Sullivan, K.M., Buckner, C.D., et al. Treatment of malignant lymphoma in 100 patients with chemotherapy, total body irradiation, and marrow transplantation. J. Clin. Oncol. 5:1340–1347, 1987.

54. Phillip, T., Armitage, J.O., Spitzer, G., et al. High-dose therapy and autologous bone marrow transplantation after failure of conventional chemotherapy in adults with intermediate grade or high-grade non-Hodgkin's lymphoma. N. Engl. J. Med. 316:1493–1498, 1987.

55. Tsuruo, T., Hamada, H., Shigeo, S., et al. Inhibition of multidrug-resistant human tumor growth in athymic mice by anti-P-glycoprotein monoclonal antibodies. Jpn. J. Cancer Res. 80:627–631, 1989.

56. Fitzgerald, D.J., Willingham, M.C., Cardarelli, C.O., et al. A monoclonal antibody — Pseudomonas toxin conjugate that specifically kills multidrug-resistant cells. Proc. Natl. Acad. Sci. USA 84:4288–4292, 1987.

57. Tong, A.W., Lee, J., and Wang, R.-M. Elimination of chemoresistant multiple myeloma clonogenic colony-forming cells by combined treatment with a plasma cell-reactive monoclonal antibody and a P-glycoprotein-reactive monoclonal antibody. Cancer Res. 49:4829–4834, 1989.

58. Safa, A.R., Glover, C.J., Sewell, J.I., et al. Identification of the multidrug resistance-related membrane glycoprotein as an acceptor for calcium channel blockers. J. Biol. Chem. 262:7887–7888, 1987.

59. Akiyama, S.-I., Cornwell, M.M., Kuwano, M., et al. Most drugs that reverse multidrug resistance also inhibit photoaffinity labeling of P-glycoprotein by a vinblastine analog. Mol. Pharmacol. 33:144–147, 1988.

60. Naito, M. and Tsuruo, T. Competitive inhibition by verapamil of ATP-dependent high affinity vincristine binding to the plasma membrane of multidrug-resistant K562 cells without calcium ion involvement. Cancer Res. 49:1452–1455, 1989.

61. Hamada, H., Hagiwara, K.-I., Nakajima, T., et al. Phosphorylation of the M_r 170,000 to 180,000 glycoprotein specific to multidrug-resistant tumor cells: effects of verapamil, trifluoperazine, and phorbol esters. Cancer Res. 47:2860–2865, 1987.

62. Zamora, J.M., Pearce, H.L., and Beck, W.T. Physical-chemical properties shared by compounds that modulate multidrug resistance in human leukemia cells. Mol. Pharmacol. 33:454–462, 1988.

63. Pearce, H.L., Safa, A.R., Bach, N.J., et al. Essential features of the P-glycoprotein

206

pharmacophore as defined by a series of reserpine analogs that modulate multidrug resistance. Proc. Natl. Acad. Sci. USA 86:5128–5132, 1989.

64. Choi, K., Chen, C., Kriegler, M., et al. An altered pattern of cross-resistance in multidrug-resistant human cells results from spontaneous mutations in the mdr1 (P-glycoprotein) gene. Cell 53:519–529, 1988.

65. Bellamy, W.T., Dorr, R.T., Dalton, W.S., et al. Direct relation of DNA lesions in multidrug-resistant human myeloma cells to intracellular doxorubicin concentration. Cancer Res. 48:6360–6364, 1988.

66. Durie, B.G.M. and Dalton, W.S. Reversal of drug-resistance in multiple myeloma with verapamil. Br. J. Haematol. 68:203–206, 1988.

67. Keilhauer, C., Emling, F., Raschack, M., et al. The use of R-verapamil (R-VPM) is superior to racemic VPM in breaking multi drug resistance (MDR) of malignant cells. Proc. Am Assoc. Cancer Res. 30:503, 1989.

68. Krishan, A., Sridhar, K.S., Davila, E., et al. Patterns of anthracycline retention modulation in human tumor cells. Cytometry 8:306–314, 1987.

69. Kokenberg, E., Sonneveld, P., Delwel, R., et al. In vivo uptake of daunorubicin by acute myeloid leukemia (AML) cells measured by flow cytometry. Leukemia 2:511–517, 1988.

70. Gruber, A., Reizenstein, P., and Peterson, C. Effect of verapamil in vitro and in vivo on the accumulation of vincristine in leukemic cells from patients with low malignant lymphoma. Anticancer Res. 9:9–12, 1989.

71. Pradhan, S.G., Basrur, V.S., Chitnis, M.P., et al. In vitro enhancement of adriamycin cytotoxicity in human myeloid leukemia cells exposed to verapamil. Oncology 41:406–408, 1984.

72. Gore, M.E., Selby, P.J., Millar, B., et al. The use of verapamil to overcome drug resistance in myeloma. Proc. Am. Soc. Clin. Oncol. 7:228, 1988.

73. Trumper, L.H., Ho, A.D., Wulf, G., et al. Addition of verapamil to overcome drug resistance in multiple myeloma: preliminary clinical observations in 10 patients. J. Clin. Oncol. 7:1578–1579, 1989.

74. Ozols, R.F., Cunnion, R.E., Klecker, R.W., et al. Verapamil and adriamycin in the treatment of drug-resistant ovarian cancer patients. J. Clin. Oncol. 5:641–647, 1987.

75. Horton, J.K., Thimmaiah, K.N., Houghton, J.A., et al. Modulation by verapamil of vincristine pharmacokinetics and toxicity in mice bearing human tumor xenografts. Biochem. Pharmacol. 38:1727–1736, 1989.

76. Cordon-Cardo, C., O'Brien, J.P., Casals, D., et al. Multidrug-resistance gene (P-glycoprotein) is expressed by endothelial cells at blood-brain barrier sites. Proc. Natl. Acad. Sci. USA 86:695–698, 1989.

77. Miller, R.L., Bukowski, R.M., Budd, G.T., et al. Clinical modulation of doxorubicin resistance by the calmodulin-inhibitor, trifluoperazine: a phase I/II trial. J. Clin. Oncol. 6:880–888, 1988.

78. Mirski, S.E.L., Gerlach, J.H., and Cole, S.P.C. Multidrug resistance in a human small cell lung cancer cell line selected in adriamycin. Cancer Res. 47:2594–2598, 1987.

79. Slovak, M.L., Hoelige, G.A., Dalton, W.S., et al. Pharmacological and biological evidence for differing mechanisms of doxorubicin resistance in two human tumor cell lines. Cancer Res. 48:2793–2797, 1988.

80. McGrath, T. and Center, M.S. Mechanisms of multidrug resistance in HL60 cells: evidence that a surface membrane protein distinct from P-glycoprotein contributes to reduced cellular accumulation of drug. Cancer Res. 48:3959–3963, 1988.

81. Miller, T.P., Lippman, S.M., Spier, C.M., et al. HLA-DR (Ia) immune phenotype predicts outcome for patients with diffuse large cell lymphoma. J. Clin. Invest. 82:370–372, 1988.

82. Grogan, T.M., Lippman, S.M., Spier, C.M., et al. Independent prognostic significance of a nuclear proliferation antigen in diffuse large cell lymphomas as determined by the monoclonal antibody Ki-67. Blood 71:1157–1160, 1988.

83. Lokhorst, H.M., Boom, S.E., Terpstra, W., et al. Determination of the growth fraction in monoclonal gammopathy with the monoclonal antibody Ki-67. Br. J. Hematol. 69:477–481, 1988.

84. Willingham, M.C., Cornwell, M.M., Cardarelli, C.O., et al. Single cell analysis of daunomycin uptake and efflux in multidrug-resistant and — sensitive KB cells: effects of verapamil and other drugs. Cancer Res. 46:5941–5946, 1986.

85. Konen, P.L., Currier, S.J., Rutherford, A.V., et al. The multidrug transporter: rapid modulation of efflux activity monitored in single cells by the morphologic effects of vinblastine and daunomycin. J. Histochem. Cytochem. 37:1141–1145, 1989.

10. DNA repair in drug resistance: Studies on the repair process at the level of the gene

Charles J. Link Jr. and Vilhelm A. Bohr

Preface

Increasing evidence shows that DNA repair processes are important in drug resistance. In this article we will review some types of DNA damage seen after chemotherapy and examine experimental results suggesting that enhanced DNA repair processes can play a role in drug resistance. We will review aspects of the DNA repair mechanisms in mammalian cells, with an emphasis on newer methodologies that allow us to study DNA damage and repair processes at the level of individual genes. It has recently become possible to quantitate various types of damage in individual genes; this includes damage and repair after treatment with cisplatin and alkylating agents, which are important drugs in anticancer therapy. Studies of this sort should broaden our understanding of the mechanisms of drug resistance. It has been known for some time that DNA-damaging agents are distributed heterogeneously in DNA, and it is now becoming apparent that DNA repair processes are also heterogeneous over the mammalian genome. For instance, active genes are preferentially repaired, i.e., repaired faster or more efficient than noncoding genomic regions and the bulk of the genome. Significant changes in the repair process at the level of important genes could be overlooked if repair is only studied at the level of the overall genome, which represents an average of all repair events. When DNA repair is increased in drug resistance, additional treatment with DNA repair inhibitors may render the chemotherapeutics more effective. We will survey agents that affect the repair processes and enzymes that could represent targets for therapy in this situation.

Introduction

The development of drug resistance in tumors is a critical problem in oncology today. Cells challenged with drug may be resistant de novo, rapidly acquire resistance, or gradually develop the resistant phenotype. Clinically the resistance manifest by poor initial response, failure to achieve a partial

Robert F. Ozols (ed.), *MOLECULAR AND CLINICAL ADVANCES IN ANTICANCER DRUG RESISTANCE. Copyright © 1991.*
Kluwer Academic Pulishers, Boston. All rights reserved. ISBN 0-7923-1212-0

or complete remission, or as an unresponsive recurrent tumor. With recent advances in molecular biology and biotechnology, many mechanisms have been found that confer cellular resistance to chemotherapeutic agents [1]. Some of the mechanisms are increased drug efflux, decreased drug influx, gene amplification, failure to metabolize the drug to an active species, increased drug metabolism to an inactive species, altered drug targets, altered nucleotide pools, and increased DNA repair.

The DNA repair processes are vital to our cells, since the genetic material is constantly exposed to endogenous and exogenous damage caused by various agents, including chemotherapeutic drugs, irradiation, and carcinogens. This damage can give rise to malignant transformation, in part via mutations at specific sites in certain oncogenes. However, most of this damage is removed by the DNA repair mechanisms, and were it not for these enzymes, we would not survive this exposure. Good evidence also supports that DNA repair plays an important role in the prevention of cancer. For example, certain human disorders with a high incidence of cancer are associated with decreased DNA repair capacity in cells from the patients. Although DNA repair is as essential to the cell as the related processes of replication and transcription, this process is not as well understood. However, lately there have been some important advances in the field of DNA repair. One of these is the increased understanding of the fine structure of the repair process.

Little is known about DNA repair mechanisms in the development of drug resistance, but there is growing interest in these processes among clinicians and others concerned about drug resistance. In the following, we will examine relevant types of DNA damage and situations where DNA repair has been associated with drug resistance. We will then briefly review basic aspects of DNA repair processes and proceed to discuss how they can be studied at the level of individual genes and why that may be important. If DNA repair enhancement plays an important role in drug resistance, it is of interest to consider whether tumors can be made more drug sensitive through inhibition of the repair processes. We will briefly discuss which compounds may be of interest in this situation.

Chemotherapeutic drugs that damage DNA

DNA damage can result from chemotherapy, environmental hazard, or arise spontaneously within the organism. Many chemotherapeutic agents cause damage to DNA, and this damage is often responsible for the cytotoxicity of the drug. Each type of DNA-damaging agent gives rise to a different spectrum of adducts in the DNA; in some cases, such as UV irradiation, this spectrum is relatively clearly defined and understood, and in other cases, such as ionizing irradiation, the spectrum of adducts is vast and not clearly defined. Some common types of DNA damage are shown in Figure 1. The figure shows a pyrimidine dimer (a covalent linkage between two adjacent

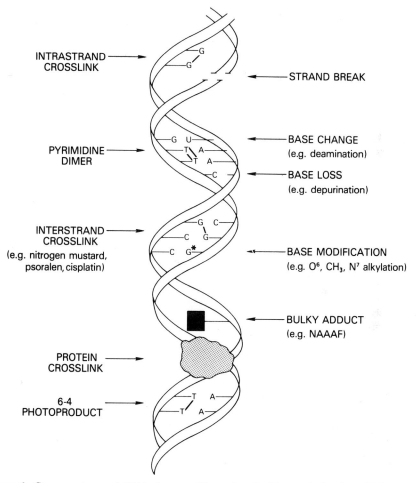

INTRASTRAND CROSSLINK

STRAND BREAK

PYRIMIDINE DIMER

BASE CHANGE
(e.g. deamination)

BASE LOSS
(e.g. depurination)

INTERSTRAND CROSSLINK
(e.g. nitrogen mustard, psoralen, cisplatin)

BASE MODIFICATION
(e.g. O^6, CH_3, N^7 alkylation)

BULKY ADDUCT
(e.g. NAAAF)

PROTEIN CROSSLINK

6-4 PHOTOPRODUCT

Figure 1. Common types of DNA damage. (Reproduced with permission from Bohr et al. [62].)

pyrimidines), which is the most common type of damage after UV irradiation (254 nm), and a 6–4 photoproduct, which is a less frequent but important photoproduct seen after UV. Intrastrand and interstrand cross links are seen after many types of damage, for example, after treatment with cisplatin or psoralen. Alkylating agents cause alterations such as guanine N^7 and O^6 alkylations. Ionizing radiation causes direct single- or double-strand breaks in DNA and base modifications. Some of the DNA damage seen after chemotherapy will now be considered.

Alkylating agents

Alkylating agents include numerous clinically useful drugs that bind covalently to DNA; examples are nitrogen mustard, cyclophosphamide,

211

ifosphamide, melphalan, chlorambucil, and busulfan. Bifunctional agents can form cross links in DNA [2]. Chloronitrosureas can form two reactive species, a chlorethyl diazohydroxide and an isocyanate group, that produce DNA alkylation and interstrand cross links [3]. Monofunctional and bifunctional nitrosureas used in clinical practice include steptozotocin, bischlorethylnitrosurea (carmustine, BCNU), cyclohexylnitrosurea (lomustine, CCNU), and methylcyclohexylnitrosurea (semustine, methyl CCNU). The alkylation at the N^7 position of guanine is the predominant product [4], but the O^6 position of guanine can also be modified by alkylating agents and represent another important target for these compounds. Many other base modifications are possible and the spectrum varies for each specific agent. Singer has presented a detailed review [4].

Cis(II)platinum diamminedichloride (cisplatin)

Cisplatin and carboplatinum are heavy metal compounds with antitumor activity. Covalent bonds are formed with DNA, and both intrastrand and interstrand cross links occur [5]. The most frequently recognized base sequences are GG, AG, and GNG (where N is any nucleotide); interstrand cross-links account for about 1% of the damage [6].

Antitumor antibiotics

Bleomycin binds preferentially to GT or GC sequences and produces free radicals, which result in single- and double-strand breaks in DNA [7,8]. Visible chromosomal breaks and deletions can occur as a result. The anthracyclines, daunomycin and adriamycin, cause single-strand DNA breaks, probably through interaction with DNA topoisomerase II [9]. Mitomycin C, another antitumor antibiotic, acts as a DNA intercalating agent after activation by the cell and can cross link DNA [10,11]. Actinomycin D inhibits RNA and DNA synthesis, and causes single-strand breaks after intercalation into DNA [12]. The epipodophyllotoxins, etoposide (VP-16) and teniposide (VM-26), can cause single- and double-strand breaks in DNA [13] through their interaction with topoisomerase II [14,15].

Antimetabolites

5-Fluorouracil can be metabolized into FdUTP, which is a toxic metabolite that can then be incorporated into DNA [16]. Another antimetabolite, cytosine arabinoside (Ara-C), functions in the cell as an analog to 2'deoxycytidine and is metabolized to Ara-CTP. Ara-CTP is an inhibitor of DNA polymerase and is also incorporated into DNA and results in slowing of DNA chain elongation [17]. The purine analogs, 6-mercaptopurine and 6-thioguanine, both require activation to monophosphates and triphosphates before they are incorporated into DNA [18].

212

Other agents

Decarbazine and 5-(3-methyl-triazeno)imidazole-4-carboxamide (MTIC) function as alkylating agents that can methylate DNA [19]. Procarbazine also probably functions as an alkylation agent [20]. Amsacrine (mAMSA) intercalates DNA to form both single- and double-strand breaks in DNA, presumably through its interaction with toposiomerase II [21].

DNA Repair mechanisms

When our cells are exposed to damage, they can deal with it in different ways. In some cases they can simply tolerate it. This important pathway is still poorly understood and in many cases involves damage bypass replication and the introduction of errors into daughter DNA. Recombination processes can be categorized both under tolerance and repair pathways.

Excision repair

DNA damage can be directly reversed only under a limited number of circumstances. These include the direct removal of UV-induced pyrimidine dimers by photolyase. Also, O^6-alkylguanine damage from various alkylation agents can be directly repaired by the mammalian O^6-alkyl transferase enzyme [22]. More often the elaborate nucleotide excision repair mechanisms are involved; this is the most general and widely characterized form of DNA repair. The sequential steps in nucleotide excision repair include: 1) pre-incision recognition of damage, 2) incision of the damaged DNA strand near the site of the defect, 3) excision of the defective site and localized degradation of the affected strand, 4) repair replication to replace the excised region with a corresponding stretch of normal nucleotides, and finally 5) ligation to join the repair patch at its 3' end to the contiguous parental DNA. Each of these steps involve specific enzymes to carry out the various functions. Only a few of the enzymes involved in the mammalian repair process have been characterized, and most of our knowledge about the repair process comes from studies in prokaryotes. Also, there is different enzymology for different kinds of damage. Some enzymes, such as the T4 endonuclease V of bacteriophage T4-infected *E. coli*, are specific for a single type of damage, in this case, cyclobutane pyrimidine dimers. The T4 endonuclease V enzyme has both recognition and incision functions [23]. An example of an enzyme with a wider range of recognition capabilities is the *E. coli* (A)BC excinuclease. The (A)BC excinuclease is a complex of three high molecular weight proteins that, in concert, are able to accomplish the first three parts of the excision repair process: recognition, incision, and excision [24]. This recognition is broad and covers a number of bulky DNA adducts, and the excision removes a 12 base segment containing the damage [24]. Both enzymes, the T4 endonuclease V and the *E. coli* (A)BC excinuclease complex, have been purified and utilized to study preferential gene repair, as discussed below.

DNA repair in drug resistance

In Table 1 we have listed a number of resistant cell lines in which altered DNA repair has been reported. In most of the situations in the table or in the discussion below, the investigators believe that the DNA repair enhancement observed is a major feature explaining the drug resistance. The investigators have often examined a number of mechanisms commonly thought to play a role in the resistance (see Introduction), as well as the DNA repair process. Here is a brief survey of some of these situations.

Alkylating agents

One mechanism of DNA repair that has been widely studied is the O^6-alkylguanine transferase enzyme (O6AGT). O^6-methylguanine is a common alkylation product, which can result in mispairs with thymidine in DNA [22,24] Increased levels of O6AGT have been found in HL60 cells resistant to nitrosureas [26], in a human glioma cell line resistant to nitrosureas [27], in a human melanoma cell line resistant to MTIC [28], in a rat brain tumor cell line selected for BCNU resistance [29], and in a lymphoblastoid cell line resistant to cell killing with carmustine [30]. Decreased O6AGT activity has been found to correlate with sensitivity to alkylating agents [27,28,30]. Increased O6AGT activity has been found in the peripheral blood lymphocytes of patients with chronic myelogenous leukemia and nonlymphocytic leukemia who became clinically resistant to nitrosureas [31]. Poly (ADP ribose) polymerase activity has also been noted to be increased in alkylation-resistant HeLa cells and in L1210-resistant lines [32].

Adriamycin

Experimental evidence reveals that resistance to adriamycin is multifactorial. By analyzing double-strand breaks by a neutral elution technique, Deffie et al. studied murine P388 leukemia cells selected for resistance. They found a number of possible mechanisms, including increased efflux protein expression, increased glutathione transferase expression, and increased DNA repair [33]. Several resistant clones showed an earlier onset of DNA repair in resistant versus sensitive cells. Other investigators have also shown more rapid DNA repair of single-strand breaks in adriamycin-resistant cells [34]. A human leukemic lymphoblast cell line isolated for adriamycin resistance also showed decreased DNA single-strand break accumulation; the same cells had decreased single-strand breaks when treated with VP-16, m-AMSA, or daunomycin [35].

214

Table 1. Drug resistant cell lines with indications of increased DNA repair

Cell Line	Cell Type	Resistance (Level of Resistance[a])	DNA Repair Finding	Reference
CCRF-CEM	Human leukemic	Adriamycin (25:1)	Decreased drug-induced strand breakage	35
P388/ADR3	Mouse leukemia	— (5:1)	Early onset of DNA repair	33
P388/ADR7	—	— (10:1)	Early onset of DNA repair	33
MM/70	Human melanoma	MTIC (10:1)	Low levels of O^6 AGT	28
SF-188	Human glioma	BCNU (5:1)	Elevated O^6 AGT	27
9L-BTRC-19	Rat brain tumor	BCNU (6:1)	Elevated O^6 AGT	29
L1210/DDP5	Murine leukemia	Cisplatin (50:1)	Increased reporter gene expression after damage	94
A2780 CP	Human ovarian carcinoma	Cisplatin (20:1)	Increased repair synthesis	36
A-253/D-10	Human head and neck squamous carcinoma	Bleomycin (9:1)	Rapid repair of x-ray damage	44
HeLa BLM^r	Human cervical carcinoma	Bleomycin (20:1)	Efficient repair of single-strand breaks	42

Cisplatin

Enhanced DNA repair is likely to be important in cisplatin resistance. Human ovarian cancer cell lines have been shown to have increased rates of DNA repair after selection for resistance to increasing amounts of drug [36]. In murine L1210 leukemia cells, a biphasic repair curve is noted, with rapid repair the first 6 hr, then slower repair rates. Cisplatin-resistant cell lines removed up to four times as many adducts during the rapid phase [37]. Elevated levels of the repair enzyme DNA polymerase beta has been found in chemoresistant cell lines, such as a cisplatin-resistant murine leukemia line [38]. It has been observed that the quantitation of cisplatin DNA adducts correlates with clinical response in patients with ovarian cancer [39]. In a cohort of patients receiving single-agent cisplatin or carboplatin chemotherapy, the level of drug binding to leukocyte DNA correlated with disease response more closely than any other clinical prognostic variable, suggesting that the drug-DNA interactions are the primary determinants of disease response and that leukocytes may serve as a surrogate marker for what occurs in tumor tissues [40]. However, there are some patients who do not respond to therapy, although they have high levels of adducts in their DNA [39,41]. Perhaps these poor correlations may be explained by the level of adducts in certain active genes in relation to response to therapy. Furthermore, preliminary data suggest that human DNA repair gene(s) may be expressed at higher levels in patients who show clinical resistance to platinum compounds [40]. Thus, cisplatin will be an important model agent for studies on specific gene repair and drug resistance.

Bleomycin

Mechanisms of resistance to bleomycin are incompletely understood but seem to involve at least decreased drug uptake, increased bleomycin hydrolase activity, and increased DNA repair activity [42,43]. Bleomycin-resistant HeLa cells with stable 20-fold increased levels of drug resistance showed about 40% decreased intercellular drug accumulation, no bleomycin hydrolase activity, but increased DNA repair rates at 30 min after damage (measured by decreased single-strand breaks) [42]. Three bleomycin-resistant sublines of a human head-and-neck cancer cell line were analyzed by Lazo et al. One cell line had increased bleomycin hydrolase, another had predominantly decreased uptake, and the third had high levels of initial damage to genomic DNA and more efficient repair when compared to the parental line [44]. Thus preliminary data from resistant cell lines implicates DNA repair contributing to bleomycin resistance.

The above data suggest a role for DNA repair in drug resistance in a number of systems studied. However, the repair studies above are all done at the level of the overall genome, thus averaging the repair events over the entire cellular DNA. We now know that there are differences in the repair process within the genome, as discussed in the following. Studies on damage formation and the repair process in individual genes provide a new and promising line of investigation in the field of drug resistance.

DNA repair at the level of the gene

It is well recognized that DNA in the nucleus of mammalian cells exists in the form of chromatin, which is organized and packaged into higher order structures. This highly complex structural organization must affect all nuclear reactions, including replication, transcription, recombination, and DNA repair. The mammalian genome contains on the order of 10^5 genes, which constitute on the order of 1% of the total DNA, the remainder being noncoding sequences. It is now possible to measure DNA repair in parts of the genome, such as individual genes.

Methodology for gene-specific damage and repair assays

Techniques have recently been developed to study damage and repair in genes and other specific sequences [45–47]. In general this approach can be used to determine the frequency of strand breaks in any genomic restriction fragment of interest. A requirement is that a strand break can be generated

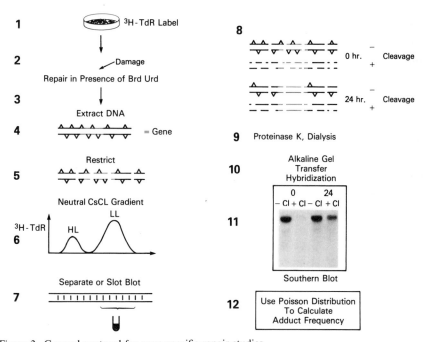

Figure 2. General protocol for gene-specific repair studies.

at the site of the DNA damage, and this is accomplished in different ways for different kinds of damage. Some agents cause strand breaks directly (e.g., ionizing irradiation and bleomycin), and in other cases the DNA lesions are detected with specific endonucleases that cleave the DNA or (in the case of alkylation) after depurination followed by alkaline hydrolysis. The frequency of strand breaks in specific restriction fragments is determined through quantitative Southern analysis and probing of denaturing gels.

The general technique is outlined in Figure 2 and will be briefly discussed. Cells are uniformly prelabeled with [^{3}H]-thymidine to tag the DNA. After damage the cells are incubated for repair in the presence of the heavy thymidine analog bromodeoxyuridine (BrdUrd); this allows us to later separate the (semiconservatively) replicated DNA from the parental. This step is required in most repair experiments, since the replicated (lesion free) DNA can mistakenly be assayed as repaired. The DNA is then isolated and restricted, and the parental DNA is separated on CsCl gradients. After DNA quantitation, strand breaks are generated by endonuclease treatment or (for alkylation) depurination followed by alkaline hydrolysis, and the DNA is electrophoresed on alkaline gels.

After transfer, the membranes are hybridized with the appropriate DNA probes and subjected to autoradiography. Bands are quantitated by densitometry or directly on the membrane using a (Betagen) blot analyzer. The number of lesions per fragment are calculated on the basis of the zero class, i.e., the fraction of fragments free of damage, using the Poisson distribution. Initially, we used a specific endonuclease (T4 endonuclease V) to detect pyrimidine dimers after UV irradiation and to generate strand breaks. We now also use the bacterial enzyme (A)BC excinuclease for studies on DNA damage and repair of bulky adducts other than pyrimidine dimers in specific genes. In another approach, strand breaks at sites of alkylation are generated by depurination followed by alkaline hydrolysis. These three different approaches are shown schematically in Figure 3.

Use of the ABC excinuclease. The *E. coli* uvr ABC gene products together form the (A)BC excinuclease, which has proven to be one of the most versatile DNA repair enzymes known [24]. It recognizes a wide variety of DNA adducts and cleaves the DNA at the site of the damage. We can study damage and repair in specific genes after treatment of cells in culture with various agents that are recognized and incised by the (A)BC excinuclease. The purified DNA is then reacted with the excinuclease to create strand breaks at sites of DNA damage.

Preferential DNA repair in active genes

Most available results on repair in specific sequences have been obtained after UV damage to the cells. It was initially demonstrated that repair of UV damage in the essential gene for dihydrofolate reductase (DHFR) in

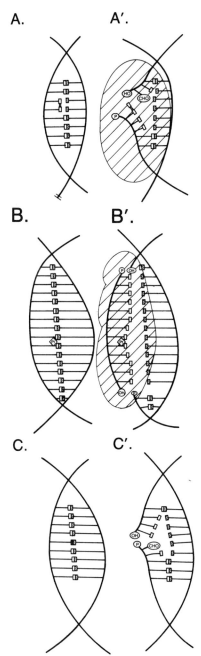

Figure 3. Methods for creating cleavage sites at locations of DNA damage. *A*: Cyclobutane pyrimidine dimer forms between adjacent thymidine residues. *A'*: T4 endonuclease V repair enzyme recognizes and binds at the site of the pyrimidine dimer then initiates 5' DNA glycosylase activity 5' from the dimer and subsequent 3' AP endonuclease function to create DNA strand break. *B*: Cisplatin induced intrastrand platinum cross link in DNA. *B'*: *E. coli* UVR(A)BC excision nuclease recognizes damaged bases, binds to DNA-damaged site, and cleaves with 5' to 3' exonuclease activity beginning 8 bases before the damage and ending 4 or 5 bases 3' of the damage site to create two strand breaks. *C*: Alkylated base represented by blackened rectangle. *C'*: Neutral depurination followed by alkaline hydrolysis creates cleavage of DNA strand.

Chinese hamster ovary (CHO) cells was much more efficient than the repair in the overall genome [45]. In normal repair-proficient human cells, the whole genome is repaired during 24 hr after UV damage. However, essential genes are repaired faster than noncoding sequences in the genome [48]. These phenomena has been termed *preferential DNA repair*. The Southern analysis for a UV damage and repair experiment in the DHFR gene in CHO cells is shown in Figure 4.

DNA repair has been studied in a number of different genes and in cells from a variety of different species. The data suggest that the preferential DNA repair of pyrimidine dimers in active genes after UV damage is not only a general phenomenon in mammalian cells, but is also seen in species as diversified as gold fish, yeast [49], *Drosophila*, and *E. coli* [50]. A DNA repair domain has been described in the CHO DHFR locus: the preferential repair of the DHFR gene is confined to a 60–80 kb region centered around the 5' end of the gene [51]. The initial frequency of pyrimidine dimers is similar in all fragments in and around the DHFR gene, whereas the repair differs considerably and is maximal at the 5' end of the gene. The size of this DNA repair domain is similar to a loop or higher order structure in chromatin and suggests a relation between DNA repair processes and chromatin structure.

Different genes within the same cell can be repaired with different efficiencies. In a study on the repair of a number of protooncogenes in mouse cells, the *c-abl* gene was found to be repaired much more efficiently than the

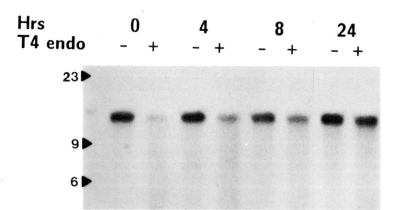

Figure 4. Typical gene-specific repair experiment after UV irradiation in the CHO DHFR gene. The number of hours after UV irradiation is given at the top of the figure; + indicates incubation with T4 endonuclease V (DNA with pyrimidine dimers is cleaved). The support membrane is probed with plasmid pMB5, which hybridizes to a 14 kb *Kpn*I fragment encompassing a 5' portion of the DHFR gene. The increasing intensity of the DHFR band in the + lane with time shows repair of the dimers, as there are less cleavage sites created by the T4 endonuclease V. Betagen blot analysis showed that 35% of the damaged sites were removed at 4 hr after damage, 72% were repaired at 8 hr, and 85% were repaired at 24 hr.

c-mos gene [52]. There are many important differences between these two oncogenes, and one is that the *c-abl* gene is actively transcribed in the cells, whereas the *c-mos* is not. These experiments suggest a correlation between the level of transcription and the efficiency of repair for a gene. This correlation was further supported by studies on the repair of UV damage in the metallothionein gene in CHO cells [53] and in human cells [54]. The repair in this gene is markedly more efficient when the gene is transcriptionally active than when inactive. These findings suggest some cellular association between the repair machinery and the transcription machinery.

Preferential DNA repair of genes might be ascribed to the more "open" chromatin structure in actively transcribed genomic regions. The recent demonstration that DNA repair shows strand specificity towards the transcribing strand [55], however, suggests that repair is directed towards certain genomic regions, rather than just being dependent upon chromatin accessibility. Repair enzymes may be linked with the transcription complex. Further studies are needed to examine the relative importance of three features: 1) local chromatin structure, 2) primary DNA sequence, and 3) function of the DNA for the efficiency of DNA repair in a given gene.

Certain protein molecules may play important roles in locating vital sequences to be dealt with early after damage by the DNA repair machinery. Also, the importance of local levels of methylation may play a role. We have recently reported [56] that demethylation of CHO cells by incubation for many generations in the presence of azacytidine enhanced the overall genome DNA repair and changed the fine structure organization of the DNA repair domain in the DHFR gene.

Different results suggest that there may be enzymatic differences between the "average" repair pathway in the cell or bulk of the DNA and that responsible for the preferential repair seen in active genes. This is currently being investigated in our laboratory.

We have been able to detect *6–4 photoproducts* in specific genes with the use of the (A)BC excinuclease [57]; this was previously not possible. UV irradiation introduces different photoproducts in the DNA, of which the major one (about 80% of total) is the (cyclobutane) pyrimidine dimer. However, other photoproducts are also formed, notably the 6–4 photoproduct. Almost all the work done on UV damage and repair is based on analysis of pyrimidine dimers, and although recent data suggest that the 6–4 photoproduct plays a major role in mutagenesis, little is known about the fate of this photoproduct [58]. We have found that the frequency of 6–4 photoproducts is about 40% of that of pyrimidine dimers in the DHFR gene and that these adducts are preferentially removed from this gene as compared to nontranscribed genomic regions [57].

We can also detect the formation and repair of adducts formed after treatment of cells with *N-acetoxy-acetaminofluorene (NAAAF)* in specific genes using (A)BC excision nuclease. NAAAF is a potent liver carcinogen that has been extensively studied. The adduct was formed with similar frequency and repaired with similar efficiency in the average, overall genome, in the DHFR gene, and in its 3′ flanking noncoding sequences [59]. Thus we found no preferential damage or repair of this adduct in expressed gene regions where the chromatin structure supposedly is less compact.

Chemotherapeutics

Only recently has the range of damage that can be studied at the gene level been expanded to include chemotherapeutic drugs. Of relevance to drug resistance is that it is now possible to detect *cisplatin adducts* in specific regions in vivo by the use of the (A)BC excinuclease complex. In addition to the assessment of the total cisplatinum adducts using (A)BC excinuclease, we also separately visualize the interstrand *cross links* in specific genes. Whereas the normal procedure for strand-break detection involves electrophoresis in alkaline gels to study single-stranded DNA, we run neutral gels in the cross-link assay. The drug treated DNA is denatured (30 mM NaOH for 15 min), allowed to reanneal briefly (10 min on ice), and then electrophoresed. We have found that the cisplatin interstrand cross links are repaired from all the genomic regions studied [59a]. The intrastrand adducts are preferentially repaired in the active DHFR gene in CHO cells, when compared to inactive genes, to noncoding genomic regions, or to the removal of cisplatin adducts from the overall genome using atomic absorption [59a]. We are presently studying the repair of cisplatin adducts and cross-links in specific genes in drug-sensitive and -resistant human cell lines. In the case of *alkylating* agents, we have studied the formation and removal of *nitrogen mustard*, *dimethyl sulphate*, and *methyl nitrosurea* in specific genes in CHO cells. For nitrogen mustard we observe that there is preferential damage formation in a noncoding genomic region compared to the active gene [59b]. This is in contrats to our previous studies on UV and cisplatin, where we found similar initial adduct frequencies in the various regions studied immediately after damage. This result is the first demonstration in our studies that drugs are preferentially localized in certain genomic regions. As yet we do not know whether this is related to base composition or sequence of the regions studied or to chromatin structural components. Whereas dimethyl sulphate is repaired with similar efficiency from an active gene and from a noncoding region, nitrogen mustard [59b] and methyl nitrosurea [59c] adducts are preferentially repaired from the active gene. Thus, related compounds can be repaired in different ways; we do not yet know how this is regulated, but it is possible that the specific chromatin structural alterations caused by these drugs is the important factor determining the repair characteristics.

These findings demonstrate that our assays may be useful in the search for *gene specific therapy*: we can look for therapeutics with high affinity for certain genes, such as oncogenes, where the expression may be undesirable (in a given disease). This affinity may be exploited to increase the therapeutic index of a given drug. We could then treat patients at lower drug levels and thus lower systemic side effects.

DNA repair inhibition

We will now discuss the possibilities for DNA repair inhibition. This can involve the use of specific inhibitors or the targeting of specific enzymes that are likely to be involved in the repair process. Again, the data below are overwhelmingly obtained at the overall genome level, and only recently are we examining the effect of specific inhibitors on the repair process at the gene level [59d]. Table 2 is an overview of the effect of some important inhibitors to be discussed. Clearly, more work is needed, particularly at the gene level.

O^6-Alkylguanine transferase

This enzyme acts by direct suicidal transfer of the alkly group to its own cysteine residue. Inhibition of this enzyme is aimed at either blocking the enzyme or depleting its level in cells. Inhibition of O6AGT has been found after incubation with O^6-methylguanine in cell lines and patients' blood

Table 2. Compounds that inhibit or modify cellular responses to DNA damage

Target	Mechanism
DNA synthesis inhibitor	
Aphidicolin	Inhibits DNA polymerase (alpha)
Ara-C	" "
Dideoxythymidine	" " (beta)
Hydroxyurea	Inhibits ribonucleotide reductase
Topoisomerase inhibitor	
Teniposide	Inhibits topoisomerase II
Novobiocin	" "
Merbarone	" "
m-AMSA	" "
Camptothecin	Inhibits topoisomerase I
Beta lapachone	Affects topoisomerase I
Alter poly (ADP-ribose) metabolism	
Nicotinamide	Inhibits poly (ADP-ribose)
3-aminobenzamide	" "
Others	
Leupeptin	Inhibits proteinase
Antipain	" "
Pepstatin	" "
Trifluoperazine	Inhibits protein kinase C
O^6 methyl guanine	Inhibits O^6 me guanine transferase
Streptozotocin	" "
Caffeine	Prevents cell-cycle delay after DNA damage
Buthione sulfoxamine	Inhibits glutamyl cysteine synthetase inhibition

samples [26]. O^6-methylguanine acts as a substrate for O6AGT and transfers a methyl group, thus inactivating the enzyme. *Streptozotocin*, also acting as a methylating agent, can biochemically modulate and deplete O6AGT activity in vivo, and possibly in patients [26,60]. These agents may prove to be clinically useful if integrated into regiments designed to take advantage of their DNA-repair-inhibiting qualities.

Topoisomerase inhibitiors

The mammalian DNA topoisomerases are involved in DNA replication and transcription [61]. There is mounting evidence that they are also involved in DNA repair [62], although their exact role is unclear. It is therefore of interest to examine these enzymes as targets of DNA repair inhibition. DNA topoisomerases I and II have been isolated and characterized, and recent evidence points to the existence of two types of topoisomerase II [63]. Topoisomerase II forms double-strand breaks in DNA through a co-valently bound topoisomerase II-DNA cleavage complex intermediate [61]. Novobiocin, a competitive inhibitor of topoisomerase II, inhibits the repair of certain types of DNA damage [64,65]. VP-16 interferes with strand break-age of the cleavage complex of topoisomerase II and has modest inhibitory effects on DNA repair [61,64]. mAMSA is a DNA intercalating agent that stimulates topoisomerase II mediated DNA cleavage and has been shown to inhibit DNA repair [61,64]. Camptothecin inhibits topoisomerase I, trapping the enzyme on DNA as drug-enzyme-DNA complexes [66]. This covalently bound cleavable complex can block progression of the DNA replication fork, with resultant cell toxicity [66]. Beta-lapachone, a possible topoiso-merase I inhibitor, enhances cell toxicity and alters DNA repair [67]. Beta-lapachone also prevents potentially lethal damage repair in human cells, probably via topoisomerase I inhibition [68]. Recent work in our laboratory has failed to identify a single topoisomerase inhibitor that could modify gene-specific repair [59d]. However, a combination of merbarone (a new inhibitor of topoisomerase II that does not create strand breaks [63]) with camptothecin (a topoisomerase I inhibitor) produced marked inhibition of DNA repair in the hamster DHFR gene after UV damage (experiments per-formed T. Stevnser). This interesting result represents a clearly documented inhibition of gene repair with pharmacologic intervention, and we have to await further experimentation to find out whether this has any clinical implications. The reason for the synergy between these two drugs that accomplishes this effect is unknown and is the subject of ongoing research in our laboratory.

Inhibition of DNA synthesis

Drugs that inhibit DNA synthesis can often modulate DNA repair functions of the cell. This alteration is most prominent with DNA polymerase inhibi-

224

tors. The DNA repair polymerase in mammalian cells has not been definitively identified. Although the notion has prevailed that the DNA polymerase beta is the main repair polymerase, it is likely that different polymerases participate in the repair processes, depending on the type of damage and cell type. Ara-C is a potent inhibitor of DNA synthesis and can inhibit the repair polymerization [69]. The compound inhibits DNA synthesis at the resynthesis step for UV, X-ray, and alkylation damage [70]. DNA polymerase alpha and delta, and to a lesser extent beta, are inhibited by ara-C when it competes with dCTP [71]. Ara-C also slows DNA chain elongation and can result in chain termination when incorporated into DNA [70]. Aphidicolin is a fairly specific inhibitor of DNA polymerase alpha and delta [72], and has been found to inhibit DNA repair of UV and X-ray irradiation in some cell systems [64,69], but not in others. Dresler et al. [73] found that aphidicolin inhibited overall genome UV repair in confluent human fibroblasts. Repair of 4-nitroquinoline-1-oxide (4NQO) is inhibited by aphidicholin [74]. Both Ara-C and aphidicolin reduce X-ray-induced chromosome exchanges [75], and ara-C inhibits some repair of cisplatin interstrand cross-links at late time points (and has enhanced cytotoxicity in this setting) [76]. Ara-C is considered a potent inhibitor of repair polymerization and is often used in combination with hydroxyurea. Hydroxyurea inhibits the ribonucleotide reductase enzyme and depletes cellular dNTP pools, resulting in DNA synthesis inhibition [69]. Although hydroxyurea has been shown to decrease the removal of cisplatin-induced interstrand cross-links [76], it is a much more effective inhibitor of the replicative than the repair synthesis. Hydroxyurea and ara-C have often been used in combination to inhibit repair polymerization and thus to examine the incision step of the repair process. Dideoxythymidine is reported to be a more specific inhibitor of DNA polymerase beta and can halt chain elongation and alter DNA repair [69]; a drawback when using this inhibitor is the requirement that it be added to permeabilized cells, since it does not readily penetrate the cell membrane.

Inhibition of ADP-ribosyl transferase

The mammalian ADP-ribosyl transferase enzyme (ADPRT) transfers the ADP-ribosyl portion of nicotinamide adenine dinucleotide (NAD) to chromatin proteins or to mono-or oligo-(ADP-ribosyl) protein to form a covalent bond [77]. The enzyme is activated by DNA strand breaks and has been implicated in the regulation of mammalian DNA repair [77]. The dynamics of (ADP-ribosyl)n processing and the half-lives of the various polymers also vary with the damaging agent [78]. Specific competitive inhibitors of ADPRT include methylxanthines, nicotinamide, benzamide, and 3-amino-benzamide (3-AB). The mechanism through which ADPRT inhibition alters DNA repair is not understood at this time. Hunting [79] found that 3-AB enhanced the accumulation of strand breaks in cultured normal human fibroblasts after UV and that the compound inhibited the ligation of the repair patch. DNA ligase II activity can be decreased after cells are exposed to 3-AB, and thus the inhibition of the ligation step of excision repair has been proposed as the mechanism [77]. However, a few studies have reported that 3-AB stimulates DNA repair measured by strand rejoining [80,81] or has no effect [82]. We have found that 3-aminobenzamide does not affect the gene-specific repair in the hamster DHFR gene after UV damage [59d].

Proteinase inhibition

Studies on the *E. coli* SOS response provide evidence that proteinase activity may be involved in regulating the cellular response to DNA damage [83]. This model of repair regulation led to the investigation of the effect that proteinase inhibitors may have on DNA repair in mammalian cells. Tumor-promoter-induced sister chromatid exchange (SCE) can be inhibited by *antipain*, a proteinase inhibitor [84]. *Leupeptin*, another proteinase inhibitor, strongly inhibits potentially lethal damage repair caused by gamma irradiation [85]. However, an extensive study of various proteinase inhibitors on different mutagens showed few effects for most, except *pepstatin*, which caused a reduced frequency of subsequent mutations [86]. These data suggest a role of proteinase inhibitors in the regulatory pathways for DNA repair of certain types of damage. At present, this class of agents are most useful for the exploration of how DNA repair is regulated by the cell, and we are aware of no clinical studies with these compounds.

Other modulators of DNA repair

Other compounds have been shown to modulate the cellular response to damage during DNA replication. A compound of obvious interest is *caffeine*, which has multitude of effects on cells and on cellular responses to damage [87]. Some of the effects of caffeine are: a reversal of alkylation and cisplatin-induced depression of DNA synthesis, reversal of inhibition by damaging agents of replicon initiation and prevention of cell-cycle delay after damage, thus preventing DNA repair synthesis. Caffeine reverses the G_2 cell cycle delay after DNA damage in many systems and must be present before the cell enters G_2 to exert its effect [87–89]. Thus caffeine has complex interactions in cells treated with DNA-damaging agents. A number of other drugs have been used in attempts to inhibit DNA repair. Inhibition of calmodulin by *trifluoperazine* decreases DNA repair after damage [64,90]. This inhibitior has also been shown to potentiate cell sensitivity to bleomycin [91]. Buthionine Sulfoximine (BSO) inhibits the gamma glutamyl cysteine synthetase enzyme and results in glutathione depletion in cells [92]. BSO decreases unscheduled DNA synthesis in cisplatin-resistant cell lines, and in combination with aphidicolin it can reverse the cisplatin-resistant phenotype

226

[92]. These compounds are entering clinical trials. The obvious hope is that future combinations of chemotherapeutic drugs can be designed to augment each other's cell-killing effects by inhibiting the cell's defenses against DNA damage.

Perspectives

Formation and repair of cisplatin and alkylation adducts can now be detected at the level of individual genes. These chemotherapeutics are frequently used in the treatment of a wide range of neoplasms. It is important that the laboratory investigations should progress simultaneously to the development of clinical protocols; for example, in small-cell lung cancer, which initially responds to cisplatin-based chemotherapy and most often relapses with a cisplatin drug-resistant phenotype. Does cisplatin resistance in this setting occur because of enhanced DNA repair? Does gene-specific repair change? Can agents that inhibit DNA repair be used either in combination with upfront therapy or at the time of relapse improve disease-free survival or relapsed disease response rates? These are questions that need to be answered in the near future and that are approachable with the present technology. Standard tumor cell line screening will not normally identify agents that affect gene-specific repair processes. Clearly, if DNA repair processes play an important role in drug resistance, selection of drugs that affect these processes may be important as a part of a combination chemotherapy. Only very recently have we found drugs that inhibit specific gene repair, and we are presently searching for more such agents. The methodology for detection of chemotherapeutic gene lesions should also be useful for following patients undergoing therapy, since damage and repair in certain important genes is likely to be a good prognostic parameter. This is suggested by previous studies on gene-specific damage and repair in mammalian cells after UV damage. It was observed that the repair of essential genes may be better related to biological endpoints, such as cellular survival, then is the average overall genome repair [93].

Acknowledgments

We wish to thank members of our laboratory group for sharing unpublished material.

References

1. Kessel, D., (ed). Resistance to Antineoplastic Drugs. CRC Press, Boca Raton, 1988.
2. Kohn, K.W. Interstrand cross-linking of DNA by 1,3-bis(2-chloroethyl)-1-nitrosourea and other 1-(2-haloethyl)-1-nitrosoureas. Cancer Res. 37:1450–1454, 1977.

227

3. Ewig, R.A.G. and Kohn, K.W. DNA damage and repair in mouse leukemia L1210 cells treated with nitrogen mustard, 1,3-bis (2-chloro-ethyl)-1-nitrosourea, and other nitrosoureas. Cancer 37:2114–2122, 1977.

4. Singer, B. The chemical effects of nucleic acid alkylation and their relation to mutagenesis and carcinogenesis. Prog. Nucleic Acids Res. Mol. Biol. 15:219–284, 1975.

5. Zwelling, L.A. and Kohn, K.W. Mechanism of action of cis-dichlorodiammineplatinum(II). Cancer Treat. Rep. 63:1439–1444. 1979.

6. Eastman, A. The formation, isolation and characterization of DNA adducts produced by anticancer platinum complexes. Pharmacol. Ther. 34:155–166. 1987.

7. Takeshita, M., Grollman, A.P., Ohtsubo, E., and Ohtsubo, H. Interaction of bleomycin with DNA. Proc. Natl. Acad. Sci. 75:5983–5987, 1978.

8. Wu, J.C., Stubbe, J., and Kozarich, J.W. Mechanism of bleomycin: evidence for 4'-ketone formation in poly (dA-dU) associated exclusively with free base release. Biochemistry 24:7569–7573, 1985.

9. Tewey, K.M., Chen, G.L., Nelson, E.M., and Liu, L.F. Intercalative antitumor drugs interfere with the breakage-reunion reaction of mammalian DNA topoisomerase II. J. Biol. Chem. 259:9182–9187, 1984.

10. Crooke, S.T. and Brander, W.T. Mitomycin C: a review. Cancer Treat. Rev. 3:121–139, 1976.

11. Dorr, R.T., Bowdan, G.T., Alberts, D.S., and Liddil, J.D. Interactions of mitomycin C with mammalian DNA detected by alkaline elution. Cancer Res. 45:3510–3516, 1985.

12. Ross, W.E., Glaubiger, D.L., and Kohn, K.W. Quantitative and qualitative aspects of intercalator-induced DNA damage. Biochim. Biophys. Acta 562:41–50, 1979.

13. Wozniak, A.J. and Ross, W.E. DNA damage as a basis for 4'-demethylepipodophyllotoxin-9(4,6-o-ethylidene-beta-D-glucopyranoside)-(etoposide) cytotoxicity. Cancer Res. 43: 120–124, 1986.

14. Dorr, R.T., Liddil, J.D., and Gerner, N.W. Modulation of etoposide cytotoxicity and DNA strand scission in L1210 and 8226 cells by polyamines. Cancer Res. 46:3891–3895, 1986.

15. Pommier, Y., Schwartz, R.E., Zwelling, L.A., Kerrigan, D., Mattern, M.R. and Charcossett, J.Y. Reduced formation of protein-associated DNA strand breaks in Chinese hamster ovary cells resistant to topoisomerase II inhibitors. Cancer Res. 46:611–616, 1986.

16. Schuetz, J.D., Collins, J.W., Wallace, H.J., and Diasio, R.B. Alteration of the secondary structure of newly synthesized DNA from murine bone marrow cells by 5-fluorouracil. Cancer Res. 46:119–123, 1986.

17. Cleaver, J.E. Mechanism of DNA repair and the structures of repaired sites in the presence of polymerase inhibitors, In: DNA Repair and its Inhibition, Collins, A., Downes, C.S., and Johnson, R.T. (eds). IRL Press, Oxford, pp. 127–141, 1984.

18. Tidd, D.M. and Patterson, A.R. Distinction between inhibition of purine nucleotide synthesis and the delayed cytotoxic reaction of 6-mercaptopurine, Cancer Res. 34:733–737, 1974.

19. Montgomery, J.A. Experimental studies at Southern Research Institute with DTIC (NSC-45388). Cancer Treat. Rep. 60:125–134, 1976.

20. Shiba, D.A., Weinkam, R.J., and Levin, M. Metabolic activation of procarbazine: activity of intermediates and the effects of pretreatment. Proc. Am. Assoc. Cancer Res. 20:173, 1979.

21. Pommier, Y., Minford, J.K., Schwartz, R.E., Zwelling, L.A., and Kohn K.W. Effects of DNA intercalators 4'-(9-acridinylamino)methanesulfon-m-anisidide and 2-methyl-9-hydroxyellipticinium on topoisomerasel-II-mediated DNA strand cleavage and strand passage. Biochemistry 24:6410–6416, 1985.

22. Pegg, A.E. Methylation of the 06 position of guanine in DNA is the most likely initiating event in carcinogenesis by methylating agents. Cancer Invest. 2:223–231, 1984.

23. Doodson, M.L. and Lloyd, R.S. Structure-function studies of the T4 endonuclease V repair enzyme. Mutation Res. 218:49–65, 1989.

24. Sancar, A. and Sancar, G.B. DNA repair enzymes. Annu. Rev. Biochem. 57:29–39, 1988.
25. Bhanot, O.S. and Ray, A. The in vivo mutagenic frequency and specificity of 06-methylguanine in X174 replicative form DNA. Proc. Natl. Acad. Sci. USA 83:7348–7352, 1986.
26. Gerson, S.L. and Trey, J.E. Modulation of nitrosourea resistance in myeloid leukemias. Blood 71:1487–1494, 1988.
27. Bodell, W.J., Tokvda, K., and Ludlum, D.B. Differences in DNA alkylation products formed in sensitive and resistant human glioma cells treated with N-(2-chloroethyl)-N-nitrosoruea. Cancer Res. 48:4489–4492, 1988.
28. Maynard, K., Parsons, P.G., Cerny, T., and Margison, G.P. Relationship among cell survival, O^6-alkylguanine-DNA alkyltransferase-activity, and reactivation of methylated adenovirus 5 and herpes simplex virus in human melanoma cell lines. Cancer Res. 49:4813–4817, 1989.
29. Linfoot, P.A., Barcellos-Hoff, M.H., Brent, T.P., Morton, L.J., and Deen, D.F. Cell-cycle, phase-specific cell killing by carmustine in sensitive and resistant cells. NCI Monogr. 6:183–186, 1988.
30. Arita, I., Tatsumi, K., Tachibana, A., Toyoda, M., and Takebe, H. Instability of mex phenotype in human lymphoblastoid cell lines. Mutation Res. 208:167–172, 1988.
31. Gerson, S.L. Modulation of human lymphocyte 06-alkylguanine-DNA by streptozocin in vivo. Cancer Res. 49:3134–3138, 1989.
32. Gorbacheva, L.B., Kukushkina, G.V., Durdeva, A.D., and Ponomarenko, N.A. In vivo damage and resistance to 1-methyl-1-nitrosourea and 1,3-bis(2-chloroethyl)-1-nitrosourea in L1210 leukemia cells. Neoplasma 35:3–14, 1988.
33. Deffie, A.M., Alam, T., Seneviratne, C., Beenken, S.W., Batra, J.K., Shea, T.C., Henner, W.D., and Goldenberg, G.J. Multifactorial resistance to adriamycin: relationship of DNA repair, glutathione transferase activity, drug efflux, and P-glycoprotein in cloned cell lines of adriamycin-sensitive and-resistant P388 leukemia. Cancer Res. 48:3595–3602, 1988.
34. Bankusli, I., Yin, M., Mazzoni, A., Abdellah, A., and Rustum, Y.M. Enhancement of adriamycin-induced cytotoxicity by increasing retention and inhibition of DNA repair in Dox-resistant P388 cell lines with the new calcium channel blocker DMDP. Anticancer Res. 9:567–574, 1989.
35. McGrath, T., Marquardt, D., and Center, M.S. Multiple mechanisms of adriamycin resistance in the human leukemia cell line CCRF-CEM. Biochem. Pharmacol. 38:497–501, 1989.
36. Lai, G., Ozols, R.F., Smyth, J.F., Young, R.C., and Hamilton, T.C. Enhanced DNA repair and resistance to cisplatinum in human ovarian cancer. Biochem. Pharmacol. 37: 4597–4600, 1988.
37. Eastman, A. and Schulte, N. Enhanced DNA repair as a mechanism of resistance to cis-diamminedichloroplatinum(II). Biochemistry. 27:4730–4734, 1988.
38. Kraker, A.J. and Moore, C.V. Elevated DNA polymerase beta activity in a cis-diammine dichloroplatinum (II) resistant P388 murine leukemia cell line. Cancer Lett. 38:307–315, 1988.
39. Reed, E., Ozols, R.F., Tarone, R., Yuspa, S.H., and Poirier, M.C. Platinum-DNA adducts in leukocyte DNA correlate with disease response in ovarian cancer patients receiving platinum based chemotherapy, Proc. Natl. Acad. Sci. USA 84:5024–5028, 1987.
40. Parker, R.J., Poirier, M.C., Bostick-Bruton, F., Vionnet, J., Bohr, V.A., and Reed, E. The use of peripheral blood leucocytes as a surrogate marker for cisplatin drug resistance-studies of adduct levels and ERCC1. In: Damage and Repair in Human Tissues. Eds., B.M. Sutherland and A.D. Woodhead, Plenum Press, N.Y., pp. 251–261, 1990.
41. Reed, E., Ostchega, Y., Steinberg, C., Yuspa, S.H., Young, R.C., Ozols, R.F., and Poirier, M.C. An evaluation of platinum-DNA adduct levels relative to known prognostic variables in a cohort of ovarian cancer patients. Cancer Res. 50:2256–2260, 1990.
42. Urade, M., Sugi, M., and Matsuya, T. Further characterization of bleomycin-resistant

HeLa cells and analysis of resistance mechanism, Cancer Res. 79:491–500, 1988.

43. Suzuki, H., Nishimura, T., and Tanaka, N. Drug sensitivity and some characteristics of a bleomycin-resistant subline of mouse lymphoblastoma L5178Y cells. J. Antibiot. 34:1210–1212, 1981.

44. Lazo, J.S., Braun, D., Labaree, D.C., Schisselbauer J.C., Meandizija, B., Newman, R.A., and Kennedy, K.A. Characteristics of bleomycin-resistant phenotypes of human cell sublines and circumvention of bleomycin resistance by liblomycin. Cancer Res. 49:185–190, 1989.

45. Bohr, V.A., Smith, C.A., Okumoto, D.S., and Hanawalt, P.C. DNA repair in an active gene: removal of pyrimidine dimers from the DHFR gene of CHO cells is much more efficient that the genome overall. Cell 40:359–369, 1985.

46. Bohr, V.A. and Okumoto, D.S. Analysis of frequency of pyrimidine dimers in specific genomic sequences. *In*: Friedberg, E.C. and Hanawalt, P.C. (eds). DNA Repair: A Laboratory Manual of Research Procedures, Vol. 3, Marcel Dekker, New York, pp. 347–366., 1988.

47. Bohr, V.A., Phillips, D.H., and Hanawalt, P.C. Heterogeneous DNA damage and repair in the mammalian genome. Cancer Res. 47:6426–6432, 1987.

48. Mellon, I., Bohr, V.A., Smith, C.A., and Hanawalt, P.C. Preferential DNA repair of an active gene in human cells. Proc. Natl. Acad. Sci. USA 83:8878–8888, 1986.

49. Terleth, C., van Sluis, C.A., and van de Putte, P. Differential repair of UV damage in *Saccharomyces cerevisiae*. Nucleic Acids Res. 17:4433–4439, 1989.

50. Mellon, I. and Hanawalt, P.C. Induction of the *E.coli* lactose operon selectively increases repair of its transcribed DNA strand. Nature 342:95–98.

51. Bohr, V.A., Okumoto, D.S., Ho, L., and Hanawalt, P.C. Characterization of a DNA repair domain containing the dihydrofolate reductase gene in CHO cells. J. Biol. Chem. 261:16666–16672, 1986.

52. Madhani, H.D., Bohr, V.A., and Hanawalt, P.C. Differential DNA repair in transcriptionally active and inactive proto-oncogenes: c-abl and c-mos. Cell 45:417–426, 1986.

53. Okumoto, D.S. and Bohr, V.A. DNA repair in the metallothionein gene increases with transcriptional activation. Nucleic Acids Res. 15:10021–10029, 1987.

54. Leadon, S.A. and Snowden, M.M. Differential repair of DNA damage in the human metallothionein gene family. Molec. Cell. Biol. 8:5331–5339, 1988.

55. Mellon, I.M., Spivak, G., and Hanawalt, P.C. Selective removal of transcription-blocking DNA damage from the transcribed strand of the mammalian DHFR gene. Cell 51:241–246, 1987.

56. Ho, L., Bohr, V.A., and Hanawalt, P.C. Demethylation enhances removal of UV damage from the overall genome and from specific DNA sequences in CHO cells. Molec. Cell. Biol. 9:1594–1603, 1989.

57. Thomas, D.C., Okumoto, D.S., Sancar, A., and Bohr, V.A. Preferential DNA repair of (6–4) photoproducts from the CHO DHFR gene. J. Biol. Chem. 264:18005–18010, 1989.

58. Mitchell, D.L. and Nairn, R.S. The biology of the (6–4) photoproduct. Photochem. and Photobiol. 49:805–819, 1989.

59. Tang, M.-S., Bohr, V.A., Zhang, X.-S., Pierce, J., and Hanawalt, P.C. Quantitation of aminofluorene adduct formation and repair in defined DNA sequences in mammalian cells using UVRABC nuclease. J. Biol. Chem. 264:14455–14462, 1989.

59a. Jones, J., Zhen, W., Reed, E., Parker, R.J., Sancar, A., and Bohr, V.A. Gene Specific Formation and Repair of cisplatin intrastrand adducts and interstrand cross links in CHO cells. J. Biol. Chem. 266:7101–7107, 1991.

59b. Wassermann, K., Kohn, K.W., and Bohr, V.A. Heterogeneity of nitrogen mustard induced damage and repair at the level of the gene following treatment of CHO cells. J. Biol. Chem. 265:13906–13913, 1990.

50c. LeDoux, S.P., Thangada, M., Bohr, V.A., and Wilson, G.L. Heterogeneous Repair of Methylnitrosurea-induced Alkali-labile sites in different DNA sequences. Cancer Research 51:775–779, 1991.

230

59d. Jones, J.C., Stevnsner, T., Mattern, M., and Bohr, V.A. Effect of specific enzyme inhibitors on replication, total genome DNA repair and on gene-specific DNA repair after UV irradiation in CHO cells. Mutation Res., DNA Repair Rep., In Press., 1991.

60. Erickson, L.C., Micetich, K.C., and Fisher, R.I. Preclinical and clinical experience with drug combinations designated to inhibit DNA repair in resistant human tumor cells, In: Mechanism of Drug Resistance in Neoplastic Cells, Wooley, P.V. and Tew, R.D. (eds). Academic Press, New York, pp. 173–183, 1988.

61. Liu, L.F., DNA topoisomerase poisons as antitumor drugs. Annu. Rev. Biochem. 58:351–375, 1989.

62. Bohr, V.A., Evans, M.K., and Fornace A.J. Jr., DNA repair and its pathogenic implications. Lab. Invest. 61:143–161, 1989.

63. Drake, F.H., Hofmann, G.A., Bartus, H.F., Mattern, M.R., Crooke, S.T., and Mirabelli, C.K., Biochemical properties of p170 and p180 forms of topoisomerase II. Biochemistry 28:8154–8160, 1989.

64. Bohr, V.A., Mansbridge, J., and Hanawalt, P.C., Comparative effects of growth inhibitors on DNA replication, DNA repair, and protein synthesis in human epidermal keratinocytes. Cancer Res. 46:2929–2935, 1986.

65. Mattern, M.R. and Scudiero, A. Characterization of the inhibition of replicative and repair-type DNA synthesis by novobiocin and nalidixic acid. Biochim. Biophys. Acta 653:248–258, 1981.

66. Hsiang, Y., Lihou, M.G., and Liu, L.F. Arrest of replication forks by drug-stabilized topoisomerase I-DNA cleavable complexes as a mechanism of cell killing by campatothecin. Cancer Res. 49:5077–5082, 1989.

67. Boorstein, R.J. and Pardee, A.B. β-lapachone greatly enhances MMS lethality to human fibroblast. Biochem. Biophys. Res. Commun. 118:828–834, 1984.

68. Boothman, D.A., Trask, D.K., and Pardee, A.B. Inhibition of potentially lethal DNA damage repair in human cells by B-lapachone, an activator of topoisomerase I. Cancer Res. 49:605–612.57, 1989.

69. Snyder, R.D., Van Horten, B., and Regan, J.D. The accumulation of DNA breaks due to incision; comparative studies with various inhibitors. In: DNA Repair and its Inhibition, Collins, A., Downes, C.S., and Johnson, R.T. (eds). IRL Press, Oxford, pp. 13–33, 1984.

70. Fram, R.J. and Kufe, D.W. The effect of inhibitors of DNA synthesis on DNA repair. In: DNA Repair and its Inhibition, Collins, A., Downes, C.S., and Johnson, R.T. (eds). IRL Press, Oxford, pp. 95–107, 1984.

71. Smith, C.A. Analysis of repair synthesis in the presence of inhibitors, In: DNA Repair and its Inhibition, Collins, A., Downes, C.S., and Johnson, R.T. (eds). IRL Press, Oxford, pp. 51–71, 1984.

72. So, A.G. and Downey, K.M. Mammalian DNA polymerases alpha and delta: current status in DNA replication. Biochemistry 27:4590–4595, 1988.

73. Dresler, S.L., Gowans, B.J., Robinson-Hill, R.M., and Hunting, D.J. Involvement of DNA polymerase delta in DNA repair synthesis in human fibroblasts at late times after ultraviolet irradiation. Biochemistry 23:6379–6383, 1988.

74. Jones, C.J., Edwards, S.M., and Waters, R. The repair of identified large DNA adducts induced by 4-nitroquinoline-1-oxide in normal or xeroderma pigmentosum groups A human fibroblasts, and the role of DNA polymerases alpha and delta. Carcinogenesis 10:1197–1201, 1989.

75. Morre, R.C., Randell, C., and Bender M.A. An investigation using inhibition of G$_2$ repair of the molecular basis of lesions which result in chromosomal aberrations. Mutation Res. 199:229–233, 1988.

76. Swinnen, L.J., Barnes, D.M., Fisher, S.G., Albain, K.S., Fisher, R.I., and Erickson. L.C., 1-B-D-arabinofuranosycytosine and hydroxyurea production of cytotoxic synergy with cis-diamminedichloroplatinum-(II) and modification of platinum-induced DNA interstrand cross-linking. Cancer Res. 49:1383–1389, 1989.

77. Shall, S. Inhibition of DNA repair by inhibitors of nuclear ADP-ribosyl transferase. In:

231

DNA Repair and its Inhibition. Collins, A., Downes, C.S., and Johnson, R.T. (eds). IRL Press, Oxford, pp. 143–192, 1984.

78. Alvarez-Gonzalez, R. and Althaus, F. Poly (ADP-ribose) catabolism in mammalian cells exposed to DNA-damaging agents. Mutat. Res. 218:67–74, 1989.

79. Hunting, D.J. and Gowans, B.J. Inhibition of repair patch ligation by an inhibitor of poly(ADP-ribose) synthesis in normal human fibroblasts damaged with ultraviolet radiation, Mol. Pharmacol. 33:358–362, 1988.

80. Bohr, V. and Klenow, H. 3-aminobenzamide stimulates unscheduled DNA synthesis and rejoining of strand breaks in human lymphocytes. Biochem. Biophys. Res. Comm. 102: 1254–1261, 1981.

81. Cleaver, J.E., Bodell, W.J., Morgan, W.F. and Zelle, B Differences in the regulation by poly CADP-ribose of repair of DNA damage from alkylating agents and ultraviolet light according to cell type, J. Biol. Chem. 258:9059–9068, 1983.

82. Burgman, P. and Konings, A.W.T. Effects of inhibitors of poly(ADP-ribose) polymerase on the radiation response of HeLa 53 cells. Radiat. Res. 119:380–386, 1989.

83. Little, J.W. and Mount, D. The SOS regulatory system of *Escherichia coli*. Cell 29:11–22, 1982.

84. Kinsella, A.R. and Radman, M. Tumor promoter induces sister-chromatid exchanges: relevance to mechanisms of carcinogenesis. Proc. Natl. Acad. Sci. (USA) 75:6149–6153, 1978.

85. Osmak, M., Korbelik, M., Suhar, A., Skrk, J., and Turk, V. The influence of cathepsin B and leupeptin on potentially lethal damage repair in mammalian cells. Int. J. Radiat. Oncol. Biol. Phys. 6:707–714, 1989.

86. Kuroki, T. and Drevon, C. Inhibition of chemical transformation in C3H10 T 1/2 cells by proteinase inhibitors. Cancer Res. 39:2755–2761, 1979.

87. Roberts, J.J. Mechanisms of potentiation by caffeine of genotoxic damage induced by physical and chemical agents. In: DNA Repair and its Inhibition, Collins, A., Downes, C.S., and Johnson. R.T. (eds). IRL Press, Oxford, pp. 193–215, 1984.

88. Boothman, D.A., Schlegal, R., and Purdee, A. Anticarcinogenic potential of DNA-repair modulators. Mutat. Res. 202:393–411, 1988.

89. Mateos, S., Pinero, J., Ortiz, T., and Cortes, F. G_2 effects of DNA repair inhibitors on chromatid-type aberrations in root tip cells treated with malic hydrazide and mitomycin C. Mutat. Res. 226:115–120, 1989.

90. Charp, P.A. and Regan, J.D. Inhibition of DNA repair by trifluoperazine. Biochim. Biophys. Acta 824:34–39, 1985.

91. Smith, P.J., Mirchesa, J.J., and Blechen, N.M. Potentiation of sensitivity to bleomycin and the drug-induced DNA damage in EMTG cells by the culmodulin inhibitor trifluoperazine. Acta. Physiol. Pharmacol. Bull. 13:41–45, 1987.

92. Lai, G., Ozols, R.F., Young, R.C., and Hamilton, T.C. Effect of glutathione on DNA repair in cisplatinum-resistant human ovarian cancer cell lines. J. Natl. Cancer Inst. 81: 535–539, 1989.

93. Bohr, V., Okumoto, D.S., and Hanawalt, P.C. Survival of UV-irradiated mammalian cells correlates with efficient DNA repair in essential gene. Proc. Natl. Acad. Sci. USA, 83:3830–3833, 1986.

94. Sheibani, N., Jennerwein, M.M., and Eastman, A. DNA repair in cells sensitive and resistant to cis-diamminedichloroplatinum (II): Host cell reactivation of damaged plasmid DNA. Biochemistry 28: 3120–3124, 1989.

11. Mechanisms of resistance to cisplatin

Alan Eastman

Introduction

Cisplatin has become a major clinical drug because of its proven efficacy against many tumors. It exhibits excellent activity against testicular tumors and is responsible for remission rates of about 50% in ovarian cancer. It is also used in combination chemotherapy for a variety of other tumors. As with all anticancer drugs, many tumors are inherently resistant to the therapy or acquire resistance after an initial treatment. Because of the high remission rate in ovarian tumors, this disease has become noted for the high incidence of recurrent tumors. It is quite possible that the mechanisms of inherent and acquired resistance are one and the same, but evidence for this requires further research.

One approach to improving therapy has been the development of new platinum analogues. Two goals have been addressed: to circumvent untoward toxicity and to overcome resistance. Analogues that have progressed to clinical trial include carboplatin, iproplatin, and tetraplatin (Figure 1). These drugs do not appear to exhibit the usual kidney toxicity of cisplatin. Carboplatin has been studied in the greatest detail so far and may even exhibit a somewhat different spectrum of therapeutic activity.

Resistance to cisplatin is not mediated through the multidrug resistance mechanism. This is important because it means cisplatin can be used against tumors that are otherwise resistant to many drugs. In addition, cisplatin-resistant cells are rarely cross-resistant to alkylating agents. Furthermore, sensitivity to cisplatin does not appear to extend to all other platinum complexes. Hence, a recent study of drug sensitivity in 10 human ovarian carcinoma cell lines demonstrated a good correlation between cisplatin, carboplatin, and iproplatin, but a significant difference between these drugs and tetraplatin [1]. This has implications not only for designing combination drug regimes, but also in understanding the mechanisms of resistance for different agents that act through the same target, DNA.

Robert F. Ozols (ed.), MOLECULAR AND CLINICAL ADVANCES IN ANTICANCER DRUG RESISTANCE. Copyright © 1991.
Kluwer Academic Publishers, Boston. All rights reserved. ISBN 0-7923-1212-0

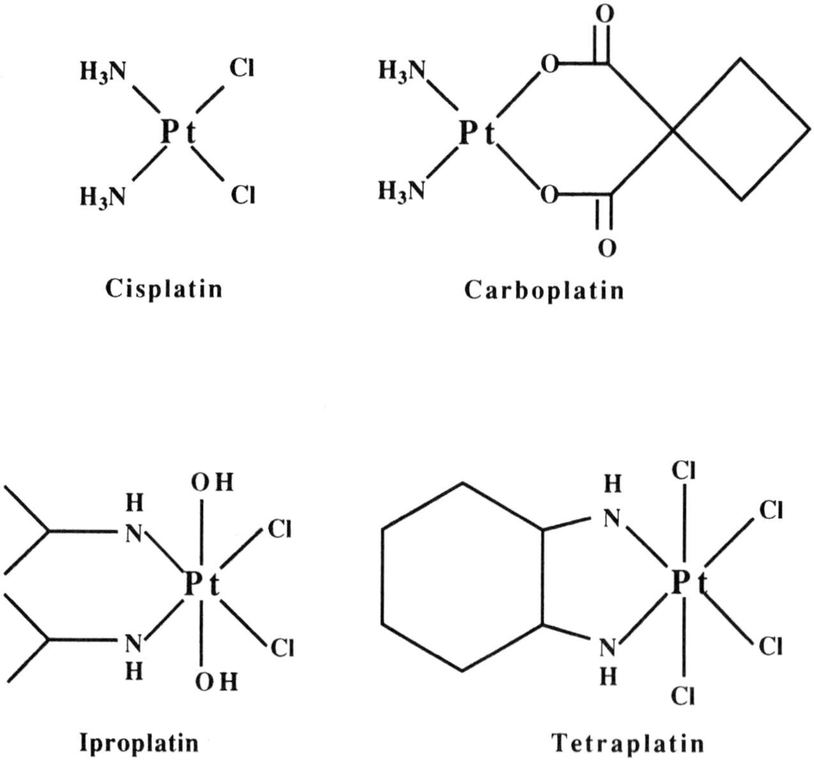

Figure 1. Structures of platinum coordination complexes.

Mechanism of action

Cisplatin is a neutral square-planar Pt(II) complex. The two chloride ligands are stable at the chloride concentration of the extracellular matrix. Upon diffusion into cells, the lower chloride concentration facilitates ligand substitution (Figure 2). In chloride-free phosphate buffer, cisplatin has a half-life of 2.4 hr [2]. One of the major differences between cisplatin and the other platinum analogues is the rate of substitution of the leaving group. For example, carboplatin is much more stable and does not appear to hydrolyze in water, although cyclobutanedicarboxylate ligand can be slowly substituted by other nucleophiles [3]. In chloride-free phosphate buffer, in which phosphate may be responsible for the substitution, the half-life of carboplatin is 268 hr [2]. Tetraplatin and iproplatin differ from the other analogues in being octahedral Pt(IV) complexes. As such, they are very unreactive and require an initial reduction to square-planar Pt(II) analogues. This is readily facilitated inside cells by agents such as glutathione [4]. The result of ligand exchange is the production of a charged electrophile that reacts with nucleophilic sites on cellular macromolecules. Extensive evidence has implicated

234

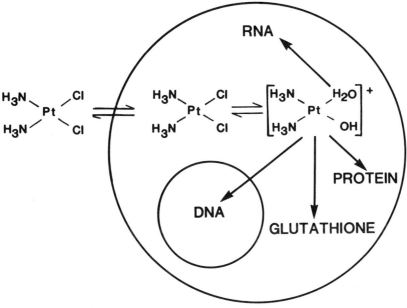

Figure 2. The interaction of cisplatin with cells.

DNA as the critical target [5]. Perhaps most convincing in this regard is the observation that DNA repair-deficient cell lines have a markedly enhanced sensitivity to cisplatin [6–8].

The types of lesions produced by cisplatin in DNA have been well characterized [reviewed in 9]. Practically all the lesions are bifunctional, although some monofunctional lesions occur as transient intermediates. This is in contrast to most alkylating agents in which reaction with water leads to inactivation of the drug and thereby inhibition of rearrangement of mono-functional to bifunctional lesions. In early studies, cisplatin-induced DNA-interstrand cross-links and DNA-protein cross-links were extensively studied, not because they represented the major lesions but rather that techniques were available for their measurement. However, these lesions represent only about 1% of the total DNA platination. Subsequently, DNA-intrastrand cross-links were identified as the major lesions. Approximately 65% of the intrastrand cross-links form between two neighboring guanines, 25% between a neighboring adenine and guanine, and about 7% between two guanines separated by one or more intervening bases (Figure 3). A further lesion has been reported whereby cisplatin mediates a cross-link between glutathione and DNA. Although the protein and glutathione cross-links are considered relatively innocuous, it is still in contention as to which of the other lesions might be more critical to the drug action.

Once the DNA has been damaged, most cells are capable of repairing the

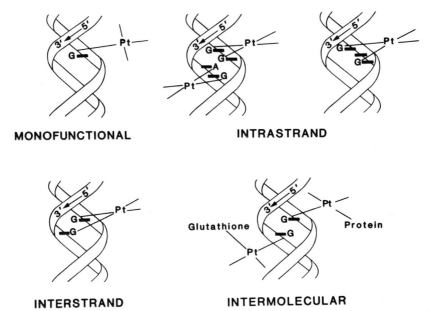

MONOFUNCTIONAL

INTRASTRAND

INTERSTRAND

INTERMOLECULAR

Figure 3. Structures of the various adducts produced in DNA by cisplatin. (Reproduced with permission from Eastman [9].)

lesions. Unrepaired lesions are responsible for the drug's effect. Xeroderma pigmentosum cells, which are deficient in their ability to repair UV-induced damage, have an increased sensitivity to cisplatin [6]. The same is true for DNA-repair-deficient mutants of Chinese hamster ovary cells [7,8]. This suggests that the damage is repaired, at least in part, by the same mechanism.

The binding of drug to DNA is not in itself sufficient to cause cell death. Cisplatin is much more toxic to dividing cells, suggesting that some cell-cycle-associated event(s) is required for toxicity [10]. Although its action is not cell-cycle phase dependent, it appears to be up to one log more toxic on cells prior to entry into the S phase [11]. It has also been shown that cytotoxicity is a function of the amount of DNA damage remaining at the time cells enter S phase [12]. Inhibition of DNA synthesis has been observed in a variety of cells following platination [13–15]. DNA synthesis has also been reported to be more sensitive to cisplatin than either RNA or protein synthesis [5]. Thus inhibition of DNA synthesis has been logically envisioned as the critical step in toxicity. However, recent work from this laboratory demonstrated that cells could die at drug concentrations that did not inhibit DNA synthesis [8,16]. DNA-repair-deficient cells that were very sensitive to cisplatin progressed at a normal rate through the S phase of the cell cycle. They arrested in the G_2 phase and subsequently died. In contrast, DNA-repair-competent cells demonstrated slowed passage through the S phase

236

but still survived. At concentrations of cisplatin that killed these cells, they also progressed through the S phase and arrested in G_2 prior to cell death. These results suggest that passage through the S phase may be necessary but not sufficient for cell death. Essential events appear to occur during the G_2 phase. There is reason to suspect that this is due to synthesis of a critical mRNA during the S phase and subsequent expression at the G_2/M transition.

Further analysis of cisplatin-induced cell death has established that many events occur that are consistent with the process of apoptosis, otherwise known as *programmed cell death* [17]. This process occurs normally during metamorphosis, differentiation, and general cell turnover [18]. Apoptosis is characterized by the requirement for new protein synthesis and by endo-nuclease degradation in the internucleosomal spacer regions of chromatin. It is a mechanism by which individual cells can actively commit suicide. Hence, the ability to commit suicide is genetically built into every cell. The current hypothesis is that incubation of cells with cisplatin, as well as with all other anticancer drugs, activates a signal transduction pathway that leads to apoptotic cell death. The details of this pathway are unknown, but the ultimate step is activation of the endonuclease that degrades genomic DNA.

Potential mechanisms of cisplatin resistance

An understanding of the mechanism of action of cisplatin permits a discussion of possible interventions by which a cell may develop resistance. Alterations in the cell membrane could decrease drug uptake or increase drug efflux. The drug could be inactivated in the cell by, for example, thiol-containing compounds such as glutathione or metallothionein. The initial monofunctional interaction of cisplatin with DNA could possibly be quenched by reaction with glutathione, thereby preventing its rearrangement to the critical bifunctional lesions. Monofunctional lesions might also be repaired more efficiently. Once the bifunctional lesions have formed, these too could be subject to enhanced DNA repair. Cells might also be more tolerant of unrepaired lesions, perhaps by alterations in replication, transcription, or in the signal transduction pathway leading to cell death.

Many of the above changes have been observed in cisplatin-resistant cells (discussed below). Hence, from an experimental point of view, it is not expected that a single mechanism will be true for all cells. An additional complication is that almost no system has been shown to exhibit a unique mechanism of resistance, rather, multiple mechanisms appear to occur in each cell system. A word of caution is warranted: many changes may occur that are not the cause of resistance but rather represent an associated event, or an event completely unrelated to the cellular resistance. For example, if a cell has enhanced DNA repair as a mechanism of resistance, then it is possible that other steps in the repair pathway may also be altered. Reported observations that DNA polymerase β is increased in certain circumstances may suggest that DNA repair is enhanced [19,20], but it does not demonstrate that the polymerase represents the critical step. If this were the case, such cells would be cross-resistant to many alkylating agents. However, this is not the case.

Development of resistance

The earliest cisplatin-resistant cells developed were murine leukemia L1210 and P388 cells. Resistant cell lines were obtained by inoculating mice with the cells and injecting cisplatin over multiple passages. L1210 cells were obtained that were up to 30-fold resistant to cisplatin and certain related analogues, but retained sensitivity to 1,2-diaminocyclohexane-Pt (DACH-Pt) complexes [21,22]. We have subsequently shown these cells to be sensitive to tetraplatin [4]. Other L1210 cells, as well as P388 cells, were developed with resistance to cisplatin [23,24]. These cells were further shown to retain sensitivity to bifunctional alkylating agents such as melphalan.

The area of cisplatin resistance was reviewed in 1986, and many of the conclusions are still pertinent [25]. That review suggested three categories of cisplatin resistance. In category I, the resistance is very specific for cisplatin and a few other closely related analogues, such as carboplatin and iproplatin. Such cells retain sensitivity to tetraplatin and other bifunctional alkylating agents. This is the pattern observed in the L1210 and P388 cells described above. Other cell lines that fit this category include a human squamous cell carcinoma [26] and an Ehrlich ascites tumor [27].

Category II was described as cell with cross-resistance to a variety of other agents, including bifunctional alkylating agents and DACH-Pt analogues. This pattern occurred in L1210 cells selected for resistance to melphalan and subsequently found to be cross-resistant with cisplatin [24]. A Burkitt lymphoma cell line (Raji) selected for resistance to chloroethylnitrosourea was also resistant to melphalan and cisplatin [26]. Hence, this category of resistance appears to occur when the selection agent is something other than cisplatin. It is also worth mentioning that not all melphalan-resistant cell lines are cross-resistant with cisplatin.

Category III occurred upon selection with heavy metals other than cisplatin, in particular cadmium, and is distinct from category II, which shows no resistance to cadmium. Human epithelial and mouse fibroblast cells resistant to cadmium were cross-resistant to cisplatin [28], while human ovarian carcinoma cells were additionally shown to be cross-resistant to melphalan [29].

There are certain limitations to a classification of this sort, because very few cell lines have been adequately tested against a comprehensive series of drugs. Another concern is the variation in the use of the term *cross-resistance*. In some cases, this may mean equal resistance to the different agents, whereas in other cases it may be used to mean that the cells have an increased, albeit a relatively low, level of cross-resistance to the other agents. This is particularly notable in category III, in which a very high resistance to cadmium is required before a low level of cross-resistance to cisplatin is observed [28]. In both categories II and III, cells generally attain only a modest level of resistance to cisplatin (two- to fivefold). In contrast, cells in category I can develop much higher levels of resistance. The L1210/DDP cells developed in this laboratory have over 100-fold resistance to cisplatin [30,31]. These cell lines were developed by stepwise exposure to increasing cisplatin concentrations for at least 5 years. The resistance was also stable after repeated passage in the absence of drug.

The L1210/DDP cells retain sensitivity to DACH-Pt complexes. In part because of this observation, a number of DACH-Pt complexes have been developed. Currently, tetraplatin is the only such drug entering clinical trials. The evidence presented above that human ovarian cells have a significantly different response to tetraplatin than to cisplatin [1] suggests that the L1210 results may be pertinent to the human situation in this regard. It seemed likely that resistance would also develop to DACH-Pt analogues. We incubated L1210 cells with increasing concentrations of DACH-Pt and a resistant line was obtained [32]. These cells were designated L1210/DACH. They exhibited about 40-fold resistance to DACH-Pt but retained sensitivity to cisplatin. In more recent studies, it has become evident that some cross-resistance exists; hence, with increasing resistance to either cisplatin or DACH-Pt, the cells begin to exhibit a low but increasing level of cross-resistance to the alternate drug [31]. We now refer to this phenomenon as cells having *preferential resistance* to each drug.

Since this early work, many cisplatin-resistant cell lines have been developed, most of them have been of human origin, with particular emphasis on ovarian carcinoma cell lines. The number of such cell lines has now become too numerous to detail individually, and as mentioned above, they have not been comprehensively tested for cross-resistance to other drugs. A couple of representative examples are worth presenting. A sevenfold resistant derivative of a human ovarian carcinoma cell line (A2780) was shown to be only slightly cross-resistant to both tetraplatin and melphalan (category 1) [33]. In contrast, a 6.4-fold resistant small-cell lung carcinoma appeared to be equally cross-resistant to both melphalan and tetraplatin (category 2) [34]. These results suggest that resistance in human cells is likely to be very complex.

Cellular accumulation of cisplatin

The mechanism by which cisplatin enters cells is still in contention. It has most frequently been assumed that entry is by passive diffusion through the lipid of the plasma membrane [35]. This is perhaps surprising, given the water solubility of cisplatin and that after a 1 hr incubation, 28% of the cisplatin remains ultrafilterable (i.e., presumably free cytosolic drug and not membrane bound) [36]. The remainder of the intracellular drug has become aquated and reacted with DNA, RNA, and protein. Changes in membrane content and fluidity were also inconsistent with the concept of passive diffusion [37]. However, a search for an alternate pathway has failed to identify any carrier-mediated transport. Cisplatin uptake was not saturable up to 3.3 mM, and the structural analogue carboplatin did not competitively inhibit accumulation of cisplatin [36]. One often cited report of a carrier-dependent pathway presented only indirect evidence that can be fully explained by cell-cycle-dependent effects [38].

It is perhaps surprising, therefore, that reduced accumulation of cisplatin is the most consistent observation in cisplatin-resistant cells. Most studies have observed only a two- to threefold reduced accumulation, even though resistance is often much greater. Unfortunately, many studies have not followed up on this observation by assessing the level of DNA platination that results. In L1210 cells, we observed an approximate twofold reduced drug accumulation [30] and a fairly comparable reduction in the level of DNA platination [39]. Increasing levels of resistance did not result in further reductions in drug accumulation. Other studies with L1210 and P388 cell lines have also reported reduced drug accumulation [40,41]. Human cell lines demonstrating reduced cisplatin accumulation include ovarian [36], squamous cell carcinoma [42], and a prostate tumor [43].

It is therefore important to resolve the question as to how cisplatin enters cells. Recent evidence has suggested that cisplatin uptake may be energy dependent [36]. Furthermore, agents that increase intracellular cyclic AMP appear to increase cisplatin uptake [44]. This suggests the involvement of protein kinase A, which is already known to modulate a variety of cellular events, including ion channels [45]. Several pieces of information suggest alterations in intracellular calcium may also affect cisplatin accumulation. Firstly, the calcium channel blocker verapamil was found to enhance cisplatin efficacy in a human neuroblastoma grown in nude mice [46]. Secondly, cisplatin-resistant L1210 cells were reported to have increased calcium-channel activity [47]. These two papers are consistent in that the former suggests that decreased calcium would increase drug accumulation, while the latter suggests that increased calcium makes cells more resistant. The potential relationship between calcium, ion channels, and cyclic AMP-dependent protein kinase still needs to be established, but it may lead to mechanisms for effectively overcoming reduced cisplatin accumulation in resistant cells.

Glutathione

Glutathione has been shown to be an important determinant of the sensitivity of cells to a wide variety of drugs [48]. In many cases, this involves the participation of glutathione transferase to conjugate glutathione to the drug.

240

However, because of its nucleophilic nature, it can also react nonenzymically with electrophilic compounds, such as the reactive intermediates of alkylating agents. Elevated glutathione has been shown to be a component of drug-resistant phenotypes that emerge in cells exposed to a number of alkylating agents, such as melphalan [49]. Sulfhydryls are also known for their potent substitution of the chloride ligands of cisplatin, however, glutathione is relatively weak in this regard. There are several steps at which glutathione could affect cisplatin toxicity; for example, by preventing it from reacting with DNA or by quenching monofunctional adducts in DNA before they rearrange to the more toxic bifunctional lesions. At least in reactions between cisplatin and DNA, both of these events have been shown to occur [50]. More recently, it has been suggested that glutathione may even play some role in modulating DNA repair [51].

Elevated glutathione has been associated with a number of cases of cisplatin resistance; for example, in mouse L1210 cells selected for resistance to either cisplatin [30,52] or melphalan (cross-resistant to cisplatin) [53], and human ovarian carcinoma cells [54,55], but not in a variety of other cell lines. Recently, we found that the elevation of glutathione in L1210 cells was dependent upon the culture medium; elevation was observed in McCoys 5A medium, which contains glutathione, but not in minimal essential medium [31]. These different culture conditions did not alter the degree of resistance.

The significance of elevated glutathione in cisplatin resistance is ambivalent. If elevated glutathione is responsible for cisplatin resistance, then experimentally lowering the glutathione concentration should reverse resistance. Buthionine sulfoximine (BSO) is the agent of choice for reducing glutathione, because it is a potent and specific inhibitor of glutathione synthesis, specifically at the γ-glutamyl cysteine synthetase step. In several reports, a reduction in glutathione resulted in sensitization of cells to cisplatin [52,55]. In other studies, little if any sensitization was observed after BSO treatment [30,54]. Andrews et al. demonstrated that only after a prolonged decrease in the glutathione levels did human ovarian carcinoma cells become sensitized to cisplatin, and this was true for both sensitive and resistant cells [56]. The apparent cross-resistance of a number of these cell lines to melphalan may indeed be associated with elevated glutathione; hence reduction in glutathione concentration does reverse melphalan resistance [53]. In L1210 cells, we observed elevated glutathione in some cisplatin-resistant cell lines, notably those that were also slightly cross-resistant to melphalan, but BSO treatment did not alter the resistance to cisplatin [30].

The intracellular concentration of glutathione is generally in the range of 0.1–10 mM. At 1 mM, we observed only a 20% reduction in the platination of DNA in an in vitro incubation [50]. At 10 mM, a 70% reduction in platination of DNA was observed. Hence, if the major role for glutathione is to reduce platination of DNA, it might be possible to modulate toxicity at the higher range of glutathione concentrations but not at intracellular concentrations less than 1 mM. This may explain the ambivalence in the results obtained in the studies to experimentally reduce glutathione concentration.

The reaction of glutathione with monofunctional adducts in DNA has been observed [50], although only very small amounts of this type of cross-link appear to occur in cells [39]. Based upon experience with the rate of substitution by thiourea [57], the rate of glutathione reaction with mono-functional adducts is likely to be faster than the reaction of glutathione with free cisplatin. The significance of this reaction depends upon the half-life of the monofunctional adducts in DNA. Intrastrand cross-links generally form immediately or within 1 hr [58], whereas interstrand cross-links continue to form for up to 12 hr [59]. Therefore, glutathione may have a greater impact on protecting against interstrand cross-links. Parenthetically, the major adduct produced by transplatin appears to be a monofunctional lesion that persists for a long period of time [60]. This lesion is rapidly modified by glutathione, which probably explains the inefficacy of this isomer. This is supported by the observation that BSO markedly sensitizes cells to trans-platin [54].

Metallothionein

Metallothioneins are small proteins that contain 30% of their amino acids as cysteine. They act as a store for a variety of metals, such as zinc, copper, or cadmium. This binding is also responsible for protection from the toxic effects of such metals. Metallothionein can also bind cisplatin [61]. Cells that have been selected for resistance to cadmium can have a high level of metallothionein and some cross-resistance to cisplatin. This phenotype has been observed in human epithelial cells [28] and human ovarian carcinoma cells [29]. However, these cases exhibit very little cross-resistance to cisplatin compared to the high level of resistance to cadmium. In most situations, cisplatin-resistant cells do not show any resistance to cadmium, suggesting that resistance is not mediated by elevated metallothionein [31]. In contrast, one survey of a number of cisplatin-resistant cell lines found many cases of elevated transcription of the metallothionein gene [62]. These cell lines were unfortunately not tested for cadmium sensitivity in that study. Several of the L1210 cell lines in our hands demonstrated no cadmium resistance [31], nor did they exhibit elevated transcription of the metallothionein gene (un-published). Several cell lines were transfected with a plasmid containing a metallothionein gene [62]. Overexpression of metallothionein led to resist-ance to cisplatin, chlorambucil, and melphalan, though apparently greater resistance to the latter drug. This cross-resistance phenotype is inconsistent with most cases of cisplatin resistance.

These results demonstrate a discrepancy between the cadmium response, the level of metallothionein, and the contribution to cisplatin resistance. Metallothionein is known as a stress protein and may be involved in the response to cisplatin, rather than as an effective protection against it. Perhaps this question will be resolved by an analysis of the level of platination of DNA: if metallothionein contributes significantly to cisplatin resistance, then a marked reduction in DNA damage should be detected.

DNA damage and repair

In many cases of cisplatin resistance, little if any reduction in DNA platination has been observed. In early studies, this involved analysis of only DNA interstrand cross-links. The results demonstrated consistently that the magnitude of such cross-links might be reduced, but not sufficiently to account for the high degree of resistance [63,64]. A more recent study found the same level of interstrand cross-links in a mouse cell line that also exhibited elevated glutathione and increased cadmium resistance [65]. A human small-cell lung carcinoma also showed elevated glutathione but no reduction in DNA intrastrand cross-links [34]. Several other reports detected no reduction in DNA damage associated with cisplatin resistance [66,67]. This type of information questions the general significance of the glutathione and metallothionein pathways for resistance, although they may be important in selected cell lines.

If cisplatin resistance cannot be adequately explained by reduced levels of DNA platination, then perhaps enhanced DNA repair could be an important determinant. Sensitivity to toxic agents is often associated with deficient DNA repair [6–8]. However, prior to 1987, neither in bacteria nor mammalian cells had an increase in DNA repair capability been reported as a mechanism of resistance, although it had frequently been suggested.

We have now demonstrated by two different methods that enhanced DNA repair is a significant contributor to cisplatin resistance in L1210 cells [39,68]. The first method required synthesis of [^{3}H]-cis-dichloro(ethylenediamine)platinum (II), an analogue of cisplatin that produces adducts at identical sites in DNA and to which the cells were equally resistant. DNA purified from treated cells was digested and the adducts were separated by HPLC. Within 6 hr of drug treatment, the sensitive cells had removed 30% of the adducts at GG sequences, whereas several resistant cell lines had removed almost 80% of these adducts. Little repair occurred after this time. The second assay involved host-cell reactivation of a platinated plasmid DNA. In this experiment, the plasmid is damaged before transfection into the cells and the level of chloramphenicol acetyltransferase (cat) coded by the plasmid is measured subsequently in cell lysates. In repair-deficient cells, one adduct per cat gene is sufficient to prevent transcription, demonstrating that intrastrand cross-links must be responsible for this inhibition. The resistant L1210 cells expressed cat activity up to considerably higher levels of cisplatin per plasmid. This can only be explained by an increased removal of cross-links from the plasmid DNA.

Enhanced DNA repair has also been demonstrated in human ovarian carcinoma cells, assayed either by unscheduled DNA synthesis [69] or by the host-cell reactivation assay [70]. Based upon this observation, attempts have been made to modulate cisplatin resistance by inhibiting the repair process, in particular, the DNA polymerase step of repair. Aphidicolin, a specific inhibitor of DNA polymerase α, inhibited both unscheduled DNA synthesis and sensitized the ovarian cells to cisplatin [69]. There is concern for the meaning of this experiment in that DNA polymerase β is more often reported to be associated with DNA repair, while DNA polymerase α is commonly associated with DNA replication. There are also reports of increased transcription of DNA polymerase β in several cases of cisplatin resistance [19, 20]. In L1210 cells, we have observed no alteration in transcript level for either of these DNA polymerases. This discrepancy has not been fully resolved, because under some circumstances both polymerases may be involved in repair, but generally DNA polymerase β is best able to fill small gaps; DNA polymerase α is more active on large gaps [71,72]. However, in neither case is the polymerase the critical step in resistance. The critical step is likely to be an earlier event, probably related to the recognition of damage in DNA. This is based on the phenotype of the cells that do not demonstrate marked cross-resistance to other alkylating agents likely to be repaired by the same excision repair pathway.

Other DNA repair genes have been investigated for their potential role in resistance. In L1210 cells, we found no difference in expression of either ERCC1 or ERCC2, the only two human repair genes currently available (unpublished). These genes were cloned by their ability to complement the repair defect in specific Chinese hamster ovary cell lines [73,74]. The functions of these proteins in repair are still unknown.

Other potential mechanisms of cisplatin resistance

We previously hypothesized that cells could become more tolerant of damage in their DNA [25]. The mechanisms could be alterations in DNA replication or postreplication DNA repair (repair of daughter strand gaps resulting from replication past adducts). To date, there are no examples of cells that have become resistant as a result of such mechanisms. However, there is one cell line that, failing all other explanations, may have become sensitive as a result of alterations of this type. A Walker rat 256 carcinoma cell line is particularly sensitive to bifunctional agents, including cisplatin. A resistant line derived from these cells appears to have reverted and demonstrates normal sensitivity [75]. These cell lines demonstrated similar levels of DNA damage and no detectable alterations in DNA repair; hence the hypothesis that alterations had occurred in a replicative or postreplicative pathway.

Several other reports of cisplatin resistance are worth noting. Increased resistance to cisplatin was observed in NIH3T3 cells transformed with the *ras* oncogene [76]. In our hands, we were unable to repeat this observation, but the difference appeared to be in the untransformed cells; our NIH3T3 cells had sensitivities equivalent to that reported for the transformed cells. We also investigated cisplatin-resistant L1210 cells but found no alteration in the transcription of *ras*.

There have also been reports of elevated expression of transcripts for a number of proteins involved in nucleotide metabolism, such as thymidylate synthetase and dihydrofolate reductase [77]. It is not clear how these could mediate resistance; rather, they could be ancillary changes associated with alterations in DNA repair or replication, or examples of unrelated changes that have occurred in specific cells. In L1210 cells, we have found no alteration of transcript levels for either of these two genes, demonstrating that the reported changes cannot be related to all cases of cisplatin resistance.

Summary

A number of changes have been detected in cisplatin-resistant cells, some of which are likely to be directly involved in the mechanism of resistance. The four most cited mechanisms are reduced accumulation, increased glutathione, increased metallothionein, and enhanced DNA repair. Of these mechanisms, reduced accumulation is probably the most common. Detoxification by glutathione or metallothionein may occur in some circumstances, but the evidence is often ambivalent. Enhanced DNA repair has been observed in several cases, but, to date, few cell lines have been adequately investigated for such changes. These observations demonstrate that multiple mechanisms of resistance exist, and often several may occur in the same cell line. To understand the significance of specific mechanisms, many laboratories are attempting to obtain genetic probes. These probes will then be used to clarify the mechanisms of resistance in fresh clinical samples and hopefully will facilitate improvements in therapeutic response.

References

1. Hills, C.A., Kelland, L.R., Abel, G., Siracky, J., Wilson, A.P., and Harrap, K.R. Biological properties of ten ovarian carcinoma cell lines: calibration *in vitro* against four platinum complexes. Br. J. Cancer 59:527–534, 1989.
2. Knox, R.J., Friedlos, F., Lydall, D.A., and Roberts, J.J. Mechanism of cytotoxicity of anticancer platinum drugs: evidence that *cis*-diamminedichloroplatinum(II) and *cis*-diammine (1,1-cyclobutanedicarboxylato) platinum(II) differ only in the kinetics of their interaction with DNA. Cancer Res. 46:1972–1979, 1986.
3. Cleare, M.J. Transition metal complexes in cancer chemotherapy. Coordination Chem. Rev. 12:349–405, 1974.
4. Eastman, A. Glutathione-mediated activation of anticancer platinum(IV) complexes. Biochem. Pharmacol. 36:4177–4178, 1987.

5. Roberts, J.J. and Thomson, A.J. The mechanism of action of antitumor platinum compounds. Prog. Nucleic Acid Res. Mol. Biol. 22:71–139, 1979.

6. Fraval, H.N.A., Rawlings, C.J., and Roberts, J.J. Increased sensitivity of UV-repair-deficient human cells to DNA bound platinum products which unlike thymine dimers are not recognized by an endonuclease extracted from *Micrococcus luteus*. Mutat. Res. 51:121–132, 1978.

7. Meyn, R.E., Jenkins, S.F., and Thompson, L.H. Defective removal of DNA cross-links in a repair-deficient mutant of Chinese hamster cells. Cancer Res. 43:3106–3110, 1982.

8. Sorenson, C.M. and Eastman, A. Influence of *cis*-diamminedichloroplatinum (II) on DNA synthesis and cell cycle progression in excision repair proficient and deficient Chinese hamster ovary cells. Cancer Res. 48:6703–6707, 1988.

9. Eastman, A. The formation, isolation and characterization of DNA adducts produced by anticancer platinum complexes. Pharmac. Ther. 34:155–166, 1987.

10. Fraval, H.N.A. and Roberts, J.J. Excision repair of *cis*-diamminedichloroplatinum(II)-induced damage of Chinese hamster cells. Cancer Res. 39:1793–1797, 1979.

11. Dornish, J.M., Pettersen, E.O., and Oftebro, R. Synergisitic cell inactivation by *cis*-dichlorodiammineplatinum in combination with 1-propargyl-5-chloropyrimidon-2-one. Br. J. Cancer 56:273–278, 1987.

12. Pera, M.F., Rawlings, C.J., and Roberts, J.J. The role of DNA repair in the recovery of human cells from cisplatin toxicity. Chem.-Biol. Interact. 37:245–261, 1981.

13. Harder, H.C. and Rosenberg, B. Inhibitory effects of anti-tumor platinum compound on DNA, RNA and protein synthesis in mammalian cells *in vitro*. Int. J. Cancer 6:207–216, 1970.

14. Howle, J.A. and Gale, G.R. *cis*-Dichlorodiammineplatinum(II) persistent and selective inhibition of deoxyribonucleic acid synthesis *in vivo*. Biochem. Pharmacol. 19:2757–1762, 1970.

15. Salles, B., Butour, J.L., and Macquet, J.P. *Cis*-Pt(NH$_3$)Cl$_2$ and *trans*-Pt(NH$_3$)Cl$_2$ inhibit DNA synthesis in cultured L1210 leukemia cells. Biochem. Biophys. Res Commun. 112: 555–563, 1983.

16. Sorenson, C.M. and Eastman, A. The mechanism of *cis*-diamminedichloroplatinum(II)-induced cytotoxicity: The role of G$_2$ arrest and DNA double strand breaks. Cancer Res. 48:4484–4488, 1988.

17. Barry, M.A., Behnke, C.A., and Eastman, A. Activation of programmed cell death (apoptosis) by cisplatin, other anticancer drugs, toxins and hyperthermia. Biochem. Pharmacol. 40:2353–2362, 1990.

18. Wyllie, A.H., Kerr, J.F.R., and Currie, A.R. Cell death: the significance of apoptosis. Int. Rev. Cytol. 68:251–306, 1980.

19. Kraker, A.J. and Moore, C.W. Elevated DNA polymerase beta activity in a *cis*-diamminedichloroplatinum(II)-resistant P388 murine leukemia cell line. Cancer Lett. 38: 307–314, 1988.

20. Scanlon, K.J., Kashani-Sabet, B.A., and Miyachi, H. Differential gene expression in human cancer cells resistant to cisplatin. Cancer Invest. 7:563–569, 1989.

21. Burchenal, J.H., Kalaher, K., O'Toole, T., and Chisholm, J. Lack of cross-resistance between certain platinum coordination compounds in mouse leukemia. Cancer Res. 37: 3455–3457, 1977.

22. Burchenal, J.H., Kalaher, K., Dew, K., Lokys, L., and Gale, G. Studies of cross-resistance, synergistic combinations and blocking activity of platinum derivatives. Biochimie 60:961–965, 1978.

23. Schabel, F.M., Trader, M.W., Laster, W.R., Wheeler, G.P., and Witt, M.H. Patterns of resistance and therapeutic synergism among alkylating agents. Antibiot. Chemotherap. 23:200–215, 1978.

24. Schabel, F.M., Trader, M.W., Laster, W.R., Corbett, T.H., and Griswold, D.P. *cis*-Diamminedichloroplatinum(II): combination chemotherapy and cross-resistance studies with tumors of mice. Cancer Treat. Rep. 63:1459–1473, 1979.

246

25. Eastman, A. and Richon, V.M. Mechanisms of cellular resistance to platinum coordination complexes. In: Biochemical Mechanisms of Platinum Antitumor Drugs, McBrien, D.C.H. and Slater, T.F. (eds). IRL Press, Oxford, pp. 91–119, 1986.

26. Teicher, B.A., Cucchi, C.A., Lee, J.B., Flatow, J.L., Rosowsky, A., and Frei, E., III. Alkylating agents: in vitro studies of cross-resistance patterns in human cell lines. Cancer Res. 46:4379–4383, 1986.

27. Seeber, S., Osieka, R., Schmidt, C.G., Achterrath, W., and Crooke, S.T. In vivo resistance towards anthracyclines, etoposide and cis-diamminedichloroplatinum(II). Cancer Res. 42:4719–4725, 1982.

28. Bakka, A., Endresen, L., Johnsen, A.B.S., Edminson, P.D., and Rugstad, H.E. Resistance against cis-dichlorodiammineplatinum(II) in cultured cells with a high content of metallothionein. Toxicol. Applied Pharmacol. 61:215–226, 1981.

29. Murphy, M.P., Andrews, P.A., and Howell, S.B. Metallothionein mediated cisplatin and melphalan resistance in human ovarian carcinoma. Proc. Am. Assoc. Cancer Res. 26:344, 1985.

30. Richon, V.M., Schulte, N.A., and Eastman, A. Multiple mechanisms of resistance to cis-diamminedichloroplatinum(II) in murine leukemia cells. Cancer Res. 47:2056–2061, 1987.

31. Eastman, A., Schulte, N., Sheibani, N., and Sorenson, C.M. Mechanisms of resistance to platinum drugs. In: Platinum and Other Metal Coordination Compounds in Cancer Chemotherapy, Nicolini, M. (ed). Martinus Nijhoff, Boston, pp. 178–196, 1988.

32. Eastman, A. and Illenye, S. Murine leukemia L1210 cell lines with different patterns of resistance to platinum coordination complexes. Cancer Treat. Rep. 68:1189–1190, 1984.

33. Behrens, B.C., Hamilton, T.C., Masuda, H., Grotzinger, K.R., Whang-Peng, J., Louie, K.G., Knutsen, T., McKoy, W.M., Young, R.C., and Ozols, R.F. Characterization of a cis-diamminedichloroplatinum(II)-resistant human ovarian cancer cell line and its use in evaluation of platinum analogues. Cancer Res. 47:414–418, 1987.

34. Hospers, G.A.P., Mulder, N.H., de Jong, B., de Ley, L., Uges, D.R.A., Fichtinger-Schepman, A.M.J., Scheper, R.J., and de Vries, E.G.E. Characterization of a human small cell lung carcinoma cell line with acquired resistance to cis-diamminedichloroplatinum(II) in vitro. Cancer Res. 48:6803–6807, 1988.

35. Gale, G.R., Morris, C.R., Atkins, L.M., and Smith, A.B. Binding of an antitumor platinum compound to cells as influenced by physical factors and pharmacologically active agents. Cancer Res. 33:813–818, 1973.

36. Andrews, P.A., Velury, S., Mann, S.C., and Howell, S.B. cis-Diammine-dichloroplatinum(II) accumulation in sensitive and resistant human ovarian carcinoma cells. Cancer Res. 48:68–73, 1988.

37. Mann, S.C., Andrews, P.A., and Howell, S.B. Comparison of lipid content, surface membrane fluidity, and temperature dependence of cis-diamminedichloroplatinum(II) accumulation in sensitive and resistant human ovarian carcinoma cells. Anticancer Res. 8:1211–1216, 1988.

38. Byfield, J.E. and Calabro-Jones, P.M. Carrier-dependent and carrier-independent transport of anti-cancer alkylating agents. Nature 294:281–283, 1981.

39. Eastman, A. and Schulte, N. Enhanced DNA repair as a mechanism of resistance to cis-diamminedichloroplatinum(II). Biochemistry 27:4730–4734, 1988.

40. Waud, W.R. Differential uptake of cis-diamminedichloroplatinum(II) by sensitive and resistant murine L1210 leukemia cells. Cancer Res. 47:6549–6555, 1987.

41. Kraker, A.J. and Moore, C.W. Accumulation of cis-diamminedichloroplatinum(II) and platinum analogues by platinum-resistant murine leukemia cells in vitro. Cancer Res. 48:9–13, 1988.

42. Teicher, B.A., Holden, S.A., Kelley, M.J., Shea, T.C., Cucchi, C.A., Rosowsky, A., Henner, W.D., and Frei, E. Characterization of a human squamous carcinoma cell line resistant to cis-diamminedichloroplatinum(II). Cancer Res. 47:388–393, 1987.

43. Metcalfe, S.A., Cain, K., and Hill, B.T. Possible mechanism for differences in sensitivity

247

to *cis*-platinum in human prostate tumor cell lines. Cancer Lett. 31:163–169, 1986.

44. Mann, S.C., Andrews, P.A., and Howell, S.B. Modulation of cisplatin accumulation by forskolin in human ovarian carcinoma cells. Proc. Am. Assoc. Cancer Res. 30:466, 1989.

45. Kume, H., Takai, A., Tokuna, H., and Tomita, T. Regulation of Ca^{2+}-dependent K^+-channel activity in tracheal myocytes by phosphorylation. Nature 341:152–154, 1989.

46. Ikeda, H., Nakano, G., Nagashima, K., Sakamoto, K., Harasawa, N., Kitamura, T., Nakamura, T., and Nagamachi, Y. Verapamil enhancement of antitumor effect of *cis*-diamminedichloroplatinum(II) in nude mouse-grown neuroblastoma. Cancer Res. 47: 231–234, 1987.

47. Vassilev, P.M., Kanazirska, M.P., Charamella, L.J., Dimitrov, N.V., and Tien, H.T. Changes in calcium channel activity in membranes from *cis*-diamminedichloroplatinum(II)-resistant and -sensitive L1210 cells. Cancer Res. 47:519–522, 1987.

48. Arrick, B.A. and Nathan, C.F. Glutathione metabolism as a determinant of therapeutic efficacy: a review. Cancer Res. 44:4224–4232, 1984.

49. Ahmad, S., Okine, L., Le, B., Najarian, P., and Vistica, D.T. Elevation of glutathione in phenylalanine mustard-resistant murine leukemia L1210 cells. J. Biol. Chem. 262:15048–15053, 1984.

50. Eastman, A. Cross-linking of glutathione to DNA by cancer chemotherapeutic platinum coordination complexes. Chem.-Biol. Interact. 61:241–248, 1987.

51. Lai, G.-M., Ozols, R.F., and Hamilton, T.C. Effect of glutathione on DNA repair in cisplatin-resistant human ovarian cancer cell lines. J. Natl. Cancer Inst. 81:535–539, 1989.

52. Hromas, R.A., Andrews, P.A., Murphy, M.P., and Burns, C.P. Glutathione depletion reverses cisplatin resistance in murine L1210 leukemia cells. Cancer Lett. 34:9–13, 1987.

53. Suzukake, K., Petro, B.J., and Vistica, D.T. Reduction in glutathione content of L-PAM resistant L1210 cell confers drug sensitivity. Biochem. Pharmacol. 31:121–124, 1982.

54. Andrews, P.A., Murphy, M.P., and Howell, S.B. Differential potentiation of alkylating and platinating agent cytotoxicity in human ovarian carcinoma cells by glutathione depletion. Cancer Res. 45:6250–6253, 1985.

55. Hamilton, T.C., Winker, M.A., Louie, K.G., Batist, G., Behrens, B.C., Tsuruo, T., Grotzinger, K.R., McKoy, W.M., Young, R.C., and Ozols, R.F. Augmentation of adriamycin, melphalan, and cisplatin cytotoxicity in drug-resistant and -sensitive human ovarian carcinoma cell lines by buthionine sulfoximine mediated glutathione depletion. Biochem. Pharmacol. 34:2583–2586, 1985.

56. Andrews, P.A., Schiefer, M.A., Murphy, M.P., and Howell, S.B. Enhanced potentiation of cisplatin cytotoxicity in human ovarian carcinoma cells by prolonged glutathione depletion. Chem. Biol. Interact. 65:51–58, 1988.

57. Eastman, A. Characterization of the adducts produced in DNA by *cis*-diammine-dichloroplatinum(II) and *cis*-dichloro(ethylenediamine)platinum(II). Biochemistry 22:3927–3933, 1983.

58. Eastman, A. Reevaluation of the interaction of *cis*-dichloro(ethylenediamine)platinum(II) with DNA. Biochemistry 25:3912–3915, 1986.

59. Eastman, A. Interstrand crosslinks and sequence specificity in the reaction of *cis*-dichloro(ethylenediamine)platinum(II) with DNA. Biochemistry 24:5027–5032, 1985.

60. Eastman, A. and Barry, M.A. The interaction of *trans*-diamminedichloroplatinum(II) with DNA: formation of monofunctional adducts and their reaction with glutathione. Biochemistry 26:3303–3307, 1987.

61. Zelazowski, A.J., Garvey, J.S., and Hoeschele, J.D. *In vivo* and *in vitro* binding of platinum to metallothionein. Arch. Biochem. Biophys. 229:246–252, 1984.

62. Kelley, S.L., Basu, A., Teicher, B.A., Hacker, M.P., Hamer, D.H., and Lazo, J.S. Overexpression of metallothionein confers resistance to anticancer drugs. Science 241: 1813–1815, 1988.

63. Zwelling, L.A., Michaels, S., Schwartz, H., Dobson, P.P., and Kohn, K.W. DNA cross-linking as an indicator of sensitivity and resistance of mouse L1210 leukemia to *cis*-

diamminedichloroplatinum(II) and L-phenylalanine mustard. Cancer Res. 41:640–649, 1981.

64. Strandberg, M.C., Bresnick, E., and Eastman, A. The significance of DNA crosslinking to *cis*-diamminedichloroplatinum(II)-induced cytotoxicity in sensitive and resistant lines of murine leukemia L1210 cells. Chem.-Biol. Interact. 39:169–180, 1982.

65. Mansouri, A., Henle, K.J., Benson, A.M., Moss, A.J., and Nagle, W.A. Characterization of a cisplatin-resistant subline of murine RIF-1 cells and reversal of drug resistance by hyperthermia. Cancer Res. 49:2674–2678, 1989.

66. Foka, M., Belehradek, J., and Paoletti, J. Interaction of *cis*-diamminedichloroplatinum(II) with sensitive and resistant L1210 cell lines. Biochem. Pharmacol. 1:3467–3472, 1989.

67. Fichtinger-Schepman, A.M.J., Vendrik, C.P.J., van Dijk-Knijnenburg, W.C.M., de Jong, W.H., van der Minnen, A.C.E., Cleassen, A.M.E., van der Velds-Visser, S.D., de Groot, G., Wubs, K.L., Steerenberg, P.A., Schornagel, J.H., and Berends, F. Platinum concentrations and DNA adduct levels in tumors and organs of cisplatin-treated LOU/M rats inoculated with cisplatin-sensitive or -resistant immunoglobulin M immunocytoma. Cancer Res. 49:2862–2867, 1989.

68. Sheibani, N., Jennerwein, M.M., and Eastman, A. DNA repair in cells sensitive and resistant to *cis*-diamminedichloroplatinum(II): host cell reactivation of damaged plasmid DNA. Biochemistry 28:3120–3124, 1989.

69. Masuda, H.,Ozols, R.F., Lai, G.-M., Fojo, A.,Rothenberg, M., and Hamilton, T.C. Increased DNA repair as a mechanism of acquired resistance to *cis*-diamminedichloroplatinum(II) in human ovarian cancer cell lines. Cancer Res. 48:5713–5716, 1988.

70. Reed, E., Budd, J., Eastman, A., and Ormond, P. Method development to assess relative carcinogen-DNA adduct repair in fresh human tissues using the model carcinogen *cis*-diamminedichloroplatinum(II) (cisplatin). In: Management of Risk from Genotoxic Substances in the Environment, Freij, L. (ed). PrintGraf AB, Stockholm, pp. 42–51, 1989.

71. Mosbaugh, D.W. and Linn, S. Excision repair and DNA synthesis with a combination of HeLa DNA polymerase β and DNase V. J. Biol. Chem. 258:108–118, 1983.

72. McBride, O.W., Zmudzka, B.Z., and Wilson, S.H. Chromosomal location of the human gene for DNA polymerase β. Proc. Natl. Acad. Sci. USA. 84:503–507, 1987.

73. van Duin, M., de Wit, J., Odijk, H., Westerfeld, A., Yasui, A., Koken, M.H.M., Hoeijmakers, J.H.J., and Bootsma, D. Molecular characterization of the human excision repair gene ERCC-1: cDNA cloning and amino acid homology with the yeast DNA repair gene RAD 10. Cell 44:913–923, 1986.

74. Weber, C.A., Salazar, E.P., Stewart, S.A., and Thompson, L.H. Molecular cloning and biological characterization of a human gene, ERCC2, that corrects the nucleotide excision repair defect in CHO UV5 cells. Mol. Cell. Biol. 8:1137–1146, 1988.

75. Roberts, J.J., Knox, R.J., Friedlos, F., and Lydall, D.A. DNA as the target for the cytotoxic and antitumor action of platinum co-ordination complexes: comparative in vitro and in vivo studies of cisplatin and carboplatin. In: Biochemical Mechanisms of Platinum Antitumor Drugs, McBrien, D.C.H. and Slater, T.F. (eds). IRL Press, Oxford, pp. 29–64, 1986.

76. Sklar, M.D. Increased resistance to *cis*-diamminedichloroplatinum(II) in NIH 3T3 cells transformed by *ras* oncogenes. Cancer Res. 48:793–797, 1988.

77. Scanlon, K.J. and Kashani-Sabet, M. Elevated expression of thymidylate synthase cycle genes in cisplatin-resistant human ovarian carcinoma A2780 cells. Proc. Natl. Acad. Sci. USA 85:650–653, 1988.

12. The role of metallothioneins in anticancer drug resistance

Robert R. Bahnson, Alakananda Basu, and John S. Lazo

Introduction

It is an unfortunate reality that many patients with solid tumors initially sensitive to anticancer chemotherapy subsequently develop recurrences that resist further treatment with these agents. This problem has fostered research efforts to define the mechanisms of resistance and to determine strategies to circumvent them. *Cis*-diamminedichloroplatinum II (cDDP) is widely used in a variety of solid tumors and has dramatically altered the survival of young men with germ-cell tumors of the testis. It also has utility in treating epithelial cancers of the head and neck and bladder, as well as in the therapy of ovarian tumors. Despite this success, the problem of intrinsic and acquired resistance to cDDP is important, and strategies to reverse it would be immensely beneficial. In the following review we will outline the role metallothionein may have in cytotoxic drug resistance, with an emphasis on its possible involvement in resistance to cDDP.

Historical aspects and biochemical features

Metallothioneins (MTs) are intracellular cysteine-rich metal-binding macro-molecules that are found throughout the animal kingdom, as well as in higher plants, microorganisms, and some prokaryotes. Metallothionein was first identified in 1957 in horse kidney cortex as a cadmium-binding protein [1] and subsequently was shown to bind other heavy metals, the biologically most common of which are Zn and Cu [2]. MTs are defined by their structural characteristics, which include a high content of cysteine, an extremely high content of heavy metals bound by clusters of thiolate bonds, and a low molecular weight, typically around 6000–7000 [3]. Each MT molecule is capable of binding seven molecules of Zn or Cu. In most mammalian tissues two major isoforms are detected; they contain either 61 or 62 amino acid residues and are designated *MT-I* and *MT-II*. In human tissue there are five known isoforms, which are distinguished by letters (e.g., MT-I_A, MT-I_E, MT-I_F, MT-I_G, and MT-II_A). The functional significance of

Robert F. Ozols (ed.), MOLECULAR AND CLINICAL ADVANCES IN ANTICANCER DRUG RESISTANCE. Copyright © 1991.
Kluwer Academic Publishers, Boston. All rights reserved. ISBN 0-7923-1212-0

Table 1. Factors that induce metallothionein synthesis

Metal ions — Cd, Zn, Cu, Hg, Au, Ag, Co, Ni, Bi	
Glucocorticoids	Phorbol esters
Estrogens	Chloroform
Progesterone	Carbon tetrachloride
Glucagon	Starvation
Catecholamines	Infection
Interleukin 1	Stress
Interferon	X-irradiation
Endotoxin	High O_2 tension
Alkylating agents	

this polymorphism has not been defined. Metallothioneins are found in most if not all organs, but are most abundant in liver, kidney, and intestine [4]. They appear to be located primarily in the cytoplasm but have been demonstrated within hepatic and renal nuclei as well [5].

Inducibility

One of the most interesting features of MTs is their inducibility. The MT content of organs, most notably liver and kidney, as well as cultured cells, can be increased by exposure to heavy metals, such as Cd, Zn, Bi, and Hg. The induction of MT in the livers of rabbits exposed to cadium was first noted in 1964 [6]. Since then the number of factors found to stimulate MT biosynthesis has increased dramatically, and many are listed in Table 1. At this time there are no known downregulators of MT.

The induction of MT by heavy metals is due to transcriptional activation of MT genes [7]. Cellular MT concentrations reach their maximum within 24–48 hr after exposure to an inducer, and the half-lives of induced MT are typically 1–4 days, although this depends on the metal state of the MT [3]. In human cells constitutive expression of MT isoforms appears to be tissue specific [8], and induction by Cu, Zn, and glucocorticoids [9] appears to be regulated differentially. For example, in a hepatoblastoma cell line human MT-II$_A$ is constitutively expressed, while MT-I$_F$ and MT-I$_G$ are not [10]. Furthermore, these three MT genes respond differently to induction with the metal ion inducers Cd, Cu, and Zn. Extensive studies of heavy metal regulation of human MT synthesis have shown that metal regulatory sequences are located in the 5' flanking region of the gene [11] and are present in multiple copies [12]. Recently, nuclear proteins that bind to these metal regulatory sequences have been identified and are postulated to play a direct role in MT gene transcription [13].

Metallothioneins are also induced by stressful conditions, such as heat, cold, and starvation, which raise circulating steroid hormone levels [14]. Glucocorticoids were first shown to regulate MT levels in cultured rat hepatocytes [15] and subsequently were found to stimulate MT synthesis in intact rodents, primarily in the liver and to a lesser extent in kidney, skeletal muscle, and spleen [16]. Glucocorticoids appear to act primarily at the level of transcriptional initiation, with a smaller effect on mRNA stability [16]. In human cells grown in culture, glucocorticoids strongly induce the MT-I_E and MT-II_A isoforms, while they only slightly induce MT-I_A and do not affect MT-I_F [8]. In addition to steroid hormones, MT synthesis in rat liver is stimulated by glucagon, angiotensin II, and by α-and β-adrenergic agonists [17].

Increased synthesis of MT has also been noted in response to inflammation. Injection of mice with bacterial endotoxin leads to increased liver and kidney MT mRNA levels [18]. The DNA sequences responsible for this inflammatory response appear to be independent of both glucocorticoid hormone and heavy-metal regulatory sequences [18]. The cytokines interferon [19] and interleukin-1 [20] have also been shown to increase intracellular MT concentration. Interleukin-I may also regulate Zn metabolism via elevated MT gene expression [21].

Finally, an increase in hepatic MT [22] and renal MT [23] has been demonstrated in rats following x-irradiation. Later reports confirmed the degree of radiation-induced MT expression is comparable to the levels achieved after treatment with heavy-metal salts, but the peak induction is delayed approximately 10 hr and remains elevated much longer than in metal-induced animal tissue [24]. Unlike previous reports, this investigation did not demonstrate an increase in renal MT mRNA or protein, nor did x-irradiation appear to induce MT-I mRNA accumulation in cultured human or rodent cells [24]. Thus, a host of agents can transiently increase MT in cells and tissues.

Physiological functions of MT

While it is quite clear that MT is a metal-binding protein, its physiologic functions have not been well defined [25]. Specific functions, which have been postulated, include heavy-metal detoxification, regulation of intracellular free Cu and Zn levels, control of fetal growth and differentiation, free-radical scavenging, and protection against ionizing irradiation. The most conclusive evidence is for a role of MT in metal detoxification. Results from several laboratories have demonstrated that: 1) cell lines that express low levels of MT are extremely sensitive to cadmium toxicity [26], 2) cells pretreated with heavy metals overexpress MT and are less sensitive to cytotoxicity to Cu, Zn, and Hg [27], 3) cell strains that are selected for cadmium resistance overexpress MT, frequently due to gene amplification [28,29], and 4) cells transfected with a bovine papilloma virus shuttle vector containing MT genes are highly resistant to cadmium due to MT overproduction [30,31]. Taken together these results suggest a prominent role for MT in heavy-metal detoxification. However, it is unlikely that this is the only biological role of MT for several reasons. First, the production of excessive amounts of cadmium containing MT has been suggested as a causative factor in kidney damage with chronic cadmium poisoning; this casts some doubt on the biological importance of MT as a specific and effective defense mechanism in animals against environmental Cd [32]. Second, in most biopsy tissue samples examined, MT is not found bound to Cd or Hg [23]. Finally, a primary protective role would imply that MT would be present in tissues only after exposure to toxic heavy metals [25]. As noted previously, MT expression is constitutively quite high in normal liver, kidney, and intestine.

Cousins has proposed a functional regulatory role for MT in Zn and Cu homeostasis [17]. It is known that the level of intestinal MT is inversely related to the absorption of Cu and Zn. This has been exploited in Wilson's disease, where intestinal MT production can be increased by oral Zn therapy with a concomitant decrease in Cu absorption [33]. The increase in intestinal MT from dietary Zn is due to an increase in MT mRNA in the intestine [17]. The involvement of MT in Zn and Cu metabolism might be particularly important, because a number of critical intercellular enzymes have Zn as an essential metal cofactor. In addition, DNA binding proteins requiring Zn or Cu have been identified, and structural motifs termed *zinc fingers* and *copper fists* have been described for regions of regulatory proteins that bind to DNA and regulate expression [34].

MT may also have an important regulatory role in growth development. This was first suggested by the observation of simultaneous, enhanced DNA synthesis and increased Zn-MT formation in livers of rats recovering from partial hepatectomy [35]. Further support of this concept stems from the finding of programmed regulation of MT mRNA levels and of MT in the course of embryogenesis [36] and in fetal [37] and perinatal [38] development. It is noteworthy that differential activation of MT isoforms in these processes has also been reported [39].

Free radicals are produced during the acute-phase response, reperfusion of hypoxic tissue, and from ionizing radiation, and there is some evidence from in vitro studies that MT can scavenge free hydroxyl ions [40]. Zn supplementation of culture medium has been reported to prevent lipid peroxidation in cultured hepatocytes, and this protection has been correlated with induction of MT [41]. Furthermore, in rodents, induction of MT by metal salts, surgical stress, and immunostimulants has been shown to confer protection against ionizing irradiation [42]. X-irradiation itself will increase MT mRNA in rat liver, kidney, and thymus [43]. These reports offer evidence of a potential protective function for MT as a scavenger of free radicals produced by infection or x-irradiation. A recent study, however, calls into question the protective effect of MT in free-radical-induced injury. Lohrer and Robson [44] have demonstrated that CHO cell lines transfected with the human MT-II_A gene integrated in a bovine papilloma vector are resistant to monofunctional alkylating and cross-linking agents, but are as sensitive as the parent cells to ionizing radiation.

Role of MT in anticancer drug resistance

The observation of protective effects of MT induction against heavy-metal toxicity led to investigations exploring the relationship between cellular MT levels and sensitivity to cDDP. Bakka et al. [45] first demonstrated that cadmium-resistant cells, which contained large amounts of MT, were resistant to cDDP. To our knowledge, every Cd-resistant cell line that has been examined subsequently has been found to be cross-resistant to cDDP. Bakka et al. [45] also found the platinum (Pt) content of the resistant cells was higher than in nonresistant cells, thus excluding decreased uptake or increased efflux as a mechanism for the observed differences in cDDP sensitivity. Moreover, the major portion of the Pt in the resistant cells was associated with MT. These results are consistent with the hypothesis that MT can act as an alternate target for cDDP and reduce DNA exposure.

More recently, additional evidence to implicate MT as a major cause of cellular resistance to cDDP and other alkylating agents has been reported. Kelley et al. [46] have shown that: 1) tumor cells with increased MT content are resistant to both alkylating agents and cDDP, 2) cells with acquired resistance to cDDP frequently have an increase in MT and overexpress MT mRNA, 3) reversal of the cDDP resistance phenotype is accompanied by a decrease in MT content, and 4) introduction of a eukaryotic expression vector encoding human MT-II$_A$ into murine cells confers the drug-resistance phenotype. Recent results from Lohrer and Robson [44] with CHO cells confirm these observations. Teicher et al. [47] isolated a human squamous carcinoma cell line stably resistant to cDDP that showed no difference in nonprotein sulfhydryl content compared to its sensitive parental line. The protein sulfhydryl levels, however, were increased two-fold in the resistant cell line. Subsequent studies using an ELISA demonstrated the increase in protein sulfhydryl in these cells was due to elevated MT [46]. These cells also were resistant to Cd. Similarly, two human ovarian cell lines resistant to both CdCl$_2$ and cDDP by stepwise selection and chronic culture in CdCl$_2$ and ZnCl$_2$ demonstrated elevated levels of cellular thiols, which were accounted for by both MT and glutathione (GSH). Cellular MT concentration was four times greater than GSH, and sensitivity to cDDP was unaffected by BSO, which depletes glutathione [48]. Finally, two murine fibroblast lines with high and low cellular levels of MT transplanted into nude mice showed low and high sensitivity to cDDP cytotoxicity, respectively [49].

Based on the available evidence, increases in MT appear to be one biochemical alteration that occurs with acquired resistance to cDDP. Not all cells with acquired cDDP resistance, however, overexpressed MT. Kelley et al. [46] noted that 1 of 5 human cell lines grown in culture with acquired resistance to cDDP had an elevated level of MT. Andrews et al. [48] noted that ovarian carcinoma cells, which were three-fold resistant to cDDP following selection with $CdCl_2$, do not overexpress MT. Certainly there are other mechanisms, which may be responsible for resistance to cDDP, including plasma membrane changes, increased cytosolic binding, decreased DNA cross-linking, and increased DNA repair [47].

In addition to cDDP resistance, normal and malignant cells with heavy-metal-induced MT display cross-resistance to alkylating agents [50]. Kelley et al. [46] reported that a transfected mouse cell line that overexpressed MT was also resistant to alkylating agents and was slightly resistant to doxorubicin and bleomycin. Webber et al. [51] found that a Cd-resistant human prostatic carcinoma cell line that overexpresses MT was resistant to doxorubicin, and when MT deinduction occurred the cell line was more sensitive to doxorubicin than either the drug-resistant or drug-sensitive parental lines. This suggests a possible role for MT in the development of resistance to doxorubicin.

Several important questions remain regarding the role of MT in the resistance phenotype. For example, it is not known how exposure to cyto-toxic drugs, specifically cDDP, increases cellular MT in a population of cells; there is no evidence for gene amplification or induction similar to that seen with heavy metals. The appearance of elevated MT in cDDP-resistant cells may reflect a selection process. In addition, it is not known which of the five major human isoforms of MT is increased within cells with acquired resistance to anticancer agents and if a specific isoform of MT is functionally more important. Understanding the circumstances under which different isoforms are overexpressed would help determine the functions of the isoforms and their regulatory mechanisms. It is also not known how MT might protect cells against the toxicity of anticancer agents. It has been suggested that elevated levels of MT can sequester electrophilic anticancer agents and reduce their cytotoxicity. More than 25% of intracellular cDDP has been found bound to MT in cells that overexpress MT, while less than 5% of cDDP was associated with MT in cells with normal levels of MT [45,52,53]. It is also possible that elevated MT may limit the available pool of intracellular Zn, an essential trace metal for numerous enzymes and macromolecules. This could produce changes in the function of these pro-teins and limit or augment anticancer-drug-related damage. The radical scavenging properties of MT could be important in the resistance that may occur to doxorubicin and x-irradiation.

The experimental observation of an association between MT and cDDP is being further examined in clinical studies. Chin et al. [54] have reported a positive correlation between cDDP exposure and MT content in a human germ-cell testis tumor cell line treated in vitro with increasing concen-trations of cDDP. Archival specimens of nonseminomatous tumors have been stained for MT by immunohistochemistry, and advanced tumors stained intensely, while low-stage tumors usually had weak staining. In addition, three patients with nonseminomatous tumors who failed first-line cDDP-containing chemotherapy had tumors that stained heavily for MT. Other investigators have sought to induce MT in normal tissues to protect animals from the toxicity of anticancer agents. In one study, pretreatment of mice with bismuth salts, which are potent MT inducers, decreased the lethality and renal, gastrointestinal, and hematopoietic toxicity of cDDP [55]. Similarly, bismuth pretreatment reduced the cardiac toxicity of doxorubicin [56]. This reduction in toxicity was unaccompanied by a loss of antitumor activity. Thus, selective induction of MT in vivo could possibly be one approach to broaden the therapeutic index of cDDP.

Conclusions

MT appears to be important in the resistance of cells to anticancer chemotherapy. It is an ubiquitous protein that is transiently induced by many factors, and it is certainly conceivable that there is transient resistance that occurs in vivo. Pharmacologic intervention could potentially increase or decrease MT in either malignant or normal tissues, with augmentation of tumor cytotoxicity or protection of nonmalignant tissues from undersirable side effects. Molecular techniques will permit the examination of MT isoform expression in response to different inducers. It is possible that the polymorphism of MT has functional significance and could be manipulated for improving the therapeutic index of cDDP and other cytotoxic drugs. Further investigation of this protein thiol will likely produce clinical strategies to overcome the important problem of tumor resistance to chemotherapy.

Acknowledgments

Dr. Bahnson is the recipient of an American Urological Association Research Scholarship from the American Foundation for Urologic Disease, 1989–1991. Dr. Lazo holds a USPHS Research Career Development Award.

References

1. Margoshes, M. and Vallee, B.L. A cadmium protein from equine kidney cortex. J. Am. Chem. Soc. 79:4813–4814, 1957.
2. Kagi, J.H.R. and Vallee, B.L. Metallothionein: a cadmium-and zinc-containing protein from equine renal cortex. J. Biol. Chem. 235:3460–3465, 1960.
3. Hamer, D.H. Metallothionein. Annu. Rev. Biochem. 55:913–951, 1986.
4. Danielson, K.G., Ohi, S., and Huang, P.C. Immunochemical detection of metallothionein in specific epithelial cells of rat organs. Proc. Natl. Acad. Sci. USA 79:2301–2304, 1982.
5. Banerjee, D., Onosaka, S., and Cherian, M.G. Immunohistochemical localization of metallothionein in cell nucleus and cytoplasm of rat liver and kidney. Toxicology 24: 95–105, 1982.

6. Piscator, M. On cadmium in normal human kidneys together with a report on the isolation of metallothionein from livers of cadmium-exposed rabbits. Nord. Hyg. Tidskr. 45:76–82, 1964.

7. Durnam, D.M. and Palmiter, R.D. Transcriptional regulation of the mouse metallothionein-I gene by heavy metals. J. Biol. Chem. 256:5712–5716, 1981.

8. Schmidt, C.J. and Hamer, D.H. Cell specificity and an effect of ras on human metallothionein gene expression. Proc. Natl. Acad. Sci. USA 83:3346–3350, 1986.

9. Richards, R.I., Heguy, A., and Karin, M. Structural and functional analysis of the human metallothionein-I$_A$ gene: differential induction by metal ions and glucocorticoids. Cell 37:263–272, 1984.

10. Sadhu, C. and Gedamu, L. Regulation of human metallothionein genes. J. Biol. Chem. 263:2679–2684, 1988.

11. Karin, M., Haslinger, A., Holtgreve, H., Richards, R., and Krauter, P. Characterization of DNA sequences through which cadmium and glucocorticoid hormones induce human metallothionein-II$_A$ gene. Nature 308:513–519, 1984.

12. Searle, P., Stuart, G.W., and Palmiter, R.D. Building a metal-responsive promoter with synthetic regulatory elements. Mol. Cell. Biol. 5:1480–1489, 1985.

13. Imbert, J., Zaf rullah, M., Culotta, V.C., Gedamu, L., and Hamer, D.H. Transcription factor MBF-I interacts with metal regulatory elements of higher eucaryotic metallothionein genes. Mol. Cell. Biol. 9:5315–5323, 1989.

14. Ryden, L. and Deutsch, H.F. Preparation and properties of the major copper binding component in human fetal liver, its identification as metallothionein. J. Biol. Chem. 253:519–524, 1978.

15. Failla, M.L. and Cousins, R.J. Zinc uptake by rat liver parenchymal cells. Biochem. Biophys. Acta 538:435–444, 1978.

16. Hager, L.J. and Palmiter, R.D. Transcriptional regulation of mouse liver metallothionein-I gene by glucocorticoids. Nature 291:340–343, 1981.

17. Cousins, R.J. Absorption, transport, and hepatic metabolism of copper and zinc: special reference to metallothionein and ceruloplasmin. Physiol. Rev. 65:238–309, 1985.

18. Durnam, D.M., Hoffman, J.S., Quaife, C.J., Benditt, E.P., Chen, H.Y., Brinster, R.L., and Palmiter, R.D. Induction of mouse metallothionein-I mRNA by bacterial endotoxin is independent of metals and glucocorticoid hormones. Proc. Natl. Acad. Sci. USA 81:1053–1056, 1984.

19. Friedman, R.L., Manly, N., McMahon, N., Kerr, I.M., and Stark, G.R. Transcriptional regulation of interferon-induced gene expression in human cells. Cell 38:745–755, 1984.

20. Karin, M., Imbra, R.J., Heguy, A., and Wong, G. Interleukin I regulates human metallothionein gene expression. Mol. Cell. Biol. 5:2866–2869, 1985.

21. Cousins, R.J. and Leinhart, A.S. Tissue-specific regulation of zinc metabolism and metallothionein genes by interleukin 1. FASEB J. 2:2884–2890, 1988.

22. Shiraishi, N., Aono, K., and Utsumi, K. Increased metallothionein content in rat liver induced by x-irradiation and exposure to high oxygen tension. Radiat. Res. 95:298–302, 1983.

23. Shiraishi, N., Yammamoto, Y., Takeda, Y., Kondoh, S., Hayashi, H., Hashimoto, K., and Aono, K. Increased metallothionein content in rat liver and kidney following x-irradiation. Toxicol. Appl. Pharmacol. 85:128–134, 1986.

24. Koropatnick, J., Leibbrandt, M., and Cherian, M.G. Organ-specific metallothionein induction in mice by x-irradiation. Radiat. Res. 119:356–365, 1989.

25. Karin, M. Metallothioneins: proteins in search of function. Cell 41:9–10, 1985.

26. Compere, S.J. and Palmiter, R.D. DNA methylation controls the inducibility of the mouse metallothionein I gene in lymphoid cells. Cell 25:233–240, 1981.

27. Durnam, D.M. and Palmiter, R.D. Induction of metallothionein-I mRNA in cultured cells by heavy metals and iodoacetate: evidence for gratuitous inducers. Mol. Cell. Biol. 4:484–491, 1984.

258

28. Beach, L.R. and Palmiter, R.D. Amplification of the metallothionein-I gene in cadmium resistant mouse cells. Proc. Natl. Acad. Sci. USA 78:2110–2114, 1981.

29. Gick, G.G. and McCarty, K.S. Amplification of the metallothionein-I gene in cadmium- and zinc-resistant Chinese hamster ovary cells. J. Biol. Chem. 257:9049–9053, 1982.

30. Schmidt, C.J., Jubier, M.-F., and Hamer, D.H. Structure and expression of two human metallothionein-I isoform genes and a related pseudogene. J. Biol. Chem. 260:7731–7737, 1985.

31. Karin, M., Cathala, G., and Nguyen-Huu, M.C. Expression and regulation of a human metallothionein gene carried on an autonomously replicating shuttle vector. Proc. Natl. Acad. Sci. USA 80:4040–4044, 1983.

32. Kagi, J.H.R. and Schaffer, A. Biochemistry of metallothionein. Biochemistry 27:8509–8515, 1988.

33. Brewer, G.J., Hill, G.M., Prasad, A.S., Cossack. Z.T., and Rabani, P. Oral zinc therapy for Wilson's disease. Ann. Intern. Med. 99:314–320, 1983.

34. Klug, A. and Rhodes, D. "Zinc fingers": A novel protein motif for nucleic acid recognition. Trends Biochem. Sci. 12:464–469, 1987.

35. Ohtake, H., Hasegawa, K., and Koga, M. Zinc-binding protein in the liver of neonatal, normal, and partially hepatectomized rats. Biochem. J. 174:999–1005, 1978.

36. Nemer, M., Travaglini, E.C., Rondinelli, E., and D'Alonzo, J. Developmental regulation, induction, and embryonic tissue specificity of sea urchin metallothionein gene expression. Dev. Biol. 102:471–482, 1984.

37. Andrews, G.K., Adamson, E.D., and Gedamu, L. The ontogeny of expression of murine metallothionein: comparison with the α-fetoprotein gene. Dev. Biol. 103:294–303, 1984.

38. Bakka, A., Samarawickrama, G.P., and Webb, M. Metabolism of zinc and copper in the neonate: effect of cadmium administration during late gestation in the rat on the zinc and copper metabolism of the newborn. Chem. Biol. evidenceact. 34:161–171, 1981.

39. Wilkinson, D.G. and Nemer, M. Metallothionein genes MT_a and MT_b expressed under distinct quantitative and tissue-specific regulation in sea urchin embryos. Mol. Cell. Biol. 7:48–58, 1987.

40. Thornalley, P.J. and Vasek, M. Possible role for metallothionein in protection against radiation-induced oxidative stress. Kinetics and mechanism of its reaction with superoxide and hydroxyl radicals. Biochem. Biophys. Acta 827:36–44, 1985.

41. Dunn, M.A., Blalock, T.L., and Cousins, R.J. Metallothionein. Proc. Soc. Exp. Biol. Med. 185:107–119, 1987.

42. Matsubara, J., Tajima, Y., Ikeda, A., Kinoshita, T., and Shimoyama, T. A new perspective of radiation protection by metallothionein induction. Pharmac. Ther. 39:331–333, 1988.

43. Shiraishi, N., Hayashi, H., Hiraki, Y., Aono, K., Itano, Y., Kosaka, F., Noji, S., and Taniguchi, S. Elevation in metallothionein messenger RNA in rat tissues after exposure to x-irradiation. Toxicol. Appl. Pharmacol. 98:501–506, 1989.

44. Lohrer, H. and Robson, T. Overexpression of metallothionein in CHO cells and its effect on cell killing by ionizing radiation and alkylating agents. Carcinogenesis 10:2279–2284, 1989.

45. Bakka, A., Endresen, L., Johnsen, A.B.S., Edminson, P.D., and Rugstad, H.E. Resistance against cis-dichlorodiammineplatinum in cultured cells with a high content of metallothionein. Toxicol. Appl. Pharmacol. 61:215–226, 1981.

46. Kelley, S.L., Basu, A., Teicher, B.A., Hacker, M.P., Hamer, D.H., and Lazo, J.S. Overexpression of metallothionein confers resistance to anticancer drugs. Science 241: 1813–1815, 1988.

47. Teicher, B.A., Holden, S.A., Kelley, M.J., Shea, T.C., Cucchi, C.A., Rosowsky, A., Henner, W.D., and Frei, E., III. Characterization of a human squamous carcinoma cell line resistant to cis-diamminedichloroplatinum II. Cancer Res. 47:388–393, 1987.

48. Andrews, P.A., Murphy, M.P., and Howell, S.B. Metallothionein mediated cisplatin

resistance in human ovarian carcinoma cells. Cancer Chemother. Pharmacol. 19:149–154, 1987.

49. Endresen, L., Schjerven, L., and Rugstad, H.E. Tumours from a cell strain with a high content of metallothionein show enhanced resistance against cis-dichlorodiammineplatinum. Acta Pharmacol. Toxicol. 55:183–187, 1984.

50. Endresen, L., Bakka, A., and Rugstad, H.E. Increased resistance to chlorambucil in cultured cells with a high concentration of cytoplasmic metallothionein. Cancer Res. 43: 2918–2926, 1983.

51. Webber, M.M., Maseehur Rehman, S.M., and James, G.T. Metallothionein induction and deinduction in human prostatic carcinoma cells: relationship with resistance and sensitivity to adriamycin. Cancer Res. 48:4503–4508, 1988.

52. Zelazowski, A.J., Garvey, J.S., and Hoeschele, J.D. *In vivo* and *in vitro* binding of platinum to metallothionein. Arch. Biochem. Biophys. 229:246–252, 1984.

53. Kraker, A., Schmidt, J., Krezoski, S., and Petering, D.H. Binding of cis-dichlorodiammineplatinum II to metallothionein in Ehrlich cells. Biochem. Biophys. Res. Commun. 130:786–792, 1985.

54. Chin, J.L., Banerjee, D., Kadhim, S., and Cherian, G. Role of metallothioneins in germ cell tumor behavior: preliminary experimental and clinical evidence. J. Urol. 143:265A, 1990.

55. Naganuma, A., Satoh, M., and Imura, N. Prevention of lethal and renal toxicity of cis-diamminedichloroplatinum (II) by induction of metallothionein synthesis without compromising its antitumor activity in mice. Cancer Res. 47:983–987, 1987.

56. Naganuma, A., Satoh, M., and Imura, N. Specific reduction of toxic side effects of adriamycin by induction of metallothionein in mice. Jpn. J. Cancer Res. 79:406–411, 1988.

13. Modulation of antitumor alkylating agents (AA)

Beverly A. Teicher and Emil Frei III

Introduction

The modulation of an antitumor agent is accomplished by a compound that modifies some aspect of the biochemical pharmacology of the anti-tumor agent in the direction of improving its therapeutic index. In the past, modulation approaches have generally involved antimetabolites, particularly 5-fluorouracil (FU). Successful clinical modulation of FU with leucovorin has recently been accomplished [1]. Leucovorin is a prodrug for 5,10-methylene-tetrahydrofolic acid, which forms the third arm of the ternary complex involving thymidylate synthase and FdUMP. As such, 5,10-methylene-tetrahydrofolic acid markedly increases the stability of the ternary complex and thus increases the effectiveness of fluoropyrimidine inhibition. This approach has proven successful in the clinic in that the addition of leucovorin to FU has substantially and significantly increased the therapeutic effect of FU in metastatic colorectal cancer in a number of comparative studies [2] and in noncomparative studies in advanced squamous-cell carcinoma of the head and neck [3] and in metastatic breast cancer. Thus there is precedent for the successful use of biochemical modulation in the clinic.

The alkylating agents (AAs) are particularly appropriate for studies involving modulation. The AAs, which include cisplatin, are the most important class of antitumor agents in terms of the magnitude and spectrum of clinical activity [4]. The demonstration that AAs are commonly non-cross-resistant [5–7] with each other would indicate a heterogeneity of mechanisms that determine sensitivity and resistance. Moreover, the AAs exhibit steep dose/response curves and most have myelosuppression as dose-limiting toxicity [8]. They are therefore ideal agents for dose intensification therapy in the bone marrow transplantation setting and other novel marrow supportive care approaches, such as with hematopoietins [9]. The purpose of this chapter is to present the current status of the determinants of AA sensitivity and resistance, with emphasis on the mechanisms of resistance and their capacity for modulation. Finally, the case will be made that resistance generally, and AA resistance particularly, is multifactorial, that is, multiple mechanisms are involved. Thus modulation, where possible,

Robert F. Ozols (ed.), MOLECULAR AND CLINICAL ADVANCES IN ANTICANCER DRUG RESISTANCE. Copyright © 1991.
Kluwer Academic Publishers, Boston. All rights reserved. ISBN 0-7923-1212-0

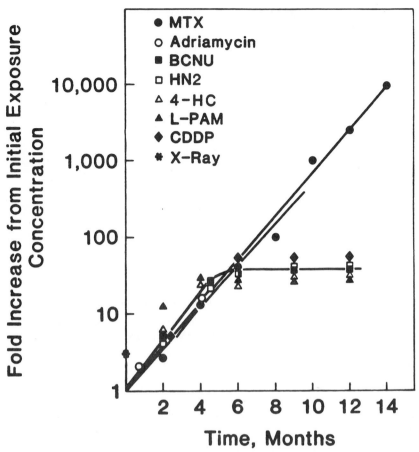

Figure 1. The development of resistance to various antineoplastic agents using selection pressure. The methotrexate line is based on data from Frei et al. [13]: The adriamycin line is based on data from Twentyman et al. [14] and Vrignaud et al. [15]. The point shown for x-rays is under hypoxic conditions. The alkylating agent line is based on the results presented in Teicher and Frei [10]. (Reprinted from Teicher and Frei [10], with permission.)

should be directed at the combination of relevant mechanisms. This will be referred to as the *multimodulation approach.*

Resistance to alkylating agents

AA resistance on the part of L1210 mouse leukemia in vivo was first demonstrated by Schabel, who observed that generally there was a lack of cross-resistance among the AA [7]. Teicher, Frei, and others [10–12] have produced resistance to AA in human tumor cells in vitro by selection pressure (Figure 1). It was found that resistance was difficult to produce,

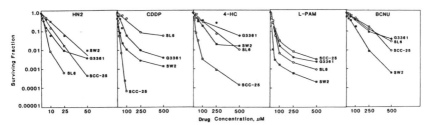

Figure 2. Survival of G3361 melanoma cells (●), SL6 lung adenocarcinoma cells (○), SW2 small-cell carcinoma cells (■), and SCC-25 head and neck carcinoma cells (□)exposed to various alkylating agents for 1 hr over a dosage range. The results are presented as the mean of three independent experiments. (Reprinted from Teicher and Frei [10], with permission.)

even after extensive, intensive selection pressure. AA-resistant human tumor cell lines were rarely more than 12-fold resistant, as compared to the parent line [10,11]. In contrast, multilog levels of resistance can be produced by the same procedure for antimetabolites, such as methotrexate, and for natural products, such as adriamycin (Figure 1). The sustained linear dose/response curves for the AAs are consistent with the aforementioned "resistance development" (Figure 2) [10]. The AAs in this regard more closely resemble radiotherapy to which resistance in the classical sense does not occur.

The relative lack of cross-resistance among AAs suggests a multiplicity of mechanisms (Table 1) [5,6,16]. This has largely been confirmed by cellular pharmacologic studies of resistance (Figure 3) [12]. In this figure, some of the described mechanisms for AA resistance are presented, starting at the level of the plasma membrane and progressing through the cytoplasm and the nucleus to the level of DNA repair.

Nitrogen mustard and phenylalanine mustard, for example, have been shown to be actively transported into cells, and some resistant cell lines are associated with a decreased capacity for active transport [16–18]. Cytotoxicity in vivo can be inhibited by the normal metabolites that compete for transport, such as choline and selected amino acids. However, it has not been possible to demonstrate that inhibition of transport will increase the

Table 1. Resistance ratios to various alkylating agents

Cell Line	HN$_2$	L-PAM	CDDP	BCNU	4-HC	TSPA	MitoC
Breast (MCF7/CDDP)	1.6	2.0	6.5	1.4	1.1	3.1	1.3
Breast (MCF7/4HC)	2.0	1.0	1.3	1.1	9.0	2.0	1.0
H&N (SCC-25/CDDP)	1.8	5.0	12.0	2.0	2.8	1.7	1.0
Lymphoma (Raji/BCNU)	1.9	4.0	4.0	5.3	1.6		
Lymphoma (Raji/HN$_2$)	6.6	1.4	2.3	1.9	2.8	1.6	1.4

Number = fold resistance.
Reprinted from Goldenberg and Alexander [16], with permission.

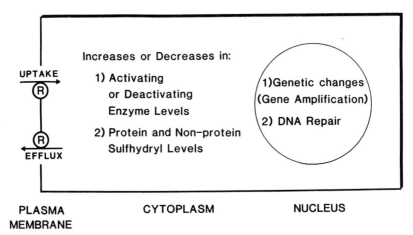

Increases or Decreases in:

1) Activating
   or Deactivating
   Enzyme Levels

2) Protein and Non−protein
   Sulfhydryl Levels

1)Genetic changes
(Gene Amplification)

2) DNA Repair

UPTAKE

EFFLUX

PLASMA
MEMBRANE

CYTOPLASM

NUCLEUS

Figure 3. Sites of biological change that can lead to alkylating agent resistance. (Reprinted from Teicher and Frei [12], with permission.)

therapeutic index, that is, an increased cytotoxicity to tumor cells as compared to normal cells.

Once an AA enters the cytoplasm, it can potentially be inactivated by the glutathione-S-transferase system. The glutathione concentration in the cytoplasm is high (2.5–10 mM), and glutathione may combine with and inactivate some AAs. Both the cellular concentration of glutathione and of the family of conjugating enyzmes (glutathione-S-transferases) may be elevated in AA-resistant cell lines [19]. Metallothionein, a protein rich in cysteines, may also be elevated in certain AA-resistant cell lines [20].

Hypoxia may contribute to resistance to radiotherapy, to oxygen-requiring antitumor agents such as bleomycin, and interestingly, to AA resistance [21–24]. The addition of the perfluorocarbon emulsion (Fluosol DA) and oxygen breathing, or the use of the oxygen mimic etanidazole, increases sensitivity to AA (see below) [25].

At the level of DNA repair, AA resistance may be associated with an increase in the levels of O^6 guanine alkyltransferase that specifically remove nitrosourea monoadducts from DNA [26,27]. Other mechanisms of repair, demonstrated by alkaline elution, may be increased in AA resistance [28].

Topoisomerase II levels have been reported to be increased in some AA-resistant tumor cell lines [29]. Topoisomerase II, by unwinding the tightly coiled DNA in the G_2 period, might increase access of repair enzymes to DNA. In any event, inhibition of topoisomerase II has been associated with increased AA activity [30,31].

DNA repair occurs primarily during the G_2 period. It has been found that methylxanthines, such as pentoxifylline, accelerate transit through the G_2 period and therefore decrease DNA repair. [32,33] Pentoxifylline produces other biochemical effects, so its mechanism of modulation in vivo is uncertain.

264

Table 2. SCC sublines with low-level MTX resistance: MTX resistance phenotype heterogeneity in human head and neck carcinoma cells

Cell Line	MTX Uptake[a]	MTX Polyglutamylation[a]	DHFR Content[b]	Generation Time[b]
SCC15/R1 (15×)[c]	Severe defect at 2.0 μM, not tested at 0.2 μM	Severe defect at 2.0 μM, not tested at 0.2 μM	Minimal change	No change
SCC25/R1 (20×)	Normal at 2.0 and 0.2 μM	Normal at 2.0 μM, moderate defect at 0.2 μM	Increase (3.5×)	No change
SCC68/R1 (13×)	Moderate defect at 2.0 and 0.2 μM	Normal at 2.0 μM, moderate defect at 0.2 μM	Increase (4.9×)	Minimal change
SCC78/R1 (6.7×)	Normal at 2.0 μM, small defect at 0.2 μM	Small defect at 2.0 and 0.2 μM	Minimal change	Increase (1.8×)

[a] The following terms are used to qualitatively describe the capacity for MTX uptake and MTX polyglutamylation in each resistant cell in comparison with its parental line: normal, <10% change in V_0 or percentage of polyglutamylation; small defect, 10–50% change; moderate defect, 50–90% change; severe defect, >90% change.
[b] Minimal change in these assays is considered to be <50%.
[c] × = fold resistance.
From Rosowsky et al. [34], with permission.

265

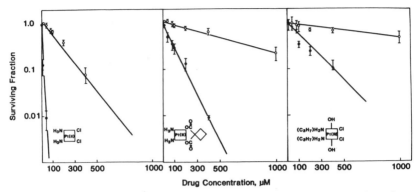

Figure 4. Survival of SCC-25 (●) and SCC-25/ CP (○) cells treated with various doses of CDDP, carboplatin, or iproplatin. Points indica means of three independent determinations ± SE (bars). (Reprinted from Teicher et al. [6], with permission.)

In summary, AA resistance can occur at many levels and by many mechanisms.

The multifactorial nature of resistance to antitumor agents

The early literature on the biochemistry of drug resistance suggested that such resistance was monofunctional. This is, in part, an artifact, since in many studies only one mechanism of resistance was analyzed. The first report that resistance is commonly multifactorial was by Rosowsky and related to methotrexate resistance (Table 2) [34]. In this study, it was found that low levels of resistance to methotrexate, that is, clinically relevant resistance levels, were most commonly associated with two or more mechanisms, that is, resistance was multifactorial [34].

Table 3. The glutathione glutathione transferase (GSH/GST) system

- General formulas — GSH + AA (alkylating agent)
- GSH Biosynthesis — inhibition
- GST isozymes
- GSH/GST — Component of overall drug activation/inactivation systems
- GSH/GST and drug resistance
- GSH conjugation with AA
- Modulation of GSH with BSO
    BSO effects:
        In vitro antitumor activity
        In vivo (experimental) antitumor activity
        Toxicology and pharmacology
        Clinical Phase I trial
- GST inhibition by ethacrynic acid
- Protection of normal tissues from AA damage GSHet, WR2721

266

GSH/GST Chemical reactions.

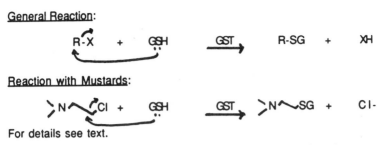

For details see text.

Figure 5. General scheme for the reaction of substrates with glutathione (GSH) as catalyzed by glutathione-S-transferase (GST).

In a study by Teicher et al. [6] of a human squamous-cell carcinoma of the head and neck rendered resistant to cisplatin in vitro, it was found that several individual mechanisms, each of which contributed relatively small changes (e.g., threefold increases in glutathione-S-transferase) led to an overall 30-fold resistance of the cell line to this drug (Figure 4) [6]. From the teleologic and evolutionary point of view, multiple mechanisms of resistance would make sense. The commonality of low levels of resistance to AAs on the part of cell lines resistant to a specific selecting alkylating agent is consistent with the multifactorial nature of resistance (see Figure 3). To the extent that resistance is in fact multifactorial, modulation by a single agent might produce a limited effect. On the other hand, a multimodulation approach would be strongly supported and is consistent with some pre-liminary data (see below).

The glutathione/glutathione-S-transferase (GSH/GST) system

An outline for this section is presented in Table 3.

The general chemical reaction catalyzed by the GSH/GST system is presented in Figure 5, where R represents an electrophilic substrate (e.g., an AA) and X is a suitable leaving group. Although reactions of this type may occur nonenzymatically, particularly at high pH (pH > 8–9), sub-stantial rate enhancement can be effected by GST enzymes. In the case of beta-chlorethyl-mustard-containing substrates (Figure 5, bottom), GST-catalyzed conjugation of GSH results in displacement of chloride ion and inactivation of the electrophilic mustard moiety. In the case of melphalan (L-phenylalanine mustard), metabolism by GSH/GST yields the inactivated mono- and di-GSH adducts, as well as a novel ring-substituted derivative, 4-(GSH) phenylalanine [35].

The biosynthesis of glutathione is presented in Figure 6. Glutamine and cysteine are conjugated enzymatically to the dipeptide glutamyl cysteine,

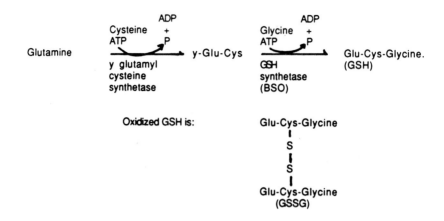

Figure 6. Biosynthesis of glutathione (GSH).

which in turn is converted by glutathione synthetase to the tripeptide gluta-thione. This second enzymatic step can be inhibited by buthionine sul-foximine (BSO), a substrate analog for that enzyme [36].

Cellular GST and GSH levels appear to be significant determinants of AA sensitivity and resistance (Table 4). GST overexpression and elevated cellular GSH levels are associated with AA resistance in a number of cell lines [19]. Conversion of the resistant cell line to sensitivity to AAs can be rendered by BSO and, in addition, BSO increases the activity of AAs against sensitive cell lines [37–39]. The contribution of glutathione-S-transferase to such resistance and such sensitivity is supported by trans-fection experiments using cloned human GST DNAs [40–42]. Melanoma cell lines (G3361) that were made resistant to AAs regularly have an increase in glutathione-S-transferase activity but were not cross-resistant. Therefore, specific isozymes of GST may be involved [19]. As above, resistance is

Table 4. GST/GSH and drug resistance

GST overexpression is associated with
  drug-resistant phenotypes
GSH ↑ associated with drug resistance
  Reversed by BSO
  BSO also ↑ activity of AAs
    against sensitive cell lines
Transfection of GST may confer resistance to AAs
Melanoma lines regularly have GST ↑
Multifactorial

Table 5. Glutathione transperase (GST) isozymes

GST enzymes utilize GSH in a broad range of cellular reactions, including:
- Conjugation of GSH to electrophilic drugs, carcinogens and endogenous steroids
- Detoxification of lipid and nucleic acid hydroperoxides

Multiple isozymes of GST, each with separate genes
Have broad range of overlapping substrates
Major isozymes can be determined by western blot analysis and include:
    a (basic) — mediates resistance to mustards
    u (neutral) — conjugates GSH to BCNU 50% of normal subects express --u (see text)
    π (acidic) prevalent in tumor tissues (marker) ?PAM resistance
Isozymes induced by substrate exposure in rodents and humans

---

commonly multifactorial, that is, GST/GSH changes may contribute part of the overall biochemical resistance.

The GST system is described in greater detail in Table 5. GSTs are Phase II drug-metabolizing enzymes that utilizes GSH in a broad range of cellular reactions, including the conjugation of glutathione to electrophilic drugs, carcinogens, and endogenous steroids. These enzymes are also involved in the detoxification of lipid and nucleic acid hydroperoxides [43].

When given by mouth, the bioavailability of BSO in the blood is very low, however, there is a comparable decrease in tissue glutathione. This suggests that major biotransformation with the first pass through the liver occurs and that a metabolite of BSO may inhibit GSH biosynthesis. There is little significant toxicity at extremely high doses of BSO in experimental animals (Table 6). Transient but inconsistent white blood cell depression and renal toxicity occurs, but again at very high doses. Most important, the normal tissue toxicity of melphalan in vivo was not altered by high doses of BSO.

BSO increases the antitumor effects of a number of agents against a number of tumor cell lines in vitro (Table 7) [38]. In vivo studies in mice indicate that BSO can increase the antitumor effects of a number of AAs in a variety of human xenografts and animal tumors, including breast cancer, ovarian cancer, bladder cancer, and brain tumors (Table 8) [39,51,52]. Interestingly, in the medulloblastoma xenograft study, BSO produced a marked decrease in GSH within the tumor, but not in normal brain tissue

Table 6. Buthionine sulfoximine (BSO): Preclinical toxicity and pharmacology in mice

---

i.v. $T_{1/2}$ initial 5 min
    $T_{1/2}$ terminal 37 min
    Plasma clearance 28 ml/min/kg
p.o. bioavailability very low
However, comparable tissue GSH ↓ with p.o. and i.v. BSO
Toxicity of high-BSO
    Transient WBC ↓
    High doses did not alter PAM toxicity
    Extremely High doses (1600 mg/kg/day × 4) BSO + PAM produced renal damage

---

Table 7. BSO antitumor effects in vitro

BSO ↑ antitumor effects of		
Drug	on	Tumors
PAM		L1210
DOX		Mult.
PAM		Mult.
PAM		Mult/R
CPA, PAM, cisplat		Human ovary/R

[53]. In general, in these in vivo studies GSH was decreased about 10-fold by BSO, both in tumors and in normal tissues. Thus the selective effect of the combination of AAs and BSO against tumor tissues as compared to normal tissues must necessitate other factors than the decrease in GSH.

Ethacrynic acid, indomethacin, and related compounds have been found to inhibit glutathione-S-transferases (Table 9) [54]. Thus ethacrynic acid will decrease GST π activity by some 50%. Ethacrynic acid can produce a 5- to 10-fold decrease in chlorambucil sensitivity in two human colon cell lines in culture [54]. In the only reported in vivo study, ethacrynic acid significantly increased the growth delay produced by phenylalanine mustard. This was at a tolerated dose of ethacrynic acid and a dose that produced a decrease in normal liver GST of some 40% [55]. Ethacrynic acid and thioTEPA are now in a Phase I clinical trial [56].

Cytosolic glutathione levels can be increased by GSH-Et, the mono-ethylester of glutathione. GSH is a polar compound and does not pass the lipid cell membrane. Esterification of glutathione in the form of GSH-Et yields a lipid-soluble compound that enters cells readily and can be hydrolyzed in the cytosol, resulting in an elevation of cytosolic glutathione levels. Toxicity, particularly liver toxicity, can be difficult, especially at transplant doses of the AAs. An analysis of the effect of this compound and the radioprotector WR-2721 on the survival of animals treated with high

Table 8. BSO antitumor effects in vivo (mice)

Drug	Tumor
MMC	EMT6 (breast)
CPA	EMT6 (breast)
PAM	Ovary
PAM	Medulloblastoma xenograft
PAM	Medulloblastoma xenograft
Marked GSH in tumor but not in normal brain	
PAM	Bladder cancer
BCNU	Bladder cancer
CPA*	Several

* Increased cardiac toxicity.

Table 9. GST inhibition by ethacrynic acid

In vitro
    Etha $\downarrow$ GSTπ activity 50+%
    Etha produced a 5–10 × $\uparrow$ in chlorambucil
        sensitivity in two human colon cell lines
In vivo
    PAM and etha in colon xenograft:
Growth delay (days)

Control	28
Etha	26
PAM	37
Etha + PAM	48

Etha dose = 10 mg/kg/day × 11
Decreased liver GST 40%

Etha = ethacrynic acid

doses of alkylating agents has therefore been carried out (Table 10) [57]. WR-2721 is relatively lipid soluble and provides a high level of intracellular organic sulfhydryls. As can be seen in Table 10, both GSH-Et particularly, and also WR-2721, provide substantial protection against the lethal toxicity of high doses of AAs. In the two studies performed to date, the mouse fibrosarcoma and the mice breast cancer (EMT6) studies, GSH-Et did not compromise the antitumor effect of AA [57].

These data suggest that BSO can decrease GSH in normal and tumor tissues, but the cytotoxicity is expressed almost exclusively in tumor tissues. On the other hand, GSH-Et will, in vitro and presumably in vivo, markedly increase GSH levels in all tissues, but would appear to provide protection of normal tissues and not tumor tissues from AA toxicity. We are in the process of extending these observations, and in particular, are analyzing the combination of BSO and glutathione monoethylester.

Metallothionein

Metallothioneins are proteins rich in cysteine residues that are increased in the cytoplasm in response to heavy-metal exposure (see Table 1) [58–61]. Thirty percent of the amino acid residues in these proteins are cysteine. In the classical study of Bakka et al., cadmium chloride was used to markedly increase metallothionein levels in cells [61]. However, such may also occur with a variety of metals and agents, but not apparently with genotoxic agents (Table 11). The increase in metallothionein with, for example, cadmium is at the transcriptional or possibly at the mRNA stabilization level [62]. Metallothionein has been found to be increased in many cisplatin and some chlorambucil-resistant cell lines [6,20,63,64]. Metallothionein could be decreased by antisense compounds. Preliminary studies indicate that metallothionein can be increased in normal organs by bismuth, which is nontoxic,

271

Table 10. Survival of animals treated with high-dose bcnu, cyclophosphamide, or mitomycin C with or without prior treatment with a potential protective agent

Drug	Dose (mg/kg)[b]	Mean Survival (Days)[a] Protective Agents (dose in mg/kg)					
		None	WR-2721 (400)	GSH (2300)	GSH (5 × 1150)	GSHet (2600)	GSHet (5 × 1300)
BCNU	150	10 ± 4	64 ± 16	35 ± 13		91 ± 27	
	125	25 ± 9	74 ± 29	54 ± 21		No deaths	
	100	84 ± 22	No deaths[c]	77 ± 29		No deaths	
	75	102 ± 24[d]	No deaths	102 ± 26		No deaths	
	5 × 50	3.0 ± 0.7[d]			3.3 ± 0.9		7.3 ± 1.4
CTX	5 × 100	65 ± 12			96 ± 36		Two of 14 died on days 98 and 130
Mitomycin C	5	88 ± 34				113 ± 42	

CTX = cyclophosphamide; GSH = glutathione; GSHet = glutathione monothyl ester.

[a] Survival is given as days ± standard error of mean. Each treatment group had seven animals, and the experiment was done twice.

[b] Drugs were administered by i.p. injection. In groups receiving the protective agent, the agent was administered 1 hr before the anticancer agent Drugs given in multiple doses were administered daily.

[c] Remaining live animals were killed on day 150.

[d] Days after completion of the treatment regimen.

TUMOR HYPOXIA - SCHEMATIC

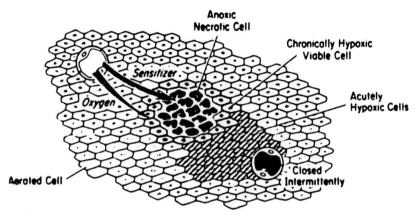

Figure 7. Schematic representation of acute and chronic hypoxia in a solid tumor mass [66].

thus protecting such organs from AA toxicity [65]. Modulation of metal-lothionein in the direction of improving the antitumor therapeutic index is a reasonable future strategy.

Tumor cell hypoxia and perfluorocarbons — oxygen

Tumor hypoxia was first recognized in the 1950s. There are two basic mechanisms (Figure 7). As tumors grow, they may outstrip their blood supply, such that hypovascularity is common in solid tumors [22,66]. Since oxygen can diffuse a maximum of 150 microns from a blood vessel, tumor cells at this limit or beyond are hypoxic. However, many remain clonogenic if the environment is corrected. In addition, hypoxia may be intermittent, i.e., may occur as arterioles open and close, a recently recognized phenomenon [67].

Table 11. Metallothionein (MT)

Protein-SH increased with heavy-metal exposure and in alkylating agent resistance
MW-6000: 30% of amino acids are cysteine
Cadmium induces 70 × ↑ in MT
Increased MT also occurs with metals, heat shock, phorbol, cAMP, endotoxin; not with genotoxic agents
↑ MT is at mRNA level: transcriptional or stabilization
MT ↑ in some cisplatin- and chlorambucil-resistant cell lines[a]
MT can be ↓ by antisense compounds (theoretical)
MT can be ↑ in normal organs by bismuth (non toxic) for protection against alkylating agents[b]

a
b

273

Table 12. Hypoxia and response to radiotherapy: Clinical studies

Response	Volume weighed pO_2 (mmHg)	Mean pO_2 Measurement (mmHg)
Complete (N = 18)	37.4 ± 8.2	20.6 ± 4.4
Partial (N = 2)	15.2 ± 4.4	8.8 ± 3.2
None (N = 11)	8.4 ± 5.1	4.6 ± 3.0

From Gatenby et al. [18], with permission.

While hypoxia is a well-known obstacle to radiotherapy in preclinical systems, clinical data is more limited, primarily for technical reasons. Table 12 represents a study by Gatenby et al. [68] indicating that almost half of his patients had tumors with severe hypoxia (less than 10 mmHg). These patients had little or no observed response to radiotherapy. Sixty percent of his patients had moderate hypoxia (in the range of 10–30 mmHg), and these patients performed substantially better in terms of their response to radiotherapy.

The perfluorochemicals are organic compounds in which the hydrogens have been replaced by fluorine atoms (Table 13). Perfluorocarbons such as perfluorodecalin readily dissolve oxygen and CO_2, and when prepared as biocompatible emulsions have been effective as red blood cell substitutes, providing oxygen-carrying capacity in vivo. The perfluorocarbon particle is less than 1% the size of a red blood cell, which gives the emulsion a much greater surface area to volume ratio and a much lower viscosity than red blood cells [69]. This permits entry of Fluosol-DA into hypoxic tumors and corrects hypoxia. Because of this, major advances in radiotherapy, and interestingly in chemotherapy, can be achieved experimentally using this compound [23,70].

In Figure 8, the correction of hypoxia in experimental solid tumors by the perfluorochemical emulsion and oxygen is presented [70]. The partial pressure of oxygen was less than 10 mmHg in 75% of the control tumors, whereas

Table 13. Perfluorocarbons: Fluosol-DA

- Tumor hypovascularity — hypoxia
- Hydrocarbons where H are replaced by F
- Dissolves O_2 & CO_2; O_2 not bound to Fluosol-DA as it is to hemoglobin.
- Volume of particle — less than 1% that of RBC
- Per packed volume Fluosol DA has >100 times more surface area than RBC
- Viscosity of Fluosol DA much less than RBC
- Therefore enters hypovascular tumors & corrects hypoxia more readily; ↓ myocardial ischemia
  Corrects hypoxia in experimental solid tumors
- Therefore increases radiation therapy effect 3–5 times
  Also ↑ activity of certain chemotherapeutic agents 3–5 times

274

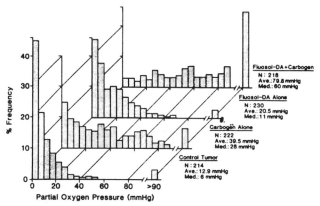

Figure 8. Frequency distribution of pO_2 in RIF-1 tumors in C3H mice under various conditions. N is the number of pO_2 determinations using 35–50 mice [70].

less than 10% of tumors in animals receiving Fluosol-DA plus oxygen breathing were severely hypoxic. That Fluosol-DA plus oxygen breathing increases the antitumor effect of radiotherapy experimentally is presented in Table 14 [23]. In this growth delay analysis of a transplantable murine Lewis lung cancer, radiotherapy was four to six times more effective when combined with oxygen breathing and Fluosol-DA [23,71].

The effect of Fluosol-DA on bleomycin-induced growth delay was minimal, but in the presence of oxygen breathing it was marked (Table 15) [24]. Bleomycin requires oxygen for its cytotoxic activity. This is not known to be the case for many of the AAs [24,72,73]. Nevertheless, it was found that for essentially all of the AAs, there was a two- to sixfold increase in antitumor activity when the AAs were delivered in the presence of Fluosol-DA and oxygen breathing (Table 15) [24]. How does one explain this effect? It is possible that AAs do require oxygen, as observed in recent studies of thioTEPA [74]. Oxygen may modify the cytokinetics of experimental tumors in the direction of an increasing growth fraction, and therefore, may im-

Table 14. Fluosol-DA increases antitumor activity of radiotherapy: Growth delay of Lewis lung tumors treated with annex solution or PFCE and carbogen breathing for 1 hr prior to and during irradiation

Treatment Condition	Growth Delay (Days)		
	10 Gy	20 Gy	30 Gy
Carbogen breathing	1.6 ± 0.5^a	6.2 ± 1.0	8.8 ± 1.0
Carbogen breathing and annex solution	3.6 ± 1.0	12.6 ± 1.5	19.7 ± 2.0
Carbogen breathing and Fluosol-DA	8.5 ± 1.5	28.5 ± 2.5	36.3 ± 2.0

[a] Mean $\pm$ S.E.
From Teicher and Rose [23], with permission.

275

Table 15. Effect of the addition of fluosol-DA/O_2 on the TGD produced by various chemotherapeutic agents

Drug	Drug Dose (mg/kg)	Treatment Schedule	TGD, Days (Tumor Growth Delay)	
			Drug/Air	Drug/Fluosol-DA/O_2
		Alkylating Agents		
Melphalan	10	Single dose	2.7 ± 0.3	9.5 ± 1.4[a]
CDDP	10	Single dose	8.0 ± 1.7	8.4 ± 2.0
Cytoxan	100	Days 7, 9, 11, 13, 15	7.98 ± 0.78	11.40 ± 3.57
Busultan	10	Days 7, 9, 11, 13, 15	1.10 ± 0.53	9.26 ± 2.14[a]
Mitomycin	2	Days 7, 9, 11, 13, 15	9.03 ± 0.72	5.33 ± 1.71
BCNU	15	Days 7, 9, 11, 13, 15	13.38 ± 1.47	26.03 ± 2.54[b]
CONU	100	Days 7, 9, 11, 13, 15	3.14 ± 0.42	12.53 ± 2.25[a]
MeCCNU	20	Days 7, 9, 11, 13, 15	1.84 ± 0.61	13.35 ± 2.27[a]
Chlorozotocin	15	Days 7, 9, 11, 13, 15	1.56 ± 0.32	8.34 ± 1.35[a]
Procarbazine	20	Single dose	0.73 ± 0.23	11.16 ± 2.40[b]
Decarbazine	400	Single dose	4.14 ± 0.63	6.8 ± 1.00
		Antibiotics and Alkaloids		
Bleomycin	10	Days 6, 10, 13, 16	2.27 ± 0.7	14.56 ± 2.97[a]
	15	Days 6, 10, 13, 16	3.66 ± 1.0	16.89 ± 2.94[a]
Vincristine	1.5	Single dose	1.86 ± 0.43	4.83 ± 1.22
VP-16	10	Days 7–12	1.84 ± 0.33	4.49 ± 1.22
	15	Days 7–12	4.89 ± 0.68	11.54 ± 2.14[a]
	20	Days 7–12	6.96 ± 1.0	21.70 ± 2.68[b]
		Antimetabolites		
Methotrexate	0.8	Days 7–12	2.23 ± 0.89	2.90 ± 0.67
5-Fluorouracil	40	Days 7–10	7.61 ± 0.56	10.47 ± 1.06

[a] $p < 0.001$.
[b]

From Teicher and Holder [24], with permission.

part greater susceptibility to antitumor agents. It is also possible that lipid-soluble AAs associate with the emulsifier surrounding the perflourocarbon particles and are thus carried into the tumor and protected from hydrolysis in the circulation [72,75,76]. Preliminary studies involving pretreatment mixing do not completely account for the perfluorocarbon effect. Thus, the explanation for Fluosol-DA oxygen breathing enhancement of the therapeutic effect of AAs remains largely unexplained.

Table 16. Nitroimidazoles: Radiation sensitizers

- Hypoxia
- Radiation damage to DNA
- Structure activity studies
- Clinical considerations and trials
- Clinical comparative study

276

X-irradiation damage to DNA.

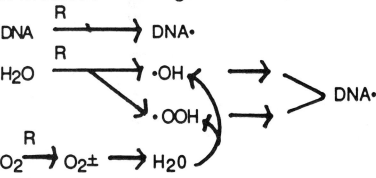

R=radiotherapy.

Figure 9. Schematic representation of the involvement of oxygen species in DNA damage by x-irradiation.

Clinical trials with Fluosol-DA oxygen breathing are underway at a Phase I/II level with radiotherapy [77] and at a Phase I level with selected chemotherapeutic agents. Preliminary results indicate that Fluosol-DA and oxygen breathing can be administered safely and that such treatment does not compromise either radiotherapy or AA chemotherapy in terms of tolerated dose and toxicity.

Nitroimidazoles: Radiation sensitizers

While Fluosol-DA oxygen breathing supplies oxygen directly to correct hypoxia, the 2-nitroimidazoles may mimic oxygen and also produce cytotoxic metabolic products [78]. A summary of the nitroimidazoles is presented in Table 16. The requirement for oxygen in X-ray cytotoxicity is depicted in Figure 9. Radiation may directly damage DNA. However, a more important mechanism is that radiation produces superoxide and hydroxyl radicals from water and from oxygen. These superoxides, or perhaps activated hydroxyl radicals, can, in turn, damage DNA. Thus oxygen is required for optimal damage to DNA by radiotherapy [79].

Figure 10 presents the metabolic transformation of the 2-nitroimidazole misonidazoles by enzymatic or chemical reduction to the radical anion, to a nitrosoderivative, to a hydroxylamine, and finally to the inactive amine represent products, which of themselves are oxygen mimics or have cytotoxic activity [22]. This process requires a hypoxic environment and thus occurs only within tumors. It should be emphasized that the precise molecular

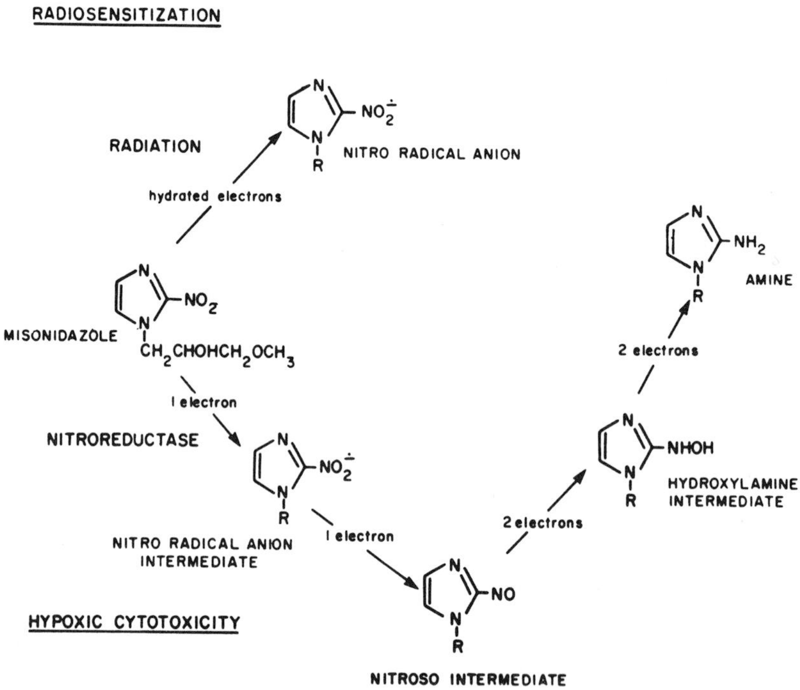

Figure 10. Activation of the radiosensitizer, misonidazole. The first step in either radiation-induced activation or metabolism by nitroreductases leads to the production of a nitro radical anion [22].

mechanism for the nitroimidazole enhancement of radiation remains obscure.

The first 2-nitroimidazole to be employed extensively in the clinic was misonidazole. Clinical trials with this compound were mostly negative, but through pharmacologic and other studies it was appreciated that the dose-limiting toxicity, specifically neurotoxicity, precluded the development of blood levels necessary, on the basis of preclinical studies, to produce a therapeutic effect [79,80].

Accordingly, structure-activity studies were conducted, with particular emphasis on lipid solubility. Thus misonidazole is substantially lipid soluble in terms of lipid-water partition studies. This might explain its retention in nervous tissue. Etanidazole or SR2508 was found to be optimal with respect to lipid-water coefficient in terms of maximizing the drug efficacy ratio. On the basis of these and other studies, etanidazole has been selected for clinical trial and is curreutly undergoing a randomized Phase III trial in head and neck cancer [81].

Clinical considerations with respect to misonidazole are presented in Table 17. It has been determined on the basis of preclinical and clinical studies that to be effective the radiosensitizer must be present at the time of

Table 17. Nitroimidazoles sensitize only hypoxic cells

Misonidazole — Clinical
Must be present at time of radiation therapy
Dose-limiting toxicity — peripheral sensory neuropathy
Total dose — 10–12 g/m^2

Etanidazole
Because the oxygen enhancement ratio is threefold greater than for misonidizole, sensitizing
  concentrations can be reached readily in the peripheral blood at doses that produce little or
  no peripheral neuropathy

Clinical trials
Miso — local control by rad. therapy in head & neck cancer
Miso — activity of melphalan in lung cancer

---

radiation therapy. As mentioned above, dose-limiting toxicity was a peripheral sensory neuropathy. Etanidazole has a sensitizer enhancement ratio comparable to misonidazole at a dose that is threefold lower than for misonidizole. Thus sensitizer concentrations can be reached readily in the peripheral blood at doses that produce little or no peripleral neuropathy [78].

In clinical trials, misonidazole in one study was found to increase local control by radiotherapy in patients with head and neck cancer. It was then subjected to a comparative study in lung cancer.

This clinical trial is presented in summary form in Table 18 [82,83]. Patients with metastatic non-small-cell lung cancer were randomally allocated to receive melphalan or melphalan plus misonidazole. Over 40 patients were entered into each treatment arm. There were no responses in the melphalan arm, and 14% of patients in the melphalan plus misonidazole arm responded (p = 0.02).

Etanidazole has been introduced into clinical trial. In Phase I studies it has been found that therapeutic blood levels can be achieved at the maximum tolerated dose with acceptable peripheral neuropathy. Etanidazole has been found in these preliminary clinical studies, not to alter the dose of the concurrently administered AA or radiotherapy or to increase the toxicity of such modalities [83].

Table 18. Nitroimidazoles: clinical

	No. Patients	Response	
NSC Lung R ⟨ Melphalan	43	0	p = 0.024
Melphalan + misonidazole	42	14% (5% CR)	
Etanidazole	Phase I studies		

Therapeutic blood levels achieved at MTD with acceptable peripheral neuropathy.

Table 19. Alkylating agents: Modulation by topoisomerase II inhibitors

Treatment Group	Tumor Growth Delay (Days)	DNA Cross-Link Factor
Novo	0	<2
cDDP	10	4
N + cDDP	29	20
BCNU	2.9	—
N + BCNU	26	—

Breast cancer (EMT6) in mice.

The repair of DNA damage

There is evidence that enhanced repair of DNA damage induced by AAs can decrease cytotoxicity. The most specific evidence for this is the increase in the O^6-methylguanine transferase that removes a monoligand of nitrosourea from DNA, thus precluding cross-linkage and DNA damage [84–88]. There is other evidence from, for example, alkaline elution studies that DNA repair augmentation might be an important mechanism for resistance [89].

Topoisomerase II inhibition may modulate DNA repair and is under study with respect to AAs (Table 19). Topoisomerase II was discovered by Wang in 1968 [90], and major contributions to the molecular biology were rendered by Liu et al. [91] In 1978, Ross et al. demonstrated that theu podophylotoxin derivative VP16 produced protein-associated DNA strand breaks, the so-called cleavable complexes [92,93]. The protein bridge was found to be topoisomerase II, suggesting that VP16 inhibited this enzyme. Topoisomerase II untangles chromosomes in the G_2 and early M period, and this may allow for an increase in DNA repair.

The mechanism of action for topoisomerase II is presented schematically in Figure 11 [94]. Thus the enzyme may encircle a DNA strand and bind to an adjacent double strand. An ATP binding site on the enzyme has been demonstrated, as well as a VP16 binding site [95]. The enzyme breaks the DNA strand, allowing for passage of the encircled strand. If fixed in this position it would represent protein-associated cleavable products. It is arrested at this level, which occurs with VP-16. In the absence of arrest, the encircled strand is passed and topoisomerase II reseals the DNA. A number of inhibitors of topoisomerase II have been identified, including particularly the intercalating agents and VP-16 (etoposide). Topoisomerase II inhibitors may indeed effectively modulate AAs, perhaps through inhibition of topoisomerase-II-mediated DNA repair [96–98].

Novobiocin has been found to be an inhibitor of topoisomerase II by inhibition the ATP binding site. At therapeutic doses, it is minimally cytotoxic. In a preclinical in vivo study in a mouse breast cancer line, novobiocin

TOPOISOMERASE II.

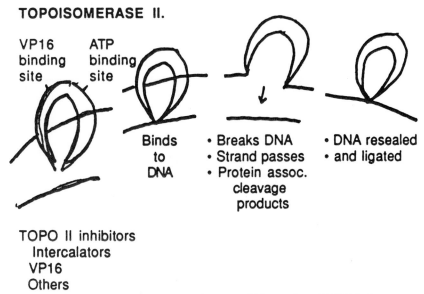

VP16 binding site   ATP binding site

Binds to DNA

• Breaks DNA
• Strand passes
• Protein assoc. cleavage products

• DNA resealed
• and ligated

TOPO II inhibitors
  Intercalators
  VP16
  Others

Figure 11. Schematic representation of topoisomerase II interaction with DNA.

was found to be inactive in terms of tumor growth delay. Cisplatin was moderately active. A combination of the two produced a highly significant increase in tumor growth delay [97]. Similarly BCNU, a nitrosourea, had a markedly enhanced antitumor effect when given with novobiocin [95,97].

This and other studies lead to a Phase I, clinical pharmacological study. The dose of the AA cyclophosphamide was kept constant, and the novobiocin dose was progressively escalated. The dose-limiting toxicity for novobiocin was nausea and vomiting. Clinical pharmacological studies found that the bioavailability of novobiocin, that is, the concentration × time in the plasma, was above that essential for in vitro activity. Noteworthy was the fact that even at maximum doses novobiocin failed to increase the toxicity or to compromise the tolerated dose of cyclophosphamide [99].

There are other clinical studies that suggest that inhibition of topoisomerase II may provide effective modulation of AAs. Thus etoposide and cisplatin have been found in some studies to be highly active in breast cancer, non-small-cell lung cancer, and small-cell lung cancer. The effect in terms of tumor progression of these two agents in combination is substantially greater than expected on the basis of their individual antitumor activity [100,101].

Further evidence that topoisomerase II inhibition is important to AA activity is the observation that topoisomerase II levels are substantially increased in some AA-resistant lines [102–104].

281

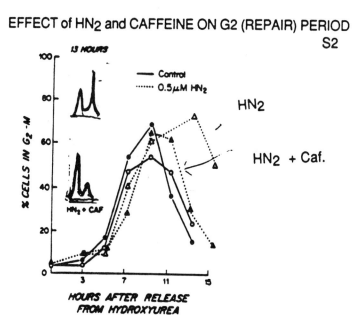

EFFECT of HN2 and CAFFEINE ON G2 (REPAIR) PERIOD
S2

Figure 12. Fraction of cells in G_2 + M phase after release from hydroxyurea. Cells were treated with 0.5 M HN$_2$ for 1 hr before release from hydroxyurea and followed by flow cytometry, as described in "Materials and Methods." Immediately after release from hydroxyurea 1 mM caffeine was added to cells with closed symbols. Inset shows typical histogram of DNA content at 13 hr: left peak, G_1 cells; right peak, G_2 + M cells.

Methylxanthines and the modulation of alkylating agents

For over 20 years it has been known that methylxanthines (MXs) such as caffeine will increase the effects of AAs and radiotherapy in in vitro systems [105]. MXs will inhibit DNA repair at several biochemical levels, and it is not clear which, if any of these, are essential to its AA modulation effect [106].

Recently it has been found that the decrease in DNA repair exhibited by methylxanthines may be due to cytokinetic effects (Figure 12) [107]. Essentially all genotoxic agents delay transit in the G_2 period of the cell cycle. From an evolutionary point of view, this would have major survival benefit, since DNA repair of DNA-damaging agents occurs largely during the G_2 period. It has been found that the MXs reverse this G_2 transit delay. In the DNA histogram insert (Figure 12), note that cells exposed to HN$_2$ show a marked increase in the G_2 plus M peak. This is largely corrected by the addition of caffeine [107–109]. The Cartesian plot in Figure 12 is also consistent with this observation, in that transit through the G_2 period is substantially longer after HN$_2$ only, as compared to nitrogen mustard plus caffeine.

The MXs also increase deformability of red blood cells (Table 20) [110,

Table 20. Methylxanthines for modulation of alkylating agents

---

- Methylxanthines (MX) (e.g. caffeine) ↑ effect of alkylating agents and radiotherapy in vitro
- MX inhibit DNA repair at several biochemical levels
- X-ray and alkylating agents arrest cells in G_2
  G_2 is DNA repair time; MX ↑ transit in G_2
- MX ↑ deformability of RBC by ATP and actin spectrin changes
  This increases entry of RBC into hypoxic areas
  Effective for peripheral and cerebrovascular disease

Pentoxifylline — a MX that is not neurotoxic

Pentoxifylline — in vitro effect
  In vivo — preclinical
  Clinical

111]. This would increase the red blood cell capacity for entry into hypo-vascular areas, such as hypoxic areas within tumors. The clinically available MX, pentoxifylline, has known clinical utility in the treatment of cardio-vascular disease associated with the decrease in blood supply [110]. The concentration of MXs required to produce red blood cell deformability is substantially lower than those required to shorten G_2 transit.

In Figure 13 survival curves after thioTEPA treatment in vitro of human

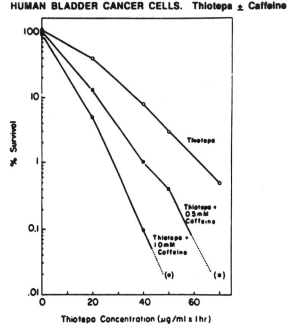

Figure 13. Enhanced lethality by caffeine (24 hr exposure) after higher concentrations of thioTEPA. No colonies were observed at lowest points (in parentheses) despite platings at multiple densities [112].

283

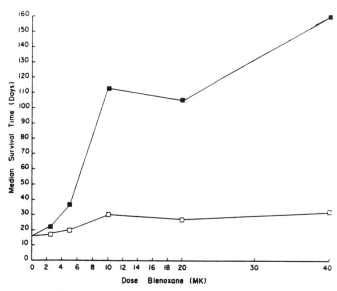

Chart 6. Effect of caffeine (874 mg/kg body weight) on MST of mice carrying Ehrlich ascites tumor and treated with Blenoxane at 5 different dose levels. □, controls (Blenoxane alone). ■, tests (Blenoxane + caffeine). MSTs are those values estimated from best-fitting survival curves (see "Appendix").

Figure 14. Effect of caffeine (874 mg/kg body weight) on MST of mice carrying Ehrlich ascites tumor and treated with Blenoxane at five different dose levels. □, controls (Blenoxane alone). ■, tests (Blenoxane + caffeine). MSTs are those values estimated from best-fitting survival curvews [113].

bladder cancer cell lines are presented [112]. Note the substantial increase in cytotoxicity when caffeine is added to the thioTEPA. The survival time of mice bearing ascites tumor as a function of treatment with bleomycin, with and without caffeine, is presented in Figure 14 [113]. The upper curve is a bleomycin plus caffeine curve, indicating substantially improving survival as a result of the concurrent use of caffeine [113].

The subrenal capsule assay allows for the evaluation of human tumor xenografts during the period before an immunologic reaction against the tumor develops. Note that the addition of pentoxifylline to thioTEPA produced a significant difference as compared to the appropriate controls (Figure 15) [114].

Table 21. Pentoxifylline — clinical studies

Phase I. TSPA (fixed dose) + pentoxyfylline po
  (escalating dose)
MTD = 1600 mg p.o. tid for 5 days
Toxicity — nausea and vomiting
No effect on toxicity of TSPA

Subrenal capsule assay.

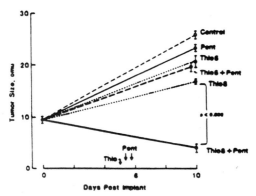

Figure 15. Enhanced in vivo activity of the combined administration of thioTEPA (Thio5; 8 mg/kg) and PENT in MX-1 human breast tumor grafts in the SRCA. Mice were immunosuppresed by CSA (80 mg/kg) given s.c. on days 2–4 and 6–9.

Pentoxifylline is a MX that is the equivalent to the caffeine prototype MX, except for central nervous system stimulation [115]. It is available commercially for the treatment of vascular disease. A Phase I clinical trial has been conducted wherein patients received a fixed standard dose of thioTEPA (TSPA) plus escalating doses of pentoxifylline orally (Table 21). The maximum tolerated dose of pentoxifylline was 1600 mg p.o. tid, and dose-limiting toxicity was exclusively nausea and vomiting. Importantly in this study, which has now been completed, there was no evidence that pentoxifylline affected the toxicity or tolerated dose of thioTEPA [116].

Miscellaneous modulating agents

Lonidamine

Lonidamine is an indazol carboxylic acid. It markedly inhibits oxygen consumption and both aerobic and anaerobic glycolysis. Based on these data, mitochondria have been considered the primary intracellular target of the drug, and more recent studies indicate that the mitochondrial membrane is the primary target. Lonidamine could be important if repair of damage by the cytotoxic agent is energy dependent. Hahn demonstrated that lonidamine inhibited the repair of potential lethal damage caused by X-ray, hyperthermia, and by the alkylating agent methylmethane sulfonate. [117] Lonidamine also enhances the toxicity of adriamycin in culture.

In Figure 16, the closed circles represent the activity of cisplatin against

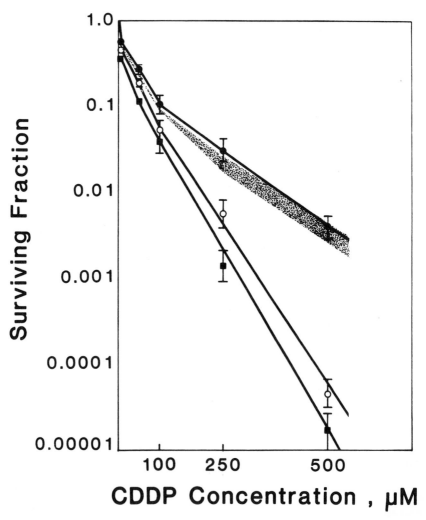

Figure 16. Survival of human MCF-7 breast carcinoma cells exposed to various concentrations of CDDP alone for 1 hr (●), with simultaneous exposure to 250 μM lonidamine for 1 hr (○), or with simultaneous exposure to 250 μM lonidamine for 1 hr followed by an additional 12-hr exposure to lonidamine. The *shaded area* is the envelope of additivity for CDDP plus either 1 hr or extended exposure to lonidamine. *Points* represent the means of three independent experiments and *bars* the SEM.

MCF7 human breast cancer cell culture. The shaded area is the area of additivity. Lonidamine alone has no activity against this cell line. The open circles and the closed squares indicate the effect of the addition of lonidamine for 1 or 12 hr, respectively. There is clearly modulation in excess of additivity. This result is repersentative of studies involving lonidamine added to other AAs and has been true for a number of tumor cell lines [118].

Lonidamine has limited but definite activity in patients with non-small-cell lung cancer [119]. It is not myelosuppressive and has neither increased toxicity nor decreased the tolerated dose of AAs. It is in Phase I clinical trial and has shown promising results as a modulator of radiation therapy and hyperthermia [120]. Clinical trials with chemotherapeutic agents are underway.

Lapachone

Lapachone is a novel inhibitor of DNA repair and has been shown experimentally to enhance the effects of radiotherapy and genotoxic therapeutic agents in a number of experimental in vitro systems. Mechanism and structure activity studies are ongoing [121].

O^6-Methylguanine

Another approach to the specific inhibition of DNA repair for nitrosoureas involves O^6-methylquanine. This material serves as a saturating substrate for the O^6-methyltransferase repair enzyme that removes nitrosoursea mono-adducts from DNA [122].

DDTC

Disulfiram, and particularly its metabolic product DDTC, may combine with AAs and thus protect normal host tissues in vivo. The AAs nitrogen mustard and cisplatin exhibit an improved therapeutic index when delivery of DDTC occurs at the appropriate interval following the alkylating agent [123].

In the biotransformation of cyclophosphamide, there is a step that involves the conversion of 4-hydroxycyclophosphamide to the inactive product carboxyphosphamide. This is mediated by the enzyme amine oxidase. This enzyme has been found to be elevated in a cyclophosphamide-resistant cell line. In preliminary studies, inhibition of this enzyme by disulfiram or other metabolites reverses the resistance [123].

Maximizing the therapeutic effects of alkylating agents by combined modulation

The following represents a summary of the status of the modulation of alkylating agents. There are at least eight major biochemical determinants of AA sensitivity. A number of these became apparent by the study of AA-resistant cell lines. A number of these determinants can be modulated on the basis of biochemical studies, and such modulation has often been substantial and significant. Many of the modulation approaches are relatively nontoxic, and the modulator does not alter the toxicity or the tolerated dose of AA.

It is proposed, therefore, that combined modulation based on the above principles should be capable of inhibiting the multiple and major sensitivity and resistance determinants of AA activity within tumor cells. Studies of combined modulation in vitro and in vivo in experimental systems are underway.

How does one select suitable combinations of modulators? An interesting approach would be to combine glutathione monoethyl ester with an inhibitor of glutathione biosynthesis, such as BSO. In the studies presented above, BSO and glutathione monoethyl ester were found not to compromise the dose of AA. In the case of glutathione monoethyl ester, there was selective protection of the host, and with BSO there was selective sensitivity of the tumor. Such studies are underway [B. Teicher, personal communication].

At the level of DNA damage, it would be interesting to know whether the combination of Fluosol-DA plus oxygen breathing and etanidazole, both of which target the hypoxic problem of tumors, are subadditive, additive, or synergistic. There is preliminary evidence with respect to radiotherapy that they are at least additive [124].

Both the methylated xanthines and topoisomerase II inhibitors are thought to exert their effects through decreasing DNA repair capacity. How would these fare in combination?

In terms of clinical strategy, Phase I studies with these agents, that is, monomodulation, must be performed initially. If the modulating agents produce acceptable dose-limiting toxicity and do not compromise the toxicity or the maximum dose of AA, they could be added to full doses of the AA. The expectation would be that they would not compromise the therapeutic effect of the AA and may, in the context of Phase II studies, augment the effect of the AA. Accordingly, it is proposed that following such Phase I studies, beginning studies of combined modulation, depending upon the preclinical results, could be undertaken in the clinic.

We are particularly impressed with the observation that the sensitivity and resistance determinants for AA action are multiple (i.e., resistance is multifoctorial) and that modulation of one mechanism may produce a limited effect, but that combined modulation might provide a major advance in AA therapy. Thus, in some instances, Phase II studies should await Phase I studies demonstrating the safety (in terms of toxicity) and effectiveness (in terms of tolerated dose of AA delivered). Where such studies are positive, Phase II, and finally, Phase III studies of combined modulation may be indicated.

If modulation of AA proves effective in the clinic, it would have major implications, considering the magnitude and disease spectrum of activity of the AA. Major effective modulation of the AA in the clinic might make some tumors that respond very well to AA but are generally short of cure (such as small-cell lung cancer, ovarian cancer, etc.) definitive.

effects of methylxanthines in human tumor cells treated with alkylating agents. Cancer Res. 46:2463–2467, 1986.

33. Fingert, H.J., Pu, A.T., Chen, Z., Googe, P.B., Alley, M.C., and Pardee, A.B. In vivo and in vitro enhanced antitumor effects by pentoxifylline in human cancer cells treated with thiotepa. Cancer Res. 48:4375–4381, 1988.

34. Rosowsky, A., et al. Phenotypic heterogeneity of cultured human head and neck cancer cells with low level methotrexate resistance. Cancer Res. 45:6205, 1985.

35. Dulik, D.M., Fenselau, C., and Hilton, J. Characterization of melphalan-glutathione adducts whose formation is catalyzed by glutathione transferases. Biochem. Pharmacol. 35:3405–3409, 1986.

36. Griffith, O.W. Mechanism of action, metabolism, and toxicity of buthionine sulfoximine and its higher homologs, potent inhibitors of glutathione synthesis. J. Biol. Chem. 257: 13704–13712, 1982.

37. Meister, A. Glutathione metabolism and its selective modification. J. Biol. Chem. 268: 17205–17208, 1988.

38. Ozols, R.F., Hamilton, T.C., Masuda, H., and Young, R.C. Manipulation of cellular thiols toinfluence drug resistance. In: Mechanisms of Drug Resistance in Neoplastic Cells, Woolley, P.V. and Tew, K.D. (eds). pp. 289–306, 1988.

39. Ozols, R.J., Louie, K.G., Plowman, J., Behrens, B.C., Fine, R.L., Dykes, D., and Hamilton, T.C. Enhanced melphalan cytotoxicity in human ovarian cancer in vitro and in tumor-bearing nude mice by buthionine sulfoximine depletion of glutathione. Biochem. Pharmacol. 36:147–153, 1987.

40. Moscow, J.A., Townsend, A.J., and Cowan, K.H. Elevation of pi class glutathione S-transferase activity in human breast cancer cells by transfection of the GST pi gene and its effect on sensitivity to toxins. Mol. Pharmacol. 36:22–28, 1989.

41. Black, S.M., Beggs, J.D., Hayes, J.D., Muramatsu, M., Sakai, M., and Wofe, C.R. Expression of human glutathione S-transferase in S. cerevisiae confers resistance to the anticancer drugs adriamycin and chlorambucil. Biochem. J., in press, 1990.

42. Puchalski, R.B. and Fahl, W.E. Expression of recombinant glutathione S-transferase pi, Ya or Ybl confers resistance to alkylating agents. Proc. Natl. Acad. Sci. USA, in press, 1990.

43. Morgenstern, R. and Depierre, J.W. Membrane-bound glutathione transferases. In: Glutathione Conjugation, Sies, H. and Ketterer, B. (eds). Academic Press, pp. 157–174, 1988.

44. Smith, M.T., Evans, C.G., Doane-Setzer, P., Castro, V.M., Tahir, M.K., and Mannervik, B. Denitrosation of 1,3-bis(2-chloroethyl)-1-nitrosourea by class Mu glutathione trans-ferases and its role in cellular resistance in rat brain tumor cells. Cancer Res. 49:2621–2625, 1989.

45. Ali-Osman, F., Caughlan, J., and Gray, G.S. Decreased DNA interstrand cross-linking and cytotoxicity induced in human brain tumor cells by 1,3-bis (2-chloroethyl)-1-nitrosourea after in vitro reaction with glutathione. Cancer Res. 49:5954–5958, 1989.

46. Seidegard, J., Pero, R.W., Miller, D.G., and Beattie, E.J. A glutathione transferase in human leukocytes as a marker for the susceptibility to lung cancer. Carcinogenesis 7: 751–753, 1986.

47. Shea, T.C., Kelley, S.L., and Henner, W.D. Identification of an anionic form of flutathione transferase present in many human tumors and human tumor cell lines. Cancer Res. 48:527–533, 1988.

48. Satoh, K., Kitahara, A., Soma, Y., Inaba, Y., Hatayama, I., and Sato, K. Purification, induction, and distribution of placental glutathione transferase: a new marker enzyme for preneopalstic cells in the rat chemical hepatocarcinogenesis. Proc. Natl. Acad. Sci. USA 82:3964–3968, 1985.

49. Eimoto, H., Tsutsumi, M., Nakajima, A., Yamamoto, K., Takashima, Y., Maruyama, H., and Konishi, Y. Expression of glutathione S-transferase placental form in human lung carconimas. Carcinogenesis 9:2325–2327, 1988.

50. Moscow, J.A., Fairchild, C.R., Madden, M.J., Ransom, D.T., Wieand, H.S., O'Brien, E.E., Poplack, D.G., Cossman, J., Myers, C.E., and Cowan, K.H. Expression of anionic glutathione S-transferase and P-glycoprotein genes in human tissues and tumors. Cancer Res. 49:1422–1428, 1989.

51. Kramer, R.A., Schuller, H.M., Smith, A.C., and Boyd, M.R. Effects of buthionine sulfoximine on the nephrotoxicity of 1-(2-chloroethyl)-3(trans-4-methylcyclohexyl)-1 nitrosourea (MeCCNU). J. Pharmacol. Exp. Therap. 234:498–506, 1985.

52. Kramer, R.A., Zakher, J., and Kim, G. Role of the glutathione redox cycle in acquired and de novo multidrug resistance. Science 241:694–697, 1988.

53. Skapek, S., Colvin, O.M., Griffith, O., Elion, G.B., Bigner, D.D., and Friedman, H.S. Enhanced cytotoxicity of melphalan secondary to BSO mediated depletion of glutathione in medulloblastoma xenografts in athymic nude mice. Cancer Res. 48:2764–2767, 1988.

54. Tew, K.D., Bomber, A.M., and Hoffman, S.J. Ethacrynic acid and piriprost as enhancers of cytotoxicity in drug resistant and sensitive cell lines. Cancer Res. 48:3622–3625, 1988.

55. Clapper, M.L., Hoffman, S.J., O'Dwyer, P.J., and Tew, K.D. Inhibition of glutathione S-transferases and sensitization of tumors to melphalan in vivo. Proc. Am. Assoc. Cancer Res. 30:530, 1989.

56. Schilder, R.J., Nash, S., Tew, K.D., Panting, L., Comis, R.L., and O'Dwyer, P.J. Phase I trial of thiotepa (TT) in combination with the glutathione transferase (GST) inhibior ethacrynic acid (EA). Proc. Am. Assoc. Cancer Res. 31:177, 1990.

57. Teicher, B.A., Crawford, J.M., Holden, S.A., Lin, Y., Cathcart, K.N.S., Luchette, C.A., and Flatow, J. Glutathione monoethyl ester can selectively protect liver from high dose BCNU or cyclophosphamide. Cancer 62:1275–1281, 1988.

58. Beach, L.R. and Palmiter, R.D. Amplification of the metallothionein-I gene in cadmium-resistant mouse cells. Proc. Natl. Acad. Sci. USA 78:2110–2114, 1981.

59. Zelazowski, A.J., Garvey, J.S., and Hoeschele, J.D. In vivo and in vitro binding of platinum to metallothionein. Arch. Biochem. Biophys. 15:246–252, 1984.

60. Durnam, D.M. and Palmiter, R.D. Induction of metallothionein-I mRNA in cultured cells by heavy metals and iodoacetate: evidence from gratuitous inducers. Mol. Cell Biol. 4:484–491, 1984.

61. Bakka, A., Endresen, L., Johnsen, A.B.S., Edminson, P.D., and Rugstad, H.E. Resistance againt cis-dichlorodiammineplatinum in cultured cells with a high content of metallothionein. Toxicol. Appl. Pharmacol. 61:215–225, 1981.

62. Karin, M. and Richards, R.I. The human metallothionein gene family: structure and expression. Environ. Health Perspect. 54:111–115, 1979.

63. Zelazowski, A.J., Garvey, J.S., and Hoeschele, J.D. In vivo and in vitro binding of platinum to metallothionein. Arch. Biochem. Biophys. 229:246–252, 1984.

64. Kraker, A., Schmidt, J., Krezoski, S., and Peterintg, D.H. Binding of cis-dichlorodiammineplatinum(II) to metallothionein in Ehrlich cells. Biochem. Biophys. Res. Commun. 130:786–792, 1985.

65. Satoh, Miura, N., Naganuma, A., Matsuzaki, N., Kawamura, E., and Imura, N. Prevention of adverse effects of gamma-ray irradiation after metallothionein induction by bismuth subnitrate in mice. Eur. J. Cancer Clin. Oncol. 25:1727–1783, 1989.

66. Coleman, C.N. Hypoxia in tumors: a paradigm for the approach to biochemical and physiologic heterogeneity. J. Nat. Cancer Inst. 80:310–317, 1988.

67. Brown, J.M. Evidence for acutely hypoxic cells in mouse tumours, and a possible mechanism of reoxygenation. Br. J. Radiol. 52:650–656, 1979.

68. Gatenby R.A., Kessler, H.B., Rosenblum, J.S., Coia, L.R., Moldofsky, P.J., Hartz, W.H., and Broder, G.H. Oxygen distribution in squamous cell carcinoma metastases and its relationship to outcome of radiation therapy. Int. J. Radiat. Oncol. Biol. Phys. 14:831–838, 1988.

69. Geyer, R.P. Substitutes for blood and its components. In: Blood Substitutes and Plasma Expanders, Vol. 19, Jamieson, G.A. and Greenwalt, T.J. (eds). Alan R. Liss, New York, p. 1021, 1978.

292

70. Hasegawa, T., Rhee, J.G., Levitt, S.H., and Song, C.W. Increase in tumor po$_2$ by perfluorochemicals and carbogen. Int. J. Radiat. Oncol. Biol. Phys. 13:569–574, 1987.

71. Teicher, B.A. and Rose, C.M. Oxygen-carrying perfluorochemical emulsion as an adjuvant to radiation therapy in mice. Cancer Res. 44:4285–4288, 1984.

72. Teicher, B.A., Herman, T.S., and Rose, C.M. Effect of Fluosol-DA on the response of intracranial 9L tumors to X rays and BCNU. Int. J. Radiat. Oncol. Biol. Phys. 15: 1187–1192, 1988.

73. Teicher, B.A., Holden, S.A., Cathcart, K.N.S., and Herman, T.S. Effect of various oxygenation conditions and Fluosol-DA on cytotoxicity and antitumor activity of bleomycin in mice. J. Natll. Cancer Inst. 80:599–603, 1988.

74. Teicher, B.A., Waxman, D.J., Holden, S.A., Wang, Y., Clarke, L., Alvarez-Sotomayor, E., Jones, S.M., and Frei, E. III. N, N′, N″-triethylenethiophosphoramide: evidence for enzymatic activation and oxygen involvement. Cancer Res. 49:4996–5001, 1989.

75. Teicher, B.A., Holden, S.A., and Jacobs, J.L. Approaches to defining the mechanism of Fluosol-DA 20%/carbogen enhancement of melphalan antitumor activity. Cancer Res. 47:513–518, 1987.

76. Teicher, B.A., Crawford, J.M., Holden, S.A., and Cathcart, K.N.S. Effects of various oxygenation conditions on the enhancement by Fluosol-DA of melphalan antitumor activity. Cancer Res. 47:5036–5041, 1987.

77. Rose, C.M., Lustig, R., McIntosh, N., and Teicher, B. A clinical trial of Fluosol-DA[R] 20% in advanced squamous cell carcinoma of the head and neck. Int. J. Radiat. Oncol. Biol. Phys. 12:1325–1327, 1986.

78. Brown, J.M. Keynote address: hypoxic cell radiosensitizers: where next? Int. J. Radiat. Oncol. Biol. Phys. 16:987–993, 1989.

79. Coleman, C.N. Modification of radiotherapy by radiosensitizers and cancer chemotherapy agents. I. Radiosensitizers. Semin. Oncol. 16:169–175, 1989.

80. Overgaard. Proceedings of the Conference in Chemical Modifiers of Cancer Treatment. Abstract FL. 1223, 1985.

81. Coleman, C.N., Halsey, J., Cox, R.S., Hirst, V.K., Blaschke, T., Howes, A.E., Wasserman, T.H., Urtasun, R.C., Pajak, T., Hancock, S., Phillips, T.L., and Noll, L. Relationship between the neurotoxicity of the hypoxic cell radiosensitizers SR 2508 and the pharmacokinetic profile. Cancer Res. 47:319–323, 1987.

82. Coleman, C.N., Friedman, M.K., Jacobs, C., Halsey, J., Ignoffo, R., Leibel, S., Hirst, V.K., Gribble, M., Carter, S.K., and Phillips, T.L. Phase I trial of intravenous L-phenylalanine mustard plus the sensitizer misonidazole. Cancer Res. 43:5022–5025, 1983.

83. Coleman, C.N., Carlson, R.W., Jalsey, J., Kohler, M., Gribble, M., Sikic, B., and Jacobs, C. Enhancement of the clinical activity of melphalan by the hypoxic cell sensitizer misonidazole. Cancer Res. 48:3528–3532, 1983.

84. Lindahl, T. DNA repair enzymes. Annu. Rev. Biochem. 51:61, 1982.

85. Frosina, G. and Abbondandolo, A. The current evidence for an adaptive response to alkylating agents in mammalian cells, with special reference to experiments with in vitro cell cultures. Mutat. Res. 154:85, 1985.

86. Sedgwick, B. and Lindahl, T. A common mechanism for repair of O^6-methylguanine and O^6-ethylguanine in DNA. J. Mol. Biol. 154:169, 1982.

87. Brent, T.P., Houghton, P.J., and Houghton, J.A. O^6-alkylguanine-DNA alkyltransferase activity correlates with the therapeutic response of human rhabdomyosarcoma xenografts to 1-(2-chloroethyl)-3-(trans-4-methylcyclohexyl)-1-nitrosourea. Proc. Natl. Acad. Sci. USA 82:2985, 1985.

88. Brent, T.P. Inactivation of purified human O^6-alkylguanine-DNA alkyltransferase by alkylating agents or alkylated DNA. Cancer Res. 46:2320, 1986.

89. Ewig, R.A.G. and Kohn, K.W. DNA damage and repair in mouse leukemia L1210 cells treated with nitrogen mustard, 1, 3-bis (2-chloroethyl)-1-nitrosourea and other nitrosoureas. Cancer Res. 37:2114, 1977.

90. Wang, J.C. DNA topoisomerases. Annu. Rev. Biochem. 54:665, 1985.

293

91. Liu, L.F., Liu, C.C., and Alberts, B.M. Cell 19:697–708, 1980.
92. Ross, W.E., Glaubiger, D.L., and Kohn, K.W. Biochim. Biophys. Acta 519:23–30, 1978.
93. Ross, W.E., Glaubiger, D.L., and Kohn, K.W. Biochim. Biophys. Acta 562:41–50, 1979.
94. Wang, J.C. Recent studies of DNA topoisomerases. Biochem. Biophys. Acta. 909:1–9, 1987.
95. Ross, W.E. DNA topoisomerases as targets for cancer therapy. Biochem. Pharmacol. 34:4191–4195, 1985.
96. Eder, J.P., Teicher, B.A., Holden, S.A., Cathcart, K.N.S., and Schnipper, L.E. Novobiocin enhances alkylating agent cytotoxicity and DNA interstrand crosslinks in a murine model. J. Clin. Invest. 79:1524–1528, 1987.
97. Eder, J.P., Teicher, B.A., Holden, S.A., Cathcart, K.N.S., Schnipper, L.E., and Frei, E. III. Effect of novobiocin on the antitumor activity and tumor cell and bone marrow survivals of three alkylating agents. Cancer Res. 49:595–598, 1989.
98. Tan, K.B., Mattern, M.R., Boyce, R.A., Hertzberg, R.P., and Schein P.S. Elevated topoisomerase II activity and altered chromatin in nitrogen mustard-resistant human cells. NCI Monogr. 4:95–98, 1987.
99. Eder, J.P., Wheeler, C.A., Teicher, B.A., and Schnipper, L.E. A phase I trial of novobiocin (N) and cyclophosphamide (CPA). Proc. Am. Assoc. Cancer Res. 31:180, 1990.
100. Cocconi, G., Gisagni, V., Delisi, G., et al. Proc Am Soc Clin. Oncol. 77:13, 1988.
101. Bononi, P., Rowland, R.M. Jr., Taylgo, S.G., Pincus, M., Reddy, S., Lee, M.S., Fuber, L.P., Warren, W., and Kutle, C.T. Breast Phase II trial of therapy in E, SFU by CI, CDDP and simultaneous split cijrca XRT in Stage III NSCLC. NCI Monogr. 331–334, 1988.
102. Tan, K.B., Mattern, M.R., Boyce, R.A., and Schein, P.S. Elevated DNA topoisomerase II activity in nitrogen mustard resistant human cells. Proc. Natl. Acad. Sci. USA 84: 7668–7671, 1987.
103. Tan, K.B., Mattern, M.R., Boyce, R.A., and Schein, P.S. Unique sensitivity of nitrogen mustard-resistant human Burkitt lymphoma cells to novobiocin. Biochem. Pharmacol. 37:4411–4413, 1988.
104. Eder, J.P., personal communication.
105. Gaudin, D. and Yielding, K.L. Response of a "resistant" plasmacytoma to alkylating agents and X-ray in combination with the excision repair inhibitors caffeine and chloroquine. Proc. Soc. Exp. Biol. Med. 131:1413–1416, 1969.
106. Lau, C.C. and Pardee, A.B. Mechanism by which caffeine potentiates lethality of nitrogen mustard. Proc. Natl. Acad. Sci. USA 79:2942–2946, 1982.
107. Fingert, J.G., Chang, J.D., and Pardee, A.B. Cytotoxic, cell cycle, and chromosomal effects of methylxanthines in human tumor cells treated with alkylating agents. Cancer Res. 46:2463–2467, 1986.
108. Grinfeld, S. and Jacquet, P. G_2 arrest in mouse zygotes after x-irradiation: reversion by caffeine and influence of chromosome abnormalities. Int. J. Radiat. Biol. 54:2567–268, 1988.
109. Schlegel, R. and Pardee, A.B. Caffeine-induced uncoupling of mitosis from the completion of DNA replication in mammalian cells. Science 232:1264–1266, 1986.
110. Aviado, D.M. and Dettelbach, H.R. Pharmacology of pentoxifylline — a hemorheologic agent for the treatment of intermittent claudication. Angiology 35:407–417, 1984.
111. Ehrly A.M. The effect of pentoxifylline on the flow properties of human blood. Curr. Med. Res. Opin. 5:608–613, 1978.
112. Fingert, J.G., Kindy, R.L., and Pardee, A.B. Enhanced lethality by methylxanthines in human bladder cancer cells treated with thiotepa. J. Urol. 132:609–613, 1984.
113. Allen, T.E., Aliano, N.A., Cowan, R.J., Grigg, G.W., Hart, N.K., Lamberton, J.A., and Lane, A. Amplification of the antitumor activity of phlemomycins and bleomycins in rats and mice by caffeine. Cancer Res. 45:2516–2521, 1985.
114. Fingert, H.J., Pu, A.T., Chen, Z., Googe, P.B., Alley, M.C., and Pardee, A.B. In vivo

and in vitro enhanced antitumor effects by pentoxifylline in human cancer cells treated with thiotepa. Cancer Res. 48:4375–4381, 1988.

115. Ward, A. and Clissold, S.P. Pentoxifylline: a review of its pharmacodynamic and pharmacokinetic properties, and its therapeutic efficacy. Drugs 34:50–97, 1987.
116. Dezube, B., personal communication.
117. Hahn, G.M., van Kersen, I., and Silvestrini, B. Inhibition of the recovery from potentially lethal damage by lonidamine. Br. J. Cancer 50:657–660, 1984.
118. Rosbe, K.W., Brann, T.W., Holden, S.A., Teicher, B.A., and Frei, E. III. Effect of lonidamine on the cytotoxicity of four alkylating agents in vitro. Cancer Chemother. Pharm. 25:32–36, 1989.
119. Evans, W.K., Murray, N., Wierzbicki, R., Shepherd, F.A., Wilson, K., Seidenfela, A., and Wilson, J. Pilot study of lonidamine in combination with chemotherapy for metastic small cell, large cell and squamous cell lung cancer.
120. Robins, H.I., Longo, W.L., Lagoni, R.K., Neville, A.J., Hugander, A., Schmitt, C.L., and Riggs, C. Phase I trial of lonidamine with whole body hyperthermia in advanced cancer. Cancer Res. 48:6587–6592, 1988.
121. Boothman, D.A., Trask, D.K., and Pardee, A.B. Inhibition of potentially lethal DNA repair in human tumor cells by B-lapachone, an activator of topoisomerase I. Cancer Res. 49:605–612, 1989.
122. Erickson, L.C. and Zlotogorski, C. Induction and repair of macromolecule damage by alkylating agents. Cancer Treat. Rev. 11 (Suppl. A):25, 1984.
123. Grates, H.E. and Valeriote, F.A. Disulfiram (DSF) and diethyldithiocarbamic acid (DDC) as potentiators of the cytotoxic effects of anticancer agents in murine leukemia models. Proc. Am. Assoc. Cancer Res. 29:476, 1988.
124. Herman, T.S., Teicher, B.A., and Pfeffer, M.R. Combined modulators (Fluosol-DA/etanidazole) of alkylating agent (AA) activity. Proc. Am. Assoc. Cancer Res. 31:407, 1990.

Index

ABC excinuclease, 14, 213, 214, 218, 221, 222
Abnormally banded regions (ABRs), 1, 3
Acetoxy-acetaminofluorene (AAAF), 29
N-Acetoxy-acetaminofluorene (NAAAF), 221–222
N-Acetyldaunorubicin, 153, 155
Acquired resistance, 109–112, 114, 187
Acridine orange, 8
Acridines, 58, 153
Acriflavine, 8
Actinomycin D, 101, 121, 171
  DNA damage and, 212
  Pgp and, 158
  topoisomerases and, 58, 62, 63, 66, 67, 68, 69, 71, 73
Acute leukemias, 1, 110, 173, 187, 202, *see also* specific types
Acute lymphoblastic leukemia, *see* Acute lymphocytic leukemia
Acute lymphocytic leukemia (ALL)
  mdr1 gene in, 105, 109, 110
  MDR in, 172, 175
  Pgp in, 187, 194, 195, 200
  topoisomerase inhibitors for, 86
Acute myelogenous leukemia (AML), 171, 172, 174
Acute nonlymphocytic leukemia (ANLL)
  mdr1 gene in, 105, 106, 109, 110
  MDR in, 172, 174
  Pgp in, 187, 194, 200
Adenine, 235
Adenine dinucleotide (NAD), 225
Adenosine deaninase gene, 5
Adenosine monophosphate (AMP), 40
Adenosine triphosphatase (ATPase), 82, 122
Adenosine triphosphate (ATP)
  in Pgp, 151, 152, 159
    immunoblot analysis and, 129
    molecular biology and, 39, 40, 41, 42, 45, 47, 48, 50
  topoisomerases and, 57, 63, 65, 66, 83, 280, 281
Adenylate cyclase, 42

ADP-ribosyl transferase enzyme (ADPRT), 225–226
Adrenergic agonists, 253
Adrenocortical carcinoma, 104, 105
Adriamycin, *see* Doxorubicin
Aflatoxin B1, 46
(Ah) gene, 30, 31
Aldosterone, 156
Alkylating agents (AAs), 261–289, *see also* specific types
  combined modulation in, 287–289
  DDI genes and, 14, 15, 16, 17, 19, 27, 31, 33
  DDTC and, 287
  DNA damage and, 74, 209, 211–212, 213, 288
  DNA repair and, 214, 222, 235, 263, 264, 280–281, 288
  GSH and, 266, 267–271, 288
  GST and, 264, 266, 267–271
  hypoxia and, 264, 273–277, 288
  lapachone and, 287
  lonidamine and, 285–287
  MDR and, 121, 174
  MTs and, 26, 252, 255, 256, 264, 271–273
  multifactoral nature of resistance to, 266–267
  MXs and, 282–285
  nitroimidazoles and, 276, 277–279
  perfluorocarbons and, 264, 273–277
  Pgp and, 155, 188–189
O⁶-Alkylguanine transferase enzyme (O6AGT), 19, 213, 214, 223–224, 264
3-Amino-benzamide (3-AB), 225–226
Amiodarone, 105, 114, 153, 175, 177, 178
Amphibians, extrachromosomal DNA in, 2
m-AMSA, 213, 224
  topoisomerases and, 58, 60–61, 62, 63, 64, 65, 67, 68, 69–70, 72, 73, 74, 75, 77, 78, 79, 81
Anionic glutathione transferase gene, 106
Anthracenediones, 58
Anthracycline analogs, 153, 154–155, 162

Anthracyclines, *see also* specific types
  DNA damage and, 212
  MDR and, 121, 171, 173, 174, 180
  mdr1 gene and, 101, 105, 106
  Pgp and, 152, 189, 200
  topoisomerases and, 58
Antibiotics, 2, 8, 153, 212, *see also* specific
    types
Antibodies, Pgp, 163, 173, *see also*
    Monoclonal antibodies
Antidepressants, 177
Antidiarrheals, 177
Antiestrogens, 153, 177
Antihistamines, 177
Antihypertensives, 153
Antimalarials, 153, 177
Antimetabolites, 174, 212, 261, 263, *see also*
    specific types
Antipain, 226
Antipsychotics, 177
Antisense oligonucleotides, 162–163
Aphidicolin, 86, 226
Apoptosis, 237
AP-1 transcription factor, 20, 22, 23, 28
Ara-CTP, 212
Astrocytomas, 105
Ataxia telangiectasis (AT), 32
Autologous bone marrow transplants, 196,
    197, 289
Azacytidine, 221
Azidopine, 158

Bacteria, DDI genes in, 13, 17, 18, 19, 24, 28
*Bam*H1-restricted DNA, 67
Base-excision repair, 15, 27
BCNU, *see* Chlorethylnitrosourea
Benzamide, 225
Benzo(a)pyrene, 30
N-Benzyladriamycin-14-valerate (AD-198),
    153
Bepridil, 176–177
*Bgl*1-restricted DNA, 67
Biological response modifiers, 189
Bisbenzylisoquinoline alkaloids, 153
Bismuth, MTs and, 252, 257, 271–273
Bladder cancer, 107, 268, 284
Bleomycin, 264, 275
  DNA damage and, 212, 218
  DNA repair and, 215, 216–217, 226
  MTs and, 256
  MXs and, 284
  topoisomerases and, 73
Bone marrow toxicity, *see* Myelotoxicity
Bone marrow transplants, 196, 197, 289
Bordetella pertussis, 42

Bovine adenylyl cyclase gene, 160
Bovine papilloma virus (BPV), 26
Brain tumors, 214, 268
Breast cancer, 101, 172, 173, 178
  AAs for, 268, 281, 288
  antimetabolites for, 261
  gene amplification and, 2
  lonidamine for, 286
  mdr1 gene in, 102, 107, 109, 110
  topoisomerase inhibitors for, 82
Bromodeoxyuridine (BrdUrd), 218
Burkitt's lymphoma, 57, 64, 81, 238
Busulfan, 212
Buthionine sulfoximine (BSO), 179, 226
  AAs and, 268–270, 271, 288
  cisplatin and, 241

c-abl gene, 220–221
CAD gene, 3, 5, 6, 8
Cadmium
  cisplatin and, 238, 239, 243
  MTs and, 26, 242, 251, 252, 253, 254, 255,
      256, 271
Cadmium chloride, 103
  MTs and, 255, 256, 271
Caffeine, 226, 282, 284, 285
Calcium, 20, 240
Calcium-channel blockers, *see also* specific
    types
  MDR and, 175, 176–177
  Pgp and, 153, 154, 156, 160, 189, 197
Calf thymus topoisomerases, 57, 76
Calmodulin-dependent protein kinase, 75
Calmodulin inhibitors
  DNA repair and, 226
  MDR and, 175, 177
  Pgp and, 153, 154, 160, 189
Calpain, 43
Camptothecin, 63, 64, 75, 82, 83–88
  activity and mechanism of, 83–84
  cell lines resistant to, 86–88
  DNA repair and, 224
  intracellular target of, 84–86
C32 antibodies, 142
C219 antibodies, 66, 122, 132, 133, 136,
      137–138, 139, 140, 142, 143, 172, 191,
      193–194, 195
  calibration of, 129–131
  properties of, 129
  radio-iodination of, 127–128
C494 antibodies, 122, 131–132, 136, 137,
      139, 140, 142, 143
  properties of, 129
  radio-iodination of, 127–128
Carbon tetrachloride, 252

Pgp and, 201
  topoisomerases and, 281
Cyclosporin A, 173, 175
  Pgp and, 153, 157–158, 159, 160
Cyclosporin C, 153
Cyclosporin G, 153
Cyclosporins, 114, 153, 155, 189, *see also*
    specific types
Cysteine, 251, 264, 267, 271
Cystic fibrosis gene, 39
Cytosine arabinoside (Ara-C), 71, 106, 212,
    225
Cytotoxic biologicals, 163
Cytotoxicity, 46, 103, 175, 176, 180
  AAs and, 263–264, 271
  DDI genes and, 18, 19, 21
  DNA damage and, 210
  DNA repair and, 225
  of nitroimidazoles, 277
  Pgp and, 156–157, 160, 162, 198, 200
  topoisomerases and, 58, 70, 71, 73, 77, 78,
    79, 80
Cytotoxicity assays, of topoisomerases, 59,
    60, 62, 80

Dactinomycin, *see* Actinomycin D
1,2-Daminocyclohexane-Pt (DACH-Pt), 238,
    239
Daunomycin
  DNA damage and, 212
  mdr1 gene and, 102, 105, 106, 174
  topoisomerases and, 58, 60, 62, 66, 67, 71,
    72, 73
Daunorubicin, 173–174, 179, 189, 200
dCTP, 225
DDIA18 gene, 25, 26, 29, 33
DDIA33 gene, 25, 26
DDR genes, 16
DDTC, 287
Decarbazine, 213
De novo resistance, *see* Intrinsic resistance
2'-Deoxycoformycin (2'-DCF), 5
2'Deoxycytidine, 212
Desethylamiodarone, 178
Detergents, 153
Dexamethasone, 112, 156, 172, 188–189, 201
Diarrhea, topoisomerase inhibitors and, 83
Dideoxythymidine, 225
Diffuse histiocytic lymphoma, 81
Diffuse large-cell lymphoma, 176, 187–188,
    203
Dihydrofolate reductase (DHFR) gene
  amplification of, 1, 2, 6, 8
  DNA repair in, 218–220, 221, 222, 224,
    226, 245

Dihydropyridines, 153, 155, 157
Diltiazem, 176, 177
Dimethyl sulphate, 222
DIN genes, 16–17
Dipyridamole, 153, 155, 157, 180
Disulfiram, 287
DNA-aneupoloid myeloma, 172
DNA damage, 220, 221, 222, 224, 225, 226,
    227, *see also* DNA repair
  AAs and, 74, 209, 211–212, 213, 288
  cisplatin and, 209, 211, 212, 243–244
  drugs causing, 210–213
  at gene level, 217–218
  mechanisms of, 213–214
  nitroimidazoles and, 277
  topoisomerases and, 73–75, 87, 212, 213
DNA-damage inducible (DDI) genes, 13–33
  in eukaryotes, 13, 16–31
    gadd genes and, 25, 26, 30, 31, 32, 33
    hybridization subtraction of, 28–29
    mammalian, 19–20, 22
    MTs and, 13, 21, 24–26
    oxidative stress and, 14, 22, 30–31
    β-polymerase and, 25, 26, 27–28, 33
    protein-kinase mediated mechanisms
      and, 20–24
    smaller varieties of, 16–18
    ubiquitin and, 17, 26–27, 33
  in prokaryotes, 13, 14–15
  resistance role of, 31–32
  topoisomerase inhibitors and, 86
  X-rays and, 16, 18, 32, 33
DNA ligase, 16, 226
DNA polymerase, *see also* specific types
  antimetabolites and, 212
  DDI genes and, 16
  DNA repair and, 216, 224–225, 237–238,
    244
  topoisomerase inhibitors and, 84, 86
DNA polymerase α, 225, 244
DNA polymerase β, 174
  DDI genes and, 25, 26, 27–28, 33
  DNA repair and, 27, 216, 225, 237–238,
    244
DNA polymerase δ, 225
DNA repair, 27, 209–227, *see also* DNA
    damage
  AAs and, 214, 222, 235, 263, 264,
    280–281, 288
  cisplatin and, 215, 216, 222, 225, 226–227,
    235–238, 243–244, 245, 281
  DDI genes and, 16, 31
  in drug resistance, 214–217
  at gene level, 209, 217–223
  GSH and, 226–227, 235, 241–242, 243

300

Interleukin-1 (IL-1), 252, 253
Interleukin-2 (IL-2), 81
Intrinsic resistance, 104–109, 114, 171, 177
Ionizing radiation, 211, 218, 254, 255
Iproplatin, 233, 234, 238
Islet cell tumors, 104
Isocyanate groups, 212
Isoprenoids, 153, 175
Isosafrole, 46

JSB-1 antibodies, 142, 191

Kanamycins, 2
kDNA, 57, 59, 60, 61, 66
Kidney cancer, *see* Renal cancer

Lapachone, 224, 287
Large-cell lung cancer, 80
Leiomyosarcomas, 82
Leishmania, extrachromosomal DNA in, 2
Leucovorin, 105, 261
Leukemias, *see also* Hematologic
    malignancies
  acute, *see* Acute leukemia
  childhood, *see* Childhood leukemias
  DNA repair and, 216
  hairy cell, 81
  lymphocytic, *see* Acute lymphocytic
    leukemia; Chronic lymphocytic
    leukemia
  MDR in, 173
  murine, *see* Murine leukemia
  myelogenous, *see* Acute myelogenous
    leukemia; Chronic myelogenous
    leukemia
  nonlymphocytic, *see* Acute
    nonlymphocytic leukemia; Chronic
    nonlymphocytic leukemia
  Pgp in, 188–189
  plasma-cell, 176
  prolymphocytic, 81
  promyelocytic, 6
  topoisomerase inhibitors for, 66, 81, 83,
    85, 86, 87
Leukopenia, daunomycin-induced, 102
Leupeptin, 226
Levamisole, 105
Lewis lung cancer, 275
lexA gene, 14
Lipid peroxidation, MTs and, 254
Liver toxicity, 270
Lonidamine, 285–287
Lung cancer
  AAs for, 263
  large-cell, 80

Lewis, 275
mdr1 gene in, 108–109
MDR in, 171, 172–173
non-small-cell, *see* Non-small-cell lung
  cancer
small-cell, *see* Small-cell lung cancer
squamous-cell, 174
topoisomerase inhibitors for, 80
Lymphomas
  Burkitt's, 57, 64, 81, 238
  diffuse histiocytic, 81
  diffuse large-cell, 186, 187–188, 203
  mdr1 gene in, 102
  murine, 75
  nodular mixed, 81
  nodular poorly differentiated, 81, 172
  non-Hodgkin's, *see* Non-Hodgkin's
    lymphoma
  Pgp in, 187, 189, 196–197, 202
  topoisomerase inhibitors for, 75, 82
Lysosomotropic agents, 153, 189
Lytic infection, 18

Magnesium, topoisomerases and, 57
malK protein, 42
Mastocytomas, 77
MDR *at*-MDR, 152
mdr gene, *see also* individual genes;
    Multidrug resistance; P-glycoprotein;
    pgp genes
  amplification of, 1, 5, 6
  human, 37, 39–41
  immunoblot detection of, 129, 132, 138
  in Pgp molecular biology, 37–43
    expression regulation of, 43–47
  rodent, 37–39, 41–42, 44
mdr1 gene, 39–41, 42, 47–48, 50, 51, 171,
    172, 173, 174, 181
  amplification of, 5, 107, 121–122, 160, 172
  DDI genes and, 24, 31
  expression of in cancer, 101–115
    acquired resistance and, 109–112, 115
    clinical studies applications of, 114–115
    evidence of drug resistance and, 102–103
    factors affecting variability of, 112–114
    intrinsic resistance and, 104–109, 115
    molecular diagnosis of, 103–104
  expression regulation of, 43, 44–45, 46, 47
  in hematologic malignancies, 189
  human, 102
  immunoblot detection of, 121–122, 129,
    130, 132, 134, 136, 137, 140, 140–141,
    142
  Pgp modulators and, 151, 152, 156, 160,
    162, 163

reversal of effects of, 178, 197
rodent, 102
topoisomerases and, 59, 62, 70
mdr1a gene, 42, 44, 51, *see also mdr3* gene
mdr1b gene, 42, 44–45, 51, *see also mdr1*
gene
mdr2 gene, 39, 41, 44, 45, 47–48, 50, *see*
also mdr3 gene
mdr3 gene, 44, 122, 129, 132, 136, 139, 141,
see also mdr1a gene; *mdr2* gene
Mechlorethamine, 111
Medulloblastomas, 268
Meiosis, topoisomerases and, 57
Melanomas, 171
AAs for, 263, 268
DDI genes and, 25
DNA repair and, 214
mdr1 gene in, 107, 108
murine, 72
Pgp in, 123, 134, 135, 136, 141
topoisomerase inhibitors for, 72
Melphalan
AAs and, 279
cisplatin and, 238, 239, 241
DDI genes and, 29
DNA damage and, 212
GSH/GST metabolism of, 267
MTs and, 242
Pgp and, 188
Merbarone, 224
6-Mercaptopurine, 212
Mercury, MTs and, 252, 253, 254
Meselsohn Sthahl technique, 5
Mesotheliomas, 107
Metallothioneins (MTs), 251–257
AAs and, 26, 252, 255, 256, 264, 271–273
biochemical features of, 251–252
cisplatin and, 26, 237, 242–243, 245, 251,
255–257, 271
in DDI genes, 13, 21, 24–26
DNA repair and, 221, 256
drug resistance role of, 255–257
inducibility of, 252
physiological functions of, 253–255
Metastasis, 85, 143, 177
Methotrexate, 1, 2, 6, 7, 8, 263
N-(*p*-Methylbenzyl) decaprenylamine, 153,
155
5,10-Methylene-tetrahydrofolic acid, 261
O^6-Methylguanine, 214, 223–224, 287
O^6-Methylguanine transferase, 280
2-Methyl-9-hydroxyellipticine, 68
Methylmethane sulfonate (MMS), 17, 24, 27,
29, 30, 31, 32, 285
Methyl nitrosourea, 222

Methylxanthines (MXs), 225, 264, 282–285,
288
met protooncogene, 39
Minute chromosomes, 1, 3
Misonidazole, 278–279
Mitomycin C (MMC), 19, 174, 212
Mitosis
DDI genes and, 30
gene amplification and, 8
topoisomerases and, 57, 76, 79
Mitoxantrone, 58, 60, 62, 65, 66, 68, 70, 71,
72, 73
MNNG, 26, 27, 58–59, 73
Monensin, 153
Monoclonal antibodies (mAbs), *see also*
specific antibodies
in *mdr1* gene analysis, 113
Pgp, 66, 114, 191–192, 193–194, 195
in immunoblot analysis, 121, 122,
127–128, 129–132, 133, 136,
137–138, 139, 140, 141–142
in immunohistochemical analysis,
141–142
in reversal of effects, 179, 196, 197
Morpholino anthracycline analogs, 154–155
MRK16 monoclonal antibodies, 114
MTIC, 213, 214, 215
Multidrug resistance (MDR), 171–181, *see*
also mdr gene; P-glycoprotein
in cell lines and tumors, 172–174
in hematologic malignancies, 189
immunoblot techniques and, 121–122
modulators of, 151–163
reversal of, 174–179
reversal of coexisting resistance
mechanisms, 179–180
topoisomerase inhibitors and, 85
Multiple myeloma, 102, 110, 112, 173, 176
Pgp in, 161–162, 188–189, 195, 200–201,
202
Murine leukemia
AAs for, 262
cisplatin for, 238
DDI genes and, 25
DNA repair and, 216
topoisomerase inhibitors for, 57, 69, 78
Murine lymphoma, 75
Murine melanoma, 72
Mutations
DDI genes and, 13, 16, 19, 21
DNA repair and, 210
in hematologic malignancies, 188
of *mdr1* gene, 121, 197
of Pgp, 50
topoisomerases and, 61, 73, 83

304

305

in hematologic malignancies, 187–203
  detection of, 190–193
  incidence of occurrence in, 193–196
  reversal of function of, 196–202
immunoblot detection of, *see* Immunoblot
  detection of Pgp
immunohistochemical analysis of, *see*
  Immunohistochemical analysis of Pgp
intrinsic resistance and, 105, 106, 107, 108,
  109
modulators of, 151–163
  action mechanisms of, 157–160
  cytotoxicity enhancement and, 156–157
  differing effectiveness of, 156
  MDR reversal by, 153–155
  rules for, 155
  structure-activity studies of, 155–156
  in vivo and clinical studies with,
    160–163
molecular biology of, 37–51
reversal of MDR associated with, 175,
  176, 177, 179
topoisomerases and, 59, 61, 66, 67, 68,
  69–70, 72, 73, 77, 82
pqp genes, 41, 42, 44–45
Phenothiazines, 46, 114, 153, 155, 157
Phenylalanine mustard, 263, 267
Phenylalkylamines, 153, 157
Pheochromocytomas, 104, 105, 109, 110, 172
Phorbol esters, MTs and, 252
Photolyase, DNA repair and, 213
6–4 Photoproducts, 221
Photorepair, enzymatic, 18–19
Phytohemagglutinin, 81
Plasma-cell leukemia, 176
Plasminogen activator, 23–24
Plasmodium falciparum, 43
Platinum, MTs and, 255
Platinum analogs, 233, 234, *see also* specific
  agents
Pleiotropic drug resistance, 121
Poly (ADP ribose) polymerase, 214
Poly (ADP ribose) synthetase, 76
Poly (ADP riobosylation), 75, 76, 77
Polyclonal antibodies, anti-topoisomerase,
  63, 64, 81
Polymerase, *see* DNA polymerase; RNA
  polymerase
P1 promoter, 46–47
P2 promoter, 47
Prednisone, 111, 189
Preferential resistance, 239
Procarbazine, 111, 213
Progesterone, 45, 153, 156, 252
Programmed cell death, 237
Prokaryotes, 13, 14–15, 42, 213

Prolymphocytic leukemia, 81
PROmace-MOPP regimen, 111
Promyelocytic leukemia, 6
Propranolol, 174
Prostate cancer, 78, 107, 240
Proteinase inhibition, 226
Protein kinase A, 240
Protein kinase C (PKC)
  DDI genes and, 17, 20, 21–24
  MDR and, 171, 180
  topoisomerases and, 75
Protein kinases, *see also* specific types
  calmodulin-dependent, 75
  cAMP-dependent, 20, 75, 240
  DDI genes and, 20–24
  topoisomerases and, 75, 76
Protooncogenes, DNA repair in, 220–221
p62 serum response factor, 20
p67 serum response factor, 20
Pseudomonas exotoxin, 114, 179, 197
pstB protein, 42
p170 topoisomerase isozymes, 64, 65, 77, 80
p180 topoisomerase isozymes, 64, 65, 77, 80
Pulse field gel electrophoresis, 5
Purine analogs, 212
Puromycin, 87
*Pvu*II-restricted DNA, 67
Pyrimidine dimers, 18–19, 210–211, 213,
  218, 220

Quinacrine, 153
Quinidine, 105, 114, 175, 177–178, 200
Quinine, 153, 200
Quinolines, 153
Quinones, 30–31, 179

RAD genes, 16, 30, 85–86
Radiation sensitizers, 276, 277–279
Radiation therapy, 210, 274, 275
  Ionidamine and, 286
  MXs and, 282
  Pgp and, 196–197
ras gene, 80, 244–245
rbsA protein, 42
*rec*A gene, 14
Renal cancer
  mdr genes in, 45, 102, 103, 104, 105, 113,
    172
  Pgp in, 123, 134, 135, 136, 137, 141
Reserpine, 153, 162, 175
Retinoic acid, 45, 102
Rhizobium heliloti, 42
Ribonucleotide reductase, 16
RNA polymerase, 84
RNase protection assays, 103, 141, 193
RNA slot blot analysis